Further Studies for Health

HILARY THOMSON

CAROLYN MEGGITT ▪ SYLVIA ASLANGUL ▪ VINCENT O'BRIEN

SECOND EDITION

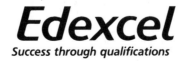

Edexcel

Success through qualifications

Hodder & Stoughton

A MEMBER OF THE HODDER HEADLINE GROUP

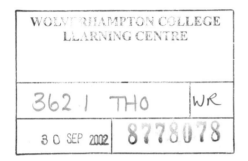
Orders: please contact Bookpoint Ltd, 130 Milton Park, Abingdon, Oxon OX14 4SB. Telephone: (44) 01235 827720, Fax: (44) 01235 400454. Lines are open from 9.00 - 6.00, Monday to Saturday, with a 24 hour message answering service.

British Library Cataloguing in Publication Data

A catalogue record for this title is available from The British Library

ISBN 0340 804238

First edition published 1996

Impression number 10 9 8 7 6 5 4 3 2 1

Year   2007 2006 2005 2004 2003 2002

This edition 2002

Cover photo from Corbis

Typeset by **Wyvern 21**

Printed in Great Britain for Hodder & Stoughton Educational, a division of Hodder Headline Plc, 338 Euston Road, London NW1 3BH by Martins the Printers, Berwick-upon-Tweed.

Contents

Acknowledgements

Crown copyright material is reproduced with the permission of the Controller of HMSO and the Queen's Printer for Scotland; the articles 'Britain ages as pregnancies fall', 'Testing the air' and 'Study finds limited Sellafield cancer link' reproduced by kind permission of The Guardian;the articles 'Rise in eating disorders blamed on media's love for thin is beautiful' by Cherry Norton and 'Watchdog cracks down on misleading claims in organic ads' by Jade Garrett reproduced by kind permission of The Independent;
'Population of the World's largest cities' from The Human Environment. Reprinted by permission of Heinemann Educational publishers;'Some tips to keep out those unwelcome creepy-crawlies' reproduced courtesy of the Okehampton Times;'Step up to safety' poster reproduced with kind permission of the Department of Trade and Industry.

Special thanks to Jatinder Bhuhi for research into the needs of asylum seekers and refugees in chapter one.

Photo credits: page 56 Wellcome Photo Library; page 121 Science Photo Library; page 122 Photofusion; page 126 Science Photo Library; page 126 National Medical Slide Bank; page 128 Science Photo Library; page 131 National Medical Slide Bank; page 138 Science Photo Library; page 139 National Medical Slide Bank; page 140 National Medical Slide Bank; page 167 Science Photo Library; page 167 Science Photo Library; page 174 Science Photo Library; page 211 Wellcome Photo Library; page 212 Wellcome Photo Library; page 215 Science Photo Library; page 216 Science Photo Library; page 228 Science Photo Library; page 231 Oxford Scientific Films; page 235 Oxford Scientific Films; page 281 Medical Photographic Library; page 282 Wellcome Photographic Library; page 290 Science Photo Library; page 294 Science Photo Library; page 299 Science Photo Library; page 302 Science Photo Library; page 308 Science Photo Library; page 310 Science Photo Library; page 319 Science Photo Library; page 320 Science Photo Library; page 325 Wellcome Photo Library.

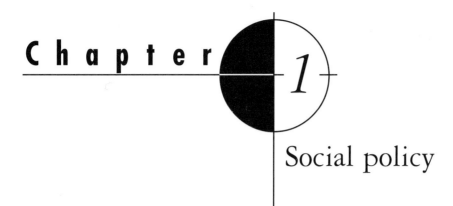

Chapter 1

Social policy

This chapter relates to Unit 9 and covers the development of social policy and social care provision in Britain. Social policy and welfare provision is developed in response to the perceived needs and problems within a society. These perceptions and needs change over a period of time and are influenced by the social, economic, political and cultural context in which they exist.

This chapter describes:

- The factors affecting social policy in the twentieth century;
- Social policy and social care services today;
- The influences on the development of social policy in the twenty first century.

This unit links to Unit 1 and Unit 5, and while you are studying this chapter it would be useful to keep your main textbook for the course available as you will need to refer to it. This icon ◇ will act as a prompt to refer to *Vocational A Level in Health and Social Care* Thomson, H. *et al* (2000) Hodder and Stoughton.

This chapter covers some of the underpinning knowledge of NVQ level 3 in Early Years and Education.

Assessment

This unit will be assessed externally and the grade you achieve in this assessment will be your grade for the unit. The test paper will include stimulus response material, including basic statistical data such as demographic trends, morbidity or mortality rates. During the chapter you will be asked to complete activities to prepare you for the test.

 Word check

Demography

The study of populations, with particular reference to their size and structure, and how and why these change over time. Demographers study birth, death and marriage rates, patterns of migration and other important factors that affect population growth or decline such as climate, food supply and the availability of employment.

Morbidity rates

Information related to the nature and extent of illness in a population. Morbidity rates can be measured using hospital admission rates, sickness rates and self-reported illness rates.

Mortality rates

The number of deaths per 1000 of the population per year. These rates are often broken down to show differences by age, gender and social class.

In the White Paper (1998) 'Our Healthier Nation', morbidity and mortality rates were the basis for deciding on the national priorities for national and local Health Improvement Programmes (HImPs) These priorities included reducing the death rates from:

- cancer;
- coronary heart disease (CHD);
- accidents;
- suicides.

Health and social care policy was developed in order to achieve these priorities.

As we can see, social policy does not come out of a vacuum. A problem is identified, data is collected and used as evidence to show the extent of the problem, and then a strategy or action plan is developed.

Social policy

What does social policy mean? Social policy covers a range of service provision in Great Britain. Traditionally, five areas have been included in social policy:

- education;
- housing;
- income maintenance (either through benefits or earned income);
- health services;
- social services.

The key legislation affecting the development of the Welfare State is presented in tables in Chapter 5 of the main text book, and it would be useful to look at this now ◇.

Historical factors affecting social policy in the twentieth century

Social policy is dependent on a range of contextual factors. During the twentieth century a variety of historical events, such as wars, changes in legislation, changes in the organisation of work and the role of Britain in the global context, have all had an effect on social policy. Many of these changes were developments of earlier social changes that had occurred in the nineteenth century. We will look at some of these in this section.

Nineteenth-Century Social Policy

The Social Conditions of Nineteenth-Century Britain

During this century the causes of poverty were seen as the result of intemperance and idleness. With the development of factories and towns, poverty became a feature of both urban and rural areas. The development of the Welfare State was a gradual process. The Poor Law Commission of 1834 resulted in the Poor Law Amendment Act of the same year. This Act was based on the belief that people were poor largely through their own fault and that to provide help would only encourage idleness. The Poor Law stated that support would only be given in the workhouse. To receive this support, the family had to leave their home and work in the workhouse for low wages. Poor Law administrators took no account of factors such as large families, old age, irregular employment or low earnings. Various charitable organisations and churches also provided support.

The workhouse test or scheme of 'less eligibility' was imposed on all those seeking help. It attempted to distinguish between the deserving and the undeserving poor. The deserving poor were the sick, the disabled, the elderly and the unintentionally unemployed. The undeserving poor were the feckless, idle and intentionally unemployed. Only those without means were offered help. The workhouses were usually segregated and families were split up, with women and children in one workhouse and men in another. Workhouses were portrayed in the literature of the time, such as Charles Dickens' *Oliver Twist*, and their strict regime meant that people tried to avoid going into them.

Activity

1   Means testing is still done today. Find a copy of the booklet 'MG 1' and identify some examples.

2   Can you think how some groups in today's society could be seen as the deserving and undeserving poor. Look at the following list and think which category these groups would fall into:

   • widows;

- teenage unmarried mothers;
- refugees and asylum seekers;
- unemployed school leavers.

The way in which society views these groups can be identified through their treatment

- in the media;
- in the benefit system.

As we have seen in this section, poverty was considered undesirable in the nineteenth century. But the poor were also seen as a threat to the social order. There had been riots against the amended Poor Law after 1834. In spite of the regime in the workhouse, the number of people in workhouses increased from 78,536 in 1838 to 197,179 in 1843 (Thompson E. (1968) *The Making of the English Working Class.* Penguin).

'Outdoor relief' still occurred in many areas as many communities did not want workhouses built in their areas, and by 1850 only 110,000 paupers out of a million were workhouse inmates, many of whom were the old and the sick who had nowhere else to go. Brendon (1994) suggests that the Poor Law Amendment Act succeeded as it brought down public expenditure from £7 million in 1834 to £4.5. million in 1844. It also brought a lasting fear of the workhouse and made poverty seem a disgrace. After the Act, as before it, poor people continued as best as they could, relying on the help of family and neighbourhood rather than on public services.

 ## Activity

Local history groups in your area may have details of workhouses, orphanages and other buildings used to support people in the nineteenth century. Your local library may have a special local history section, or books about local conditions in your area. If you have time, it may be useful to look at these or to ask a member of the local historical society to give a talk to your group. Many libraries keep old maps of the area, which are another useful source of information.

Apart from workhouses other large buildings were developed in the latter part of the century. Charities built hospitals, residential homes (Dr Barnardo's) and hostels. These large institutions reflected the view that certain groups of people should be excluded from living in the community, such as those with mental health problems, learning and physical disabilities, and older people.

Developments in Social Policy in the Early Twentieth Century

The Liberal Government of 1905 laid some of the foundations for the post-1942 welfare state. Lloyd George (who was Chancellor of the Exchequer in 1908 and Prime Minister, 1916–1922) advocated social reforms which included:

- infant welfare clinics;
- school meals for children;
- medical examinations of children in elementary school;
- juvenile employment bureaux to help school leavers find suitable jobs;
- introduction of borstals and probation courts for young offenders;
- old age pensions to the over 70s paid in weekly payments from post offices;
- national insurance schemes against unemployment or sickness.

The main Liberal legislation and administration changes, 1908–1914

- Education Acts of 1907 and 1908;
- Children's Act, 1908;
- Old Age Pensions Act, 1908;
- Trade Boards from 1909 onwards;
- Labour Exchange Act, 1909;
- National Insurance Act, 1911.

These reforms were brought about through the influence of several factors including:

- an ideological belief in the need for reform on the part of the 'New Liberals' such as Churchill and Lloyd George;
- a political need to boost support for the Liberal party, following defeats in by-elections in 1908;
- the threat of the socialist reforms by the Labour Party gaining popular support if the Liberals failed to act.

We can see from the last example that pressures on policy makers can come from both ideological and practical influences.

The impact of the First World War

By 1914, the working class had more support from the state. Many more people were insured, and council housing and a hospital system were being developed. The First World War had stimulated a desire for national efficiency in two ways:

1 There was a concern to maximise output in the war industries. Factory Acts were suspended so that women and young people could work longer hours in factories.

2 There was a concern to preserve 'the national stock' by protecting the health of mothers and children (war officials had been concerned at the poor standard of health and fitness of recruits to the Boer War).

Local councils were encouraged to improve their services for mothers and babies by setting up clinics, home visitors, and hospital treatment and food for the needy. A Ministry of Reconstruction was set up in 1917, which brought together Poor Law provision, public health and education authorities, and insurance commissions. The Ministry focused on four key areas of welfare:

1 *Housing:* "Homes fit for heroes." The 1919 Housing Act authorised local councils to build as many houses as possible. New housing estates were built outside large towns. By 1939, one million new homes had been built by the public sector.

2 *Unemployment:* This was a major problem after the war. By 1921, two million people were out of work. Unemployment insurance was extended to everyone earning less than £5 a week, except for farm labourers, domestic servants and civil service employees. Means testing was still used to determine how much assistance should be given.

3 *Health:* More effective health care provision was developed.

4 *Education:* The Fisher Education Act of 1918 established the principle that all children and young people should have access to education.

During this time, although local government still played a major role in the implementation of social policies, there was more centralised control and new ministries and government departments began to develop. Pressure groups such as the trade unions, and professional groups, such as the British Medical Association (BMA) also exerted pressure on the Government.

Activity

Look at the 4 key areas. Can you identify key initiatives that are being developed by the Labour government in 2001?

Comment

1 Housing: The need to build more affordable housing, especially for health and care workers is one of the key issues in the twenty-first century.

2 Unemployment: The New Deal initiative is a contemporary example.

3 Health: National Service Frameworks for Coronary Heart Disease and Mental Health.

4 Education: The discussion over loans and grants for university students.

We can see from the above examples that certain key areas are the concerns of government throughout the twentieth and twenty-first centuries. Factors affecting the development of these policies can be:

• economic: the need to reduce state spending;

- demographic changes: the increase in the numbers of people over 75 and a reduced birth rate;
- social: changes in family forms and expectations of certain life styles;
- ideological: ideas about who is responsible for providing support – the state or the individual and family members.

Voting rights

In 1918, the government passed the Representation of the People Act. This gave the vote to all men over 21 if they had been living in the same area for six months (peers, lunatics and criminals were excluded from voting). Women over 30 were also given the vote if they or their husbands owned or occupied any property or land. This meant that out of a total electorate of 21 million, 8.5 million women had the right to vote for the first time. In 1918, women could become MPs; in 1919 they could hold government posts; and in 1928, the right to vote was extended to all women over 21.

The changes affecting the position of women were brought about by a variety of factors:

- the influence of war, when many women worked in munitions factories and assisted the war effort;
- the influence of the Suffragette movement;
- the need to attract women as voters to support the government.

The impact of the Second World War

Just as the First World War had brought about changes in attitudes to the working class and to women, so, too, did the Second World War. Many women contributed to the war effort at home and in the forces. Evacuation of children from the cities into the country brought different groups of people into contact for the first time, and the deprivation of poor urban families could not be ignored. There was a fear that some of the problems experienced after the First World War would occur again, especially with the large-scale bombing of cities that led to a shortage of housing.

The Beveridge Report

In 1941, the government ordered a special commission of inquiry to undertake a survey of the existing national scheme of social insurance to make recommendations for future policy. The chair of the commission was Sir William Beveridge. In 1942, the recommendations were set out in the Beveridge Report. These recommendations proposed measures to deal with the five 'giants' on the road to reconstruction and social progress.

1 *Want:* A complete system of social insurance for all citizens would be set up. In return, if they were sick, unemployed or retired they would receive flat-rate benefits – means testing would be abolished.

2 *Disease:* A New National Health service would be established, free at the point of delivery.

3 *Squalor:* More and better housing would be developed.

4 *Ignorance:* More and better schools, with free secondary education for all up to the age of 15 (to be extended to 16 at a later date).

5 *Idleness*: Unemployment would be reduced by tighter government control of trade and industry.

These recommendations formed the basis for many reforms following the end of the war in 1945. Detailed discussion of these changes are to be found in Chapter 5 of the main text book.

Civil Rights and Civil Liberties

Since the 1970s, the concept of citizenship has had an important influence on social policy in the UK:

- *civil rights* to individual freedom, to free speech and thought, the right to own property and the right to justice;
- *political rights* to vote and to participate in the democratic process;
- *social rights* to economic welfare and security, including the right to education, work and health care.

The early civil rights movements in the USA in the 1960s were concerned with the rights of black Americans and of women, and resulted in Equal Opportunities Legislation outlawing discrimination based on gender, race and age. The Women's Movement of the 1970s in the UK also resulted in legislation, including the Equal Pay Act (1970) and the Sex Discrimination Act (1975). Various Race Relations Acts were passed (1965, 1968, 1976) and the 1976 Act has recently been amended (2000). Other legislation covering the rights of certain groups includes the Disability Discrimination Act and the Human Rights Act, which are covered in the main text book. ◇

Feminism and social policy

The suffragette movement in the early part of the twentieth century was a factor in widening the franchise to all women in 1928. However, women have not benefited from recent welfare development because of their traditional roles as wives and mothers.

1 **Child care.** Britain is still behind the rest of Europe in relation to the provision of child care. Table 1.1 shows the number of day care places available for children. What level of provision is provided by the state?

2 **The 1990 NHS and Community Care Act.** Under this Act many large institutions were closed down and people with mental health problems, learning and physical disabilities were to be cared for in the community. Women in the family were seen as their natural carers. Changes in surgery meant that people stayed in hospital for shorter periods and were cared for at home, again by women. As the population becomes increasingly older, women will become the main carers, either unpaid or as low paid workers.

3 **Work.** Many women would like to return to work once they have had children but there is a lack of child care at an affordable level. Single mothers are being encouraged to return to work to reduce the state benefits they are receiving, through such initiatives as the New Deal, but many women would prefer to stay at home with their children.

Table 1.1 Day care provided for children under the age of 8 (under the age of 12 in N. Ireland)

England, Wales & Northern Ireland					Thousands
	1987	1992	1997	1998	1999
Day nurseries					
Local authority provided[1]	29	24	20	19	16
Registered	32	98	184	216	235
Non-registered[2]	1	1	2	1	12
All day nursery places	62	123	206	236	263
Childminders					
Local authority provided[1]	2	2	4	4	9
Other registered	159	275	398	403	360
All childminder places	161	277	402	407	369
Playgroups					
Local authority provided	4	2	2	2	3
Registered	434	450	424	423	383
Non-registered[1]	7	3	3	1	3
All playgroup places	445	455	429	426	389
Out of school clubs[2]	–	–	–	97	119

1 England and Wales only.
2 England only.
Source: Social Trends 2001, HMSO

Activity

Look at Figure 1.1 and answer the following questions.

1 What method do you think was used for obtaining these responses?

2 Why do you think you need to be careful when reading the results and the reasons given by women for not working?

Great Britain

Percentages

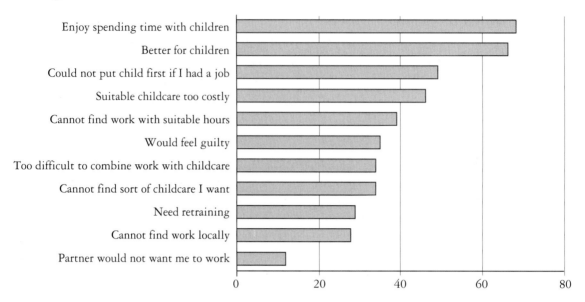

Figure 1.1 Reasons given for mothers not working 1998
Source Social Trends 2001, HMSO

Ethnic minorities and Civil Rights

Minority ethnic groups experience poorer health, more unemployment, lower incomes and poorer housing. Under Section 71 of the Race Relations Act, 1996, local councils were required to take steps to tackle racial discrimination in the provision of services. Black and Asian groups appear to be under-represented as clients of welfare agencies, but higher numbers of children from Afro-Caribbean families are taken into care. More black children are referred to local councils because of family relationships, marital breakdown and financial problems.

Age discrimination

Civil rights affecting older people are being promoted, although there is no legislation in the UK protecting people from discrimination based on age. Under the National Service Frameworks (NSFs) for Older People, health and social care agencies have to check their policies and criteria for care, in order to ensure that there is no age bias.

Disability Rights

Disability Rights groups have been very active since the 1970s. The Disability Discrimination Act, 1995, covers aspects of health and care, particularly with regard to access to services. From 1999, service providers were required to make reasonable adjustments to policies, procedures and practices that exclude disabled people such as excluding guide dogs from restaurants or shops. Service providers had to provide auxiliary aids and services, such as providing information on a cassette or installing an induction loop, to enable it to make it easier to use a service. Where a physical feature is a barrier to a service, providers have to find an alternative method of delivering the service such as low level taxi cabs that have access for wheelchairs.

From 2004, service providers will have to take reasonable steps to remove, alter or avoid physical features that make it difficult or impossible to access a service. Public transport is one of the key areas that disabled action groups have been demonstrating about, and we are now seeing the influence of this in the provision of low access public vehicles in some trains and buses. Various allowances for disabled people have been developed, allowing people to remain independent. Apart from the Disability Living Allowance for people under 66, there are other benefits such as the Direct Payments Scheme, which allows people to organise and pay for their own care. New Deal projects that encourage disabled people into the work force are another initiative that is part of the process of recognising the needs of disabled people and assisting them to take an active and independent part in society.

In this historical overview we have seen examples of policies that have been developed as a reaction to social, economic and political factors. However, another factor affecting the development of policy is related to ideology. An ideology is a set of structured ideas that form a particular perspective or view. The post-World War II legislation and style of government was based on principles of universal provision of public services, free at the point of delivery. Means testing was seen as divisive and time-wasting to administer. The role of the state was to support all its citizens and to reduce inequalities. Bevan talked about the role of the state as supporting people 'from the cradle to the grave'.

Development of Social Policy from 1945 to the present time

The terms 'Right', 'Left' or 'Centre' are used to identify the ideology of a particular political party. Different parties can be described as right-wing or left-wing. The type of social policy that is developed by a political party is affected by ideas about:

- the role and function of the State;
- the model of social welfare provision that is seen as appropriate;
- what criteria are used to identify those who are in need.

Terms related to Models of Welfare

Residual Model of Welfare: The State should provide welfare if the individual, family or private sector is unable to do so. The State should provide a safety net for those most in need.

Institutional Model of Welfare: Mixed economy of welfare that sees welfare provision as an important aspect of society, but this will be provided by a range of agencies. A combination of private, voluntary and statutory services will provide cost-effective care.

Universal Model of Welfare: Welfare services should be available to all by right. The state is responsible for all its citizens.

Table 1.2 The Key Ideologies related to Social Policy and Welfare Provision

	New right/Anti-collectivist/individualist/market models	Collectivist Old Labour	Reluctant collectivist New Labour	Feminist critique	Anti-racist critique
Core values	• Family values • Market economy • Law and order • Residual welfare	• Equality • State provision • Control of services • Universal welfare model	• Family • Equal opportunities • Consultation • Mixed economy	Equality and redistribution of power between men and women needed	Equality and redistribution of power between cultures and races needed
Role of the State	State intervention must be limited	State needs to intervene to ensure stability in society	Two pillar approach; mixed economy; state and private sector	Acts in interests of men; male dominated patriarchal	Acts in interest of white majority; discriminatory
Provision of welfare services	A range of providers would ensure effective delivery of services	State should provide services and support, voluntary and self-help groups	Mixed economy approach using a range of providers	Needs to reflect needs of women and be anti-discriminatory	Welfare services reflect institutionalised racism
Means testing	Efficient way to target those most in need	Stigmatising, bureaucratic, inefficient; universal provision supported	Used to provide services for those most in need	May adversely affect women who are not married	Stigmatising and degrading
Universal provision of services by the State	Inefficient; encourages increased demand and dependence	Committed to universal access and equality	Residual model used; target those most in need	Reflects traditional views of women as wives and mothers dependent on men	Services do not reflect needs of minority groups
Voluntary agencies	One of the providers of services	Supported by State but their main role should be to act as pressure groups	An important provider of services	Useful resource to help women; need to be led by women	Useful resource to help minority groups but need to be *led* by minority groups
Private sector	Encourages choice and competition, leading to efficient services	Choice for well-off; leads to divisions between rich and poor	One of the two pillars in Welfare State	Increases inequality because of women's economic position	Another example of divisions in society
Self-help	Should be encouraged; people should be independent and responsible for their own care	State still takes major role but provides support for self-help groups	Personal responsibility encouraged	Collective work by women useful	Collective approach useful

State intervention in the UK

1945 to the 1970s

The main approach during this time followed social reformist or collectivist views that maintained the State should control and provide welfare provision, using the Universal Model of Welfare.

1979 to 1997

The Conservatives came to power in 1979, and one of their key aims was to reduce government spending on welfare provision. It followed the Residual Model of Welfare and encouraged a mixed economy of welfare provision using State, private and voluntary agencies.

1997 onwards

Since the Labour government took office in 1997, there has been a development of the approach called the 'Third Way', in which State intervention has increased in some instances, such as setting NHS Targets, and has been reduced in others through the involvement of the private and voluntary sector working in partnership. This fits in more closely with the Institutional Model of Welfare. Table 1.2 identifies the key ideologies related to social policy and welfare.

 Activity

Look at the following quotations and choose the ideology which fits each one best (in some cases two ideologies could be relevant).

1 'People have a responsibility to look after themselves.'

2 'Instead of having a second holiday, use the money to have your varicose veins done privately.'

3 'Filling in forms is wasteful of time. It costs more in the end to the government.'

4 'Child benefit should be given to everyone, no matter what their level of income is.'

5 'The Partnership approach is important if we are to provide services that are relevant to local communities.'

6 'Giving young people housing support encourages them to leave home and depend on State handouts.'

7 'In this area we make sure that the antenatal clinics are staffed by female doctors.'

8 'It is important to support an interpreting service for our clients and provide information for them in their first language.'

Criticisms of the organisation of welfare provision

The feminist critique

Feminists suggest that welfare policies tend to reflect the patriarchal attitudes in society. Until recently, the caring role of women as mothers and as carers for the disabled or older family members meant that these women were not financially supported by the state. Instead they were used as unpaid workers. Recently, there has been additional legislation and support for carers ◇ but many carers feel the payments do not reflect the true cost of caring.

The anti-racist critique

This perspective identifies the welfare state as part of institutionalised racism in society which denies black and minority ethnic groups access to welfare provision in all aspects, including health care, benefits, housing and access to employment. The welfare state is used to control immigrants and refugees, and the police are seen as racist, failing to protect people who are from minority ethnic groups.

Table 1.3 Public choices for extra government spending in order of importance

Great Britain				Percentages
	1986	1991	1996	1999
Health	47	48	54	47
Education	27	29	28	34
Housing	7	8	4	4
Public transport	–	1	2	4
Help for industry	8	4	4	3
Police and prisons	3	2	3	3
Roads	1	1	1	3
Social security benefits	5	5	3	2
Overseas aid	1	1	–	1
Defence	1	2	1	1
All	100	100	100	100

Source Social Trends 2001, HMSO

Table 1.4 Government spending 1987–1999

United Kingdom					£ billion at 1999 prices	
	1987	1991	1996	1997	1998	1999
Social protection	102	115	140	140	137	137
Health	35	39	47	46	48	50
Education	33	35	39	39	39	40
Defence	32	32	25	25	26	26
Public order and safety	12	16	17	18	18	20
General public services	10	14	16	16	17	18
Housing and community amenities	11	12	7	7	5	5
Recreation, culture and religion	4	5	5	4	5	3
Other economic affairs and environmental protection*	26	27	29	24	23	25
Gross debt interest	32	23	30	32	31	26
All expenditure	297	318	355	351	349	350

*Includes expenditure on transport and communication, agriculture, forestry and fishing, mining, manufacture, construction, fuel and energy services.

Source Social Trends 2001, HMSO

Social expectations

During the twentieth century, the standard of living has increased, people are living longer and health care has advanced so that many illnesses are now treated successfully. The general health of the population has increased, the level of home ownership has increased and working hours have decreased. Leisure activities have expanded, and many people can retire early and look forward to an active retirement with enough money to support them as they get older. Many older people have contributed to the State National Insurance scheme since they began working and they expect to be cared for by the State as they get older.

Expectations for free long-term care for older people were raised by the recommendations made by the Royal Commission on Long Term Care (1998). The government in England and Wales has been slow to respond. In Scotland the recommendations were accepted and the Scottish parliament pledged its support. However, the costs of free long-term care would increase the social protection budget significantly, so there is a concern about how this money would be raised. Table 1.3 shows the areas in which people feel the government should increase its spending, but the government is wary about raising this extra money by increased taxation. Table 1.4 shows the expenditure of central government in 1999.

Word check

Social protection
Refers to the range of benefits, pensions and other payments made by the state.

Activity

Look at Tables 1.3 and 1.4 in turn and answer the following questions:

1 What is the source of the data for each table?

2 How was the data collected?

3 What years does the data cover?

4 What is the difference between the terms 'Great Britain' and 'United Kingdom'?

5 How are the figures in the tables shown (percentages, £s, millions, etc.)?

6 How much difference is there between the priorities given in Tables 1.3 and 1.4?

Can we infer from the information that public opinions and public expectations have an influence on policy decisions?

Public opinion

Public opinion can be assessed by using surveys such as the British Attitudes Survey or other surveys administered by a range of agencies such as Gallop Poll. Importance is given to public consultation about proposed changes to service provision, and the organisation and delivery of care services. Results from consultations are fed back to the relevant national or regional department. Telephone surveys, group meetings, patient participation groups and other focus groups are all being used to generate a response from the public. Some newspapers and TV programmes also offer people an opportunity to express their views. Websites have been set up by local and national government departments on which people can express their opinions.

Examples of how the pressure of public opinion can influence policy include:

- The poll tax riots that led to the reorganisation of collecting community rates in 1993.
- The murder of Jonathan Zito, led to changes in the support of people in the community with severe mental illness. All people with severe mental illness now have to be recorded on a SMI (Severe Mental Illness Register), available to Health and Social Care Services.
- The deaths of babies undergoing heart surgery at a Bristol hospital led to tighter controls over specialist consultants, and their clinical expertise has to be updated on a regular basis.

In many instances, public opinion may be more effective if it is focused through developing a pressure group or using an established pressure group to raise issues of concern such as Age Concern, who raised awareness of age discrimination taking place in the NHS through lobbying Parliament and the Department of Health. As a result, the new NSF for Older People contains a specific reference to removing age as a criteria for health care.

Major pressure groups in the UK

Trade unions

The membership of trade unions has fallen in recent years from 57% of all workers in 1979 to 30% in 1999. The main reason for the decline in membership is the legislation passed during the Conservative term of government that reduced union powers and limited their activities such as balloting members and secondary picketing.

UNISON is one of the largest unions and was formed in 1993 by the amalgamation of NALGO (union for local government officers) NUPE and COHSE (unions for health workers and other public employees). The major unions are affiliated to the Trades Union Congress (TUC). Trade unions exert pressure on the government especially on policy that relates to health and employment. For example, unions influenced the implementation of the national minimum wage.

Business

The CBI (Confederation of British Industry) is another important influence on government social policy. Eleven thousand individual businesses belong to the CBI, as well as 200 representative organisations, including trade associations and employers' associations. Issues that concern the CBI include the privatisation of services and state control. At the 2001 CBI conference in Birmingham, the Transport Secretary, Stephen Byers, was criticised for his department's approach to state involvement in the railway service – Railtrack.

Media

Britain has the highest number of newspaper readers in Europe – 66% of the population read a national daily paper regularly, although this number is declining because of television and the Internet. Most newspapers follow a particular political stance:

- *The Sun*, *The Times*, *The Sunday Times* and the *News of the World* are owned by the Murdoch organisation and tend to have a right-wing approach.

- *The Mirror, the Sunday Mirror, The People* and the *Daily Record* (Scotland) are owned by *The Mirror* group and tend to have a left-wing approach.

In 2000, *The Sun* had the largest circulation figures of 3.7 million whereas *The Mirror* had 2.3 million and the Mail 2.4 million. Newspapers can raise important issues, exerting pressure on the government; some carry out surveys of their readers' views.

Television

With the development of cable TV, many channels are available to viewers. However, the main terrestrial channels of BBC 1 and 2, ITV and Channel 4, all cover social policy issues through national news items, discussion programmes such as *Question Time*, and viewers can also send their views by letter or e-mail. Although there has been a great deal of research into the influence of the media on public opinion, it has been difficult to establish a causal link. In the same way, it is difficult to establish how far the government has an influence on media output. The Prime Minister's Press Secretary, Alistair Campbell, holds regular briefing sessions with the press on government matters, but some newspaper editors maintain they have an influence on government decisions.

Power of the professionals

In the last 25 years the power of professionals has been eroded. Professional groups who could be expected to have an influence on social policy such as teachers, doctors, social workers and lawyers, have all been affected by government legislation and state control, which has reduced their influence. Since 1979 centralised control by the government over these occupational groups has increased. Examples of this increased control include:

- Contracts for GPs (in 2001 these contracts were redesigned by central government). Although the British Medical Association (BMA) was seen as an effective pressure group in the past, various scandals (such as the Shipman Murders, and the Bristol baby deaths) have affected the status of the profession.
- The National Curriculum in Education, whereby teachers have to follow set guidelines and prepare children for SATs.
- The development of Ofsted, which inspects schools. It can put poorly-run schools on special measures and private agencies can be brought in to run a failing school.
- The Social Service Inspectorate (SSI) audits and inspects local government services and has the power to put departments on 'special measures'.

Social policy and social care services today

Care workers need to have a good understanding of the general nature of social care provision and factors that influence its development.

Population changes

One of the key factors affecting social policy and the provision of care services is related to the demography of the UK. The speed of population change depends on the net natural change – the difference between the numbers of births and deaths, and the net effect of people migrating

Table 1.5 Population change in the UK 1901–2021

United Kingdom						Thousands
			Average annual change			
	Population at start of period	Live births	Deaths	Net natural change	Net migration and other	Overall change
Census enumerated						
1901–1911	38,237	1,091	624	467	−82	385
1911–1921	42,082	975	689	286	−92	194
1921–1931	44,027	824	555	268	−67	201
1931–1951	46,038	785	598	188	25	213
Mid-year estimates						
1951–1961	50,287	839	593	246	6	252
1961–1971	52,807	963	639	324	−12	312
1971–1981	55,928	736	666	69	−27	42
1981–1991	56,352	757	655	103	43	146
1991–1997	57,808	754	640	113	87	200
Mid-year projections						
1997–2001	59,009	719	634	85	69	154
2001–2011	59,618	690	624	66	65	131
2011–2021	60,929	694	628	66	65	131

Source Social Trends 2001, HMSO

to and from the country. Most of the population growth in the UK during the 20th century can be attributed to these changes. See Table 1.5. However in recent years, net inward migration has become an increasingly important determinant of population growth, and is now matching the net natural change.

Figure 1.2 shows the rates for births and deaths from 1901 to the predicted figures for 2021. When birth rates and death rates remain the same, the population is said to be stable. However,

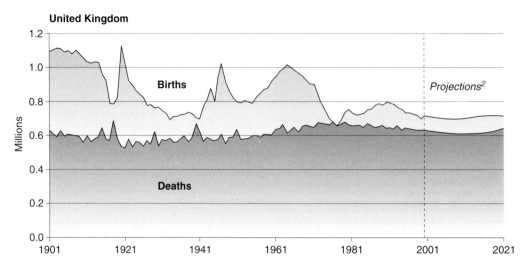

Figure 1.2 Births and deaths from 1901 to 2021 (predicted.)

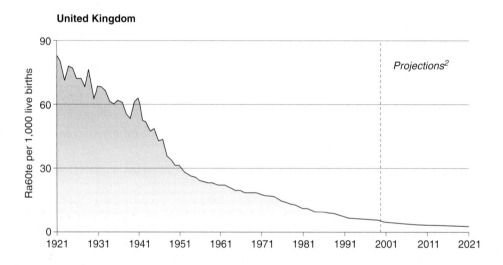

Figure 1.3 Infant mortallity rates

if the death rate remains the same and the birth rate increases, as during the birth bulge years of the post World War II period and again in the 1960s, this can also have implications for the planning of organisation of health and care services for children and mothers. More maternity services, primary schools and other health and social care services will be needed for this increase. Thus, an awareness of changes in the population is very significant when planning services.

Death rates also include infant mortality rates – deaths in children under one year old per 1000 live births. Figure 1.3 shows how infant mortality rates have fallen since 1921, with projections for the twenty-first century.

Activity

Look at Figure 1.3 and discuss factors that may have reduced infant mortality.

Infant mortality rates are an indicator of the standard of living in a country. If you look at some global statistics you will see that there are many countries in Africa, Asia and South America that have a very high rate of infant mortality. Although immunisations may play a part, many analysts believe that general standards of hygiene and the provision of a clean water supply are key factors, and that many childhood illnesses are the result of poverty.

The health of the population

The White Paper, *Our Healthier Nation* (1998), gave many statistics on the differences in health in certain groups and in different areas. As a result of the White Paper, Health Improvement Programmes (HImPs) have been set up nationally and locally to improve the nation's health.

The statistics on mortality and morbidity in the UK are discussed at length in Chapter 5 of the main text book so we will cover this briefly in this chapter.

Activity

Figure 1.4 shows the death rates for people aged under 65 in the UK between 1971 and 1997. Look at the statistics and answer the following questions:

1 What was the main cause of death for men and women in 1997?

2 Do the tables show any increase or decline in different causes of death?

Comment

The number of premature adult deaths has reduced considerably over the last 25 years. The most common cause of death for men is coronary heart disease, although the death rate has dropped by more than half since the 1970s. Cancer is the most common cause of death for women below the age of 65, with breast and lung cancer being the main cancers that affect women of this age. Suicide rates have generally fallen across the UK over the last 15 years, except among men aged 15 to 44. For both men and women aged 15 to 44, and 45 and over, suicide rates in Scotland were higher than the rest of the UK. In England and Wales, in all age groups, suicides are more common among men than women. Men aged 15 to 44 are almost four times as likely to commit suicide as women of the same age.

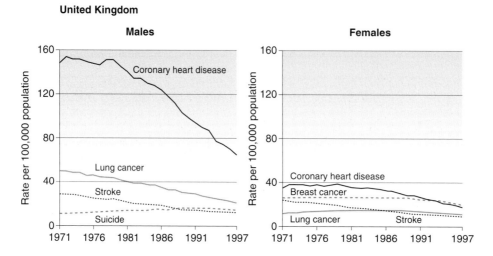

Figure 1.4 Death rates for people under 65 by gender and selected cause of death

Table 1.6   Suicide rates by region, gender, and age 1992–96

Rate per million population

	Males		Females	
	15–44	45 and over	15–44	45 and over
England & Wales	195	178	50	69
North East	198	192	55	65
North West (GOR)	233	176	64	69
Merseyside	208	164	52	53
Yorkshire & the Humber	201	178	53	71
East Midlands	192	171	45	64
West Midlands	181	170	45	63
Eastern	171	175	39	60
London	182	178	56	74
South East (GOR)	181	181	48	81
South West	196	187	50	76
Wales	247	186	42	62

Source Social Trends 2001, HMSO

Activity

1   Look at Table 1.6 (suicide rates) and describe the regional variations.

2   Read the following statistic. "A person's social class affects their likelihood of committing suicide. In 1991–93 the suicide rate among unskilled men aged 20 to 64 was more than three times higher than among professional men."

Can you think of any reasons for these variations?

Infant mortality rates

Birth weights vary by social class and low birth weight has a strong association with infant mortality. Since 1981 the infant mortality rate has nearly halved, from 11.2 deaths per 1000 live births to 5.9. deaths per 1000 live births in 1997. However, differences still occur between different groups.

Activity

Look at Table 1.7, showing infant mortality rates by social class and answer the following questions:

1   What general patterns do you notice:

   •   between 1981 and 1996;

   •   between social class groups;

   •   inside and outside of marriage;

2   What type of health programme might you develop if you were working as a health worker in an area where the infant mortality rate was high?

As the result of studying morbidity and mortality statistics, the Department of Health has agreed national targets to reduce deaths from cancer, coronary heart disease (CHD) and stroke, suicide and accidents. Local health authorities and primary care organisations have had to draw up plans outlining how these targets will be met. National Service Frameworks (NSFs) for CHD and mental health have also been produced to improve the quality of service to these groups.

By 2010 the following targets in reducing the annual death rate should be achieved:

Cancer: In people under 75 by a fifth (from 69,000 in 1997 to 55,000) in 2010.

Coronary heart disease and stroke: In people under 75 by at least two-fifths (from 69,000 in 1997 to 41,000 in 2010).

Accidents: By at least one-fifth (from 10,000 in 1997 to 8,000 in 2001) and to reduce the rate of serious injury by at least one-tenth.

Mental Health: By at least one-fifth (from 4,500 in 1997 to 3,600 in 2010).

Table 1.7 Infant mortality by social class 1981–1996

United Kingdom	Rates per 1,000 live births		
	1981	1991	1996
Inside marriage			
Professional	7.8	5.0	3.6
Managerial and			
technical	8.2	5.3	4.4
Skilled non-manual	9.0	6.2	5.4
Skilled manual	10.5	6.3	5.8
Semi-skilled	12.7	7.2	5.9
Unskilled	15.7	8.4	7.8
Other	15.6	11.8	8.3
All inside marriage	10.4	6.3	5.4
Outside marriage			
Joint registration	14.1	8.7	6.9
Sole registration	16.2	10.8	7.2
All outside marriage	15.0	9.3	7.0

Source Social Trends 2001, HMSO

Teenage pregnancies

The teenage pregnancy rate in the UK is the highest in Europe (see Figure 1.8) and this is another health statistic that is being monitored carefully. Every local health authority is producing programmes to reduce this rate.

Live births per 1,000 women

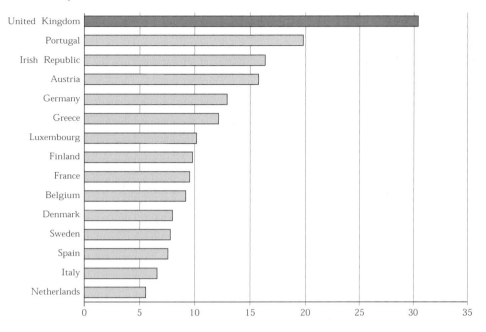

Figure 1.5 Teenage births 1996
Source Social Trends 2001, HMSO

Activity

Can you think of ways in which everyone involved with young people could work in a programme to reduce the pregnancy rate among teenagers? Some authorities have used a 'love bus', touring areas with advice on contraception. The main problem that health workers have encountered is how to involve young men in any programme. What ideas do you have on what could be done?

The role of government and others in the policy-making process

Since 1997 there has been a tremendous increase in legislation affecting health and social care. The key themes underpinning many of the changes have been partnership working, user participation and involvement, and quality of outcomes. For example, prior to the White Paper, 'Our Healthier Nation', there was a Green Paper entitled 'Saving Lives'. The Green Paper was a consultation document that encouraged members of the public, voluntary organisations, and professional health and social care workers to respond. The Health Strategy Unit at the Department of Health studied the responses, and these shaped the final White Paper.

The main piece of legislation that is concerned with the restructuring of the NHS is the Health Act of 1999. This included the White Paper proposals of the 1997 White Paper, 'The New NHS'.

Each piece of legislation has to go through a particular process before becoming law. The process takes a long time.

1 After passing through the Green Paper and the White Paper stage, a Bill is formally introduced in the House of Commons at the 'First Reading'.
2 At the 'Second Reading' the general principles of the Bill are debated and voted upon.
3 At the 'Committee Stage' each clause of the Bill is debated and voted upon.
4 At the 'Report Stage', the Bill is considered as it was reported by the committee and it is decided whether to make further changes in individual clauses.
5 At the 'Third Reading', the Bill as amended is debated and a final vote taken.
6 Next, the Bill then has to pass through the House of Lords, and the same stages are repeated there.
7 Finally, the Queen then gives her Royal Assent to the Bill which then becomes law as an Act of Parliament.

In the run up to the general election in 2001 a new NHS Bill was being debated, which proposed the abolition of the CHCs, as well as other proposals to include patient participation in the health service. Because of the pressures of the election, the Bill did not become law, but further legislation is being developed. Your local Community Health Council (CHC) may be able to advise you about any legislation that is currently being processed.

The European Dimension

The Council of Ministers is the main decision-making body within the European Union, and consists of representatives from each of the member states. The European Social Fund (ESF) provides funding for a wide variety of projects related to supporting people who are disadvantaged. Examples include:

- providing child care for single parents who wish to go back to work;
- offering skills training for people with learning difficulties;
- providing life long learning for socially excluded groups.

The ESF was set up to remove barriers to education, training and employment. There is a web site www.esfnews.org.uk that gives details about the Fund and also gives links to British government departments.

Impact of key inquiries

In recent years there have been several enquiries into health and social care services, which have resulted in changes of practice. These include:

The Bristol Hospital Enquiry, which covered the deaths of babies after heart surgery. As a result, surgeons are now more closely scrutinised and have their competence revalidated in performing certain procedures.

The Waterhouse Inquiry, which investigated irregularities in child care, is another example that will result in changes in the regulations of practice.

The Waterhouse Inquiry

The Waterhouse Inquiry was set up in 1996 to:

- inquire into the abuse of children in care in Wales since 1974;
- examine whether the agencies and authorities responsible for care could have prevented abuse or detected its occurrence at an earlier stage;
- examine the response of authorities to allegations of abuse made by people, including children formerly in care;
- consider what recommendations should be made for future practice.

Background

Internal investigations of abuse had been carried out in the 1970s and 1990s. One member of staff, Alison Taylor, raised her concerns in 1986 and, through media coverage, a major police investigation started in 1991. As a result, six former care staff were convicted.

Findings

Widespread sexual and physical abuse had occurred in several children's homes and in foster homes. Poor management and the lack of a proper complaints system added to the problems. The local authorities and the police were also criticised for failing to act promptly.

Recommendations

1 An Independent Children's Commissioner for Wales should be appointed to ensure that children's rights are respected, and to publish annual reports on the service.
2 Every social services authority in the UK should appoint an appropriately qualified children's complaints officer.
3 Clear whistle-blowing procedures should be set up.
4 Abuse awareness training for all staff would be implemented.
5 All incidents should be reported and records kept at a local police station with social services having access.
6 Inspection of all homes should be carried out by an independent agency.

Many of these recommendations are also included in the 'Modernising Social Services' White Paper (1998) and in the Consultation Document for Children, 'Working Together to Safeguard Children' (2000). Both Papers are discussed in the main textbook. ◇

Comment

As in the Welsh inquiry, many investigations start off as a result of 'whistle-blowing'. Alison Taylor went to the press to express her concerns. However, whistle-blowing is seen by some people as being disloyal to their colleagues. Because of the recent investigations, all social service and health organisations have a whistle-blowing policy that protects the employee from action against them by the organisation they are criticising. The doctor who was the whistle-blower at Bristol could no longer find work in the UK. He moved to Australia because he was seen to have betrayed his colleagues. By having a whistle-blowing policy in place, it is hoped that workers will feel more able to express their concerns about poor practice in future.

Financial constraints that influence design and delivery of services

Social services

Table 1.8 The proposed government budget 2001–2002

Government income and expenditure, 2001–2

Income (£bn)		Expenditure (£bn)	
income tax	104	Social Security	109
VAT	61	NHS	59
National Insurance	63	Education	50
Excise duties	37	Debt interest	23
Corporation Tax	38	Defence	24
Business rates	17	Law & order	23
Council tax	15	Industry, Agriculture & employment	16
Other	64	Housing & environment	18
		Transport	10
		Other expenditure	62
Total	£399 bn.	**Total**	£394 bn.

Source *Guardian* Newspaper 8/3/2001

The government operates a budget that includes the costing of health and social care expenditure. Table 1.8 shows the total government expenditure planned for 2001–2. Organisations have to operate on the principle of 'best value'; services have to reflect efficient use of scarce resources. The local social services budget is partly dependent on a central government grant. Its level depends upon various factors, such as the composition of the local population and the level of deprivation. If a local authority overspends its budget, it will not be 'bailed out' by central government but will have to make cuts in its budget for some services. Every financial year your local council undertakes a spending review, and it has to estimate how savings could be made. In some areas, the council has a public meeting to discuss these issues, and often unpopular decisions have to be made.

Activity

Find a copy of your local council's annual report. This should include details of the annual budget.

Identify the key areas of local government spending.

Health services

Every health authority (HA) has a statutory duty to balance its budget in the local health area. The HAs give money to local hospitals and these hospitals are responsible for keeping within the budget. If a hospital trust overspends, the deficit will pass to the health authority. The HA may be able to transfer the debt to the following year, but neither the HA nor the trust will be able to apply for additional funds. This means that the pressure is on all health organisations, including Primary Care Groups (PCGs) and Primary Care Trusts (PCTs) to keep within their budgets. As with the local councils, cuts may be made in services to keep within budget so hospital managers have to decide the priorities, such as choosing between redecorating the outside of the hospital or closing a ward. Because of these financial pressures, health and social care services are always reviewing services to see how efficiency can be maintained

Regulatory inspection

The Commission for Health Improvement (CHI) is the inspection body for clinical standards of the NHS in England and Wales. CHI started work in April 2000 and is a statutory body under the 1999 Health Act. It will visit every NHS Trust and health authority, including all primary care organisations, every four years and prepares a report. CHI also investigates serious failures in the NHS. CHI's work is based on the following principles. It will:

* put patient's experience at the heart of its work by asking them for their views of the service;
* be independent and fair;
* use a developmental approach to help the NHS improve;
* base its work on evidence not opinion;
* be open and accessible.

A Clinical Standards Board in Scotland provides the same kind of service. CHI has inspected several hospitals since it was set up. It presents a report and the hospital has to respond by drawing up an action plan to show how it will improve those services that are seen to be below standard. The CHI website is www.chi.nhs.uk, if you want further information about inspections in your area.

Inspection and regulation in social care

The Social Services Inspectorate (SSI) is responsible for inspecting services. As a result of the proposals made in the White Paper, 'Modernising Social Services', The Care Standards Act was passed in 2000. This will reform the regulatory system for England and Wales and will come into effect from April 2002. The National Care Standards Commission will inspect all residential and nursing homes, domiciliary care agencies, and private and voluntary care services. At present, inspection units are attached to local councils, which means that the council could be inspecting its own services. By developing a totally independent inspection regime, it is hoped that the quality of services will improve and reach a high national standard.

The main features of contemporary social care provision

This is covered in detail in Chapter 5 of the main text book ◇ Since the NHS and Community Care Act (1990), a mixed economy of care has developed. This means that the role of the public (or statutory) sector has decreased, and the role of private and voluntary organisations has increased. Many local authority care homes have been taken over by private or voluntary (non-profit making) agencies. Social services purchase social care from a range of providers – for example, day centre provision for older people, home care, meals on wheels and other services. Social services also purchase beds in residential care. With the development of closer working with the health service some provision – like intermediate care, is purchased through a pooled budget, where both partners contribute funds.

The voluntary sector also provides services for social care, through service level agreements that may be for one year or longer, or for particular projects that are national priorities, such as work with older people. Because voluntary organisations are dependent on contracts with local councils, this may reduce their role as a pressure group. Self-help groups are an important aspect of social care. As local councils' resources become more restricted, many groups form to help themselves. Young mothers and toddler groups, refugee groups and others join together to share a particular problem. The website www.self-help.org.uk lists self help groups in Great Britain.

Constraints of economic and resource factors

 # Case study

In South London there are two hospitals, both offering kidney transplant services. It is proposed by the Health Authority that the service should be centralised at one centre for the following reasons:

1 There is a national shortage of specialist nephrology (kidney) consultants and clinical staff.

2 Consultants who specialise in this area have to undertake a certain number of operations each year in order to be accredited as competent. By concentrating the service at one hospital this will make it easier for surgeons to be accredited.

As part of the NHS's commitment to involving patients in consultation about possible changes to service provision, the health authority had various meetings with patient groups Patient Action to Retain Transplant Services (PARTS) – at both hospitals. Patients were concerned about travelling longer distances for transplant surgery and relatives would also have a longer journey when visiting. However, the Health Authority has made an interim decision that the transplant service will be retained at one site, but there will be life-long nephrology support on both sites and continuing care on whichever site the patient receives replacement therapy. As we can see from this example, decisions about centralising services have to take account of using scarce resources in a cost effective way, even if this means longer journeys for patients.

Other examples of this kind include centralising cleft lip and palate services in London as hospitals offering this service will be reduced in future, and rationalising ambulance service provision. In Wiltshire the three emergency services, Fire, Police and Ambulances will be based in a joint headquarters. In Cleveland a joint control centre for the three emergency services is already in operation.

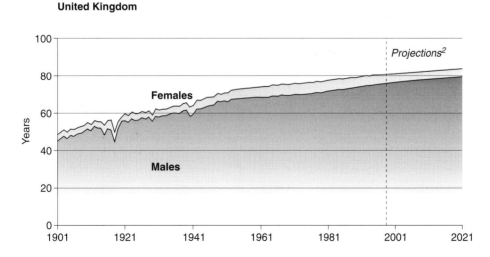

Figure 1.6 Expectations of life at birth 1901–2021

Demographic factors influencing social policy in the next 20 years

Life expectancy is increasing (see Figure 1.6) and we can see from the predicted population figures that the proportion of older people in the UK population is likely to continue to increase. The following is an excerpt from the Office of National Statistics Monthly Digest for October 2001.

Population

Mid-2000 UK population estimates have been released by the ONS. Key findings include:

- The mid-2000 UK population is estimated at 59,755,700, a rise of 3.4 per cent since mid-1991.
- The largest rises were seen in the population of working age of 30 and over (30 to 64/59 for men and women respectively) and the 85 and over age group which increased by 13.6 per cent and 29.5 per cent respectively between 1991 and 2000.
- Although the UK population increased overall, there were decreases in some age groups. The largest decrease occurred in the number of people aged 16 to 29. This group was estimated at 10,645,700 in 2000 which is a fall of 13.9 per cent since 1991.

Source ONS Monthly Digest August 2001, HMSO

Activity

Look at the population changes that are identified and think about the implications of these for welfare policy, especially in the following age groups

- 16–29;
- over 85.

Britain ages as pregnancies fall

Retirement at 72 needed to keep workforce balance

John Carvel
Social affairs editor

The average retirement age would have to rise to 72 to maintain the present balance between the working population and numbers of older dependants, according to demographic forecasts published yesterday by the office for national statistics.

If there is no corresponding increase in the birth rate in the future, there will be fewer economically active adults paying direct taxation and national insurance contributions. Some analysts put forward the view that the retirement age in the future will need to be raised to 72 to pay for the benefits for the older groups (see the excerpt from *The Guardian*). Current predictions suggest that the number of people who are over 75 will increase and this will have an impact on all aspects of welfare.

Housing

More supported housing units will be needed to encourage older people to remain in their own homes. As many of these people will be in single households, which are also predicted to increase in the next century, this may mean a more efficient use of limited housing resources and a greater role taken by local councils in directly providing housing services.

Health

If there is an increase in the over 75s in the twenty-first century, there will be increased demand for those services that are currently provided.

 Activity

Look at Table 1.9 and identify the pattern of age to service use.

The additional use of health services will lead to the development of more intermediate care beds, chiropody and other community services, and specific clinical support for diabetes, osteo-arthritis, cardiac problems and ophthalmology. Additional staff will be needed in these areas. The drugs budget will also increase. Recruiting staff to work in health and social care may be a problem if there are fewer young people in the population as a whole.

Education

The predicted fall in 16–29 year-olds will mean fewer places in further and higher education. This may also have an effect on the numbers of people entering teacher training courses.

Employment

Fewer school leavers will be entering employment. Employers may need to recruit older people into work previously done by young people. There may be an increase in older people in their 50s and 60s working full-time or part-time to make up the shortfall.

Benefit system

More benefits will be needed to be paid to older people in order to maintain their independence in the community and also to contribute to the cost of residential care. Because the numbers of economically active people will decrease because of the decline in the younger age groups, indirect taxation may need to increase, as there will be fewer workers paying tax and national insurance on their income.

Table 1.9 Use of health services by gender & age 1998–99

United Kingdom								Percentage
							75 and	All aged 16 and
	16–24	25–34	35–44	45–54	55–64	65–74	over	over
Males								
Consultation with GP[1]	7	9	10	12	16	17	21	12
Outpatient visit[2]	12	14	13	15	20	25	29	17
Casualty visit[2,3]	7	7	5	4	3	3	3	5
Females								
Consultation with GP[1]	15	18	16	19	17	19	21	18
Outpatient visit[2]	13	13	12	17	19	21	26	17
Casualty visit[2,3]	6	4	3	3	3	3	3	4

1 Consultations with an NHS GP in the last two weeks.

2 In the last three months; includes visits to casualty in Great Britain only.

3 The question was only asked of those who said they had an outpatient visit.

Source Social Trends 2001, HMSO

Word check

Indirect taxation

Taxation that is paid indirectly on goods and services that people buy, such as VAT.

Direct taxation

Taxation that is paid directly out of income, either earned or unearned.

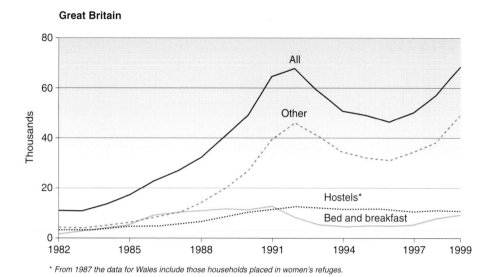

Great Britain

* From 1987 the data for Wales include those households placed in women's refuges.

Figure 1.7 Homeless households in temporary accommodation

Key Issues in the Twenty-First Century

The homeless

Since 1982 there has been an increase in the homeless in Great Britain. In Wales three out of 10 households accepted as homeless in 1999, stated that they were homeless as a result of a breakdown of a relationship with a partner. In Scotland almost a third of homeless households were homeless because they did not wish to remain with friends or family. Figure 1.7 shows the numbers of households in temporary accommodation between 1982 and 1999. When a homeless household makes an application for housing, the local housing authority must decide whether the applicant is eligible for assistance, is unintentionally homeless or is in a priority need group. If these conditions are met in England and Wales, the council must provide sufficient advice and assistance to the applicant. Suitable accommodation should be provided for up to two years. During this time the council may offer a secure council tenancy. In England the main reason for an increase in homelessness is related to the increase in housing costs in London and the south-east and to asylum seekers. Across Great Britain one in seven households in temporary accommodation were housed in hostels (including women's refuges) and one in seven were in bed and breakfast accommodation. The Rough Sleepers Unit (RSU) was established in 1999 as part of the Government's social exclusion policy of 1998. By June 2000, the number of people sleeping rough in England on any one night was estimated to be about 1.2. million

Activity

1 Look at figure 1.7 and describe the main patterns you see.

2 You are a government minister responsible for reducing homelessness. If you were taking a New Right approach whom would you see as responsible for the increase in homelessness and what solutions would you propose? If you were from the Collectivist approach, how would you differ in the causes you would identify and the approach you would use? Use Table 1.2 here.

Refugees and asylum seekers

Britain has had a long tradition of supporting immigrants, from the Huguenots in the seventeeth century to the Jews in the twentieth century. Nationals from the European Economic Area have the right to reside in the UK provided they are working or are able to provide for themselves. Nearly all other overseas nationals wishing to live in the UK require Home Office acceptance for settlement. Immigration controls were set up in 1962. The number of people accepted for settlement in the UK increased by 27,000 to 97,000 between 1998 and 1999. This increase was partly due to people seeking asylum from Yugoslavia and Turkey.

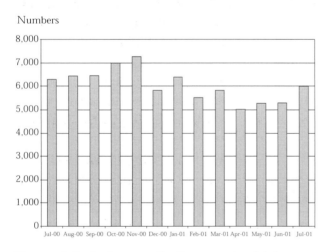

Numbers

Figure 1.8 Asylum applications received July 2000–July 2001
Source Home Office July 2001

There have also been a high percentage of refugees from Asia and Africa – some are seeking asylum, while others are married to spouses already in the UK. The Home Office required applicants to prove they had not married primarily in order to gain entrance to the UK. The latest asylum figures published by the Home Office in July 2001 show that applicants from Afghan nationals remained the highest applicant nationality for the fifth consecutive month (Figure 1.8).

Welfare and refugees

The costs of asylum in 2000 are shown in Figure 1.9. Welfare arrangements have been criticised as being degrading and ineffective. Local authorities have had to find accommodation and pay subsistence to refugees. Problems were experienced in arranging benefits for refugees because they did not have a permanent address. A local study into the experience of refugees found the following:

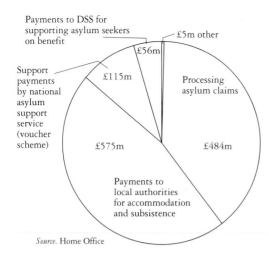

Payments to DSS for supporting asylum seekers on benefit

£5m other

£56m

£115m

Support payments by national asylum support service (voucher scheme)

Processing asylum claims

£575m

£484m

Payments to local authorities for accommodation and subsistence

Source. Home Office

Figure 1.9 The cost of asylum 2000 Source Home Office

- problems for children gaining access to schools;
- lack of support for adults and children with physical and mental difficulties;
- difficulty of access to health and dental services;
- access to housing;
- racist attacks and discrimination;
- little or no interpreting support;
- poverty related to the voucher system, which meant that there was no cash for bus fares or other activities and personal items;
- social exclusion.

Following continued criticism, David Blunkett, Secretary of State for the Home Office, announced the following changes:

- The voucher system will be replaced by Smart ID cards. These cards will include photograph and fingerprint data, and will become cash debit cards to replace vouchers from autumn 2002.
- The value of vouchers will go up in value from £10 to £14 to reflect the overall increase in income support.
- A small network of induction centres near Heathrow and Croydon will replace the use of emergency bed and breakfast accommodation. Asylum seekers will stay at these centres for up to two weeks, and during this time they will be provided with food and accommodation. Centres will not be locked.
- Reporting centres – those refugees who have been dispersed around the UK will be required to report at these centres so that they can be informed of decisions about their application. Those who are told they cannot be accepted will be put in police cells until they are taken to a removal centre.
- Accommodation centres – about four centres will be set up across the UK. They will provide a range of services including basic health care, education for children, leisure activities and access to legal advice and interpreters.
- Appeals – the back log of appeals will be cleared so that 6000 decisions a month can be made by November 2002.
- Removal centres – the network of detention centres across the UK will be enlarged to provide 4000 places by November 2002. The use of prisons for asylum seekers will cease in 2002.
- Refugee resettlement – a new programme that will arrange safe transport to Britain for those groups that are recognised by the United Nations as being in danger in their country of origin.

Activity

1 Look at Figure 1.9 and describe what you see.

2 Look carefully at David Blunkett's proposals. Can you think of possible problems with:

   • their implementation;

   • their effects on local communities in the UK;

   • additional provision that may be needed for children and families;

   • employment and integration issues?

3 Traditionally, right-wing theorists discouraged immigration and initiated tight controls. What type of ideology do you think is influencing this current policy towards refugees and asylum seekers?

Poverty

Table 1.10 Examples of recent government welfare policy related to poverty

Health	Low income	Education/employment	Support and community regenerat
<u>NHS plan</u> reform of NHS	<u>Working Families</u> <u>Tax Credit</u> To support families	Extra funding for education and <u>Life Long Learning</u>	<u>Sure Start</u> programmes increased
<u>National Service</u> <u>Frameworks (NSFs)</u> For Mental Health, CHD, older people	<u>Sure Start maternity grant</u> For pregnant and nursing mothers	<u>New Deal</u> <u>Programme extended for</u> disabled people	<u>Neighbourhood Renewal</u> Programmes in poor communities <u>New Deal for Communities</u> Covering poor neighbourhoods
Improving local services with the development of primary care trusts	<u>Income support</u> Increased for families	<u>Securing Health Together</u> Reducing occupational ill-health and disability	<u>The UK Fuel Poverty Strategy</u> Helping pensioners and other vulnerable groups
<u>Health action zones</u> Improving health of disadvantaged groups	<u>Minimum income</u> <u>guarantee</u> For pensioners		<u>Network of Healthy Living Cent</u> to strengthen community initiativ health, education and environmen
	Increasing the <u>National Minimum Wage</u>		<u>Rough Sleepers Unit</u> Developing programmes to reduce the number of people sleeping rou
	<u>Children's tax credit</u> Baby credit for a child in the first year of life		

Source. Tackling Health Inequalities. Consultation Paper (2001), DOH

Another key issue related to social welfare is the need to reduce the numbers of people in poverty. Table 1.10 shows the various welfare programmes that are running in 2001 and many of these will be extended in the future. Poverty is still seen as a major issue, especially when related to children and older people. 'Tackling Health Inequalities' (DoH 2001) identifies six priority themes for future social policy.

1 Providing a sure foundation for life through a healthy pregnancy and childhood.

2 Improving opportunities for children and young people.

3 Improving the NHS Primary Care services.

4 Tackling the major killers – Coronary Heart Disease and Cancer.

5 Strengthening disadvantaged communities.

6 Tackling the wider causes of health inequalities.

The identified national policies are directed to reducing health inequalities and to tackling the root causes of poverty and material disadvantage. They aim to:

- improve the income and material conditions of the poorest by continuing reform of the tax and benefit system;

- continue to improve the position of poorest families by increasing the National Minimum Wage;

- address inequalities in the most disadvantaged communities through implementing the National Strategy for Neighbourhood Renewal;

- reduce the risk of ill health and cut the numbers of excess winter deaths among the most vulnerable groups by implementing the UK Fuel Poverty Strategy;

- address the housing needs of deprived areas by bringing all social housing up to set standards by 2010;

- provide targeted help for those without work, and to find and retain jobs through the New Deal programmes, employment zones and Action Teams for jobs;

- help people of working age by introducing Jobcentre Plus to deliver an efficient labour market and benefit service;

- reduce work-related ill-health, and increase opportunities for rehabilitation through the occupational health strategy, 'Securing Health Together'.

There are a number of websites that are relevant to this section. They include:

http://www.inlandrevenue.gov.uk/nwm/index.htm

http://www.defra.gov.uk/environment/consult/fuelpov/index.htm

http://www.doh.gov.uk/healthinequalities

 ## Activity

There are many leaflets outlining some of these policies available at post offices and public libraries. See what you can find out. It may also be useful to collect a file of newspaper articles and headlines related to current policy.

Technological developments in the delivery of health and social care

The development of Information technology means that many people will have access to medical help and advice via the Internet in the future. With direct booking of hospital out-patient appointments and day surgery by the GP, waiting lists should be reduced. Continued development of surgical techniques for operations such as cataracts, kidney stones, gallstones and cardiac surgery, means that patients can be treated as day cases. Telemedicine is another example of changes to delivery of care, with the transfer of information via an Internet or video link. These approaches speed up diagnosis and treatment of cardiac conditions. There have been recent examples of operations being undertaken by robots, so perhaps this will be another development in the future. Specialist training is needed to use these developing techniques.

Some GPs are being trained to perform scans and other procedures so that the patient can be treated locally. Blood pressure machines and ECG machines that patients can wear as they go about their daily routine is another way of diagnosing conditions without the need to go to hospital (these machines are used for 24 hours and can be useful for detecting abnormalities that a blood pressure check or ECG carried out in the surgery would not identify). As these different approaches become better known, demand is expected to increase. New technology can cause its own problems as many GPs have been confronted by patients who have diagnosed their condition on the Internet and bring the printout to the surgery!

Scientific Developments in Health and Social Care

Transplant services

NHS transplant services started in the UK in the 1960s with kidney grafting. Heart, liver, lung, pancreas, small bowel, cornea, heart valve and bone transplants are now routine, and skin is grafted to treat severe burns. In the last 25 years over one million people have benefited from a transplant.

The UK Transplant Service Authority (UKTSSA) was set up as a Special Health Authority in 1991 and was renamed UK Transplant in 2000. It provides a 24-hour support service for the matching, allocation and distribution of donor organs. It is accountable to the Secretary of State for Health. In 1998 the Government launched an organ donation publicity campaign in order to increase the number of donors and £3 million was put into the plan in 2001 in order to:

- double the number of those on the organ donation register from 8 million to 16 million by 2010;
- develop a National Service Framework for patients with kidney failure to establish national standards and improve services;
- increase the kidney transplant rate by almost 100% by 2005;
- increase heart, lung and liver transplant by 10% by 2005.

In July 2000, Boots the Chemists launched a scheme for Advantage card customers (their loyalty card) to join the NHS organ donor register. Boots invested £500,000 in the scheme and promotes it by using leaflets in their stores.Other credit card companies are also inviting card holders to join the NHS Organ Donor Register from January 2001.

Activity

Visit your local Boots store to find the leaflets. Use the websites related to organ donation to access up to date information on the statistics related to organ donation and for general information.

www.uktransplant.org.uk provides information on the work of the UK Transplant and other general information.

The NHS organ donor website – www.nhs.uk/organdonor provides statistics.

Transplant surgery is seen as a specialist area and one of the key issues related to ensuring the continued quality of its provision is the development of specialist centres of excellence.

Potential scientific developments and their influence on social care services

There has been a great deal of discussion in the media and among the medical profession about many of the developments in this area because of the ethical issues that are raised.

Cloning of body parts

Although human cloning is banned in Britain at the moment, scientists are looking at ways of replacing diseased or failing organs with cloned cells acceptable to the immune system. In 1998, scientists in Scotland identified and managed to grow in laboratory dishes the stem cells or master cells that make all the other cells in the body – such as for skin, blood and bone. This development could mean that damaged tissues could be repaired, whether it is neurons for Parkinson's disease, damaged cartilage cells, heart muscle cells or white blood cells.

Scientists answered MPs' questions about these new developments at a meeting in November 2000. Stem cell therapy is one area that could be developed to treat a range of conditions but concern was raised that these cells would be obtained from week-old foetuses. This research would be controlled by the 1990 Human Fertilisation and Embryology Act, which prevents human embryos beyond 14 days being used. In August 2001, bone marrow stem cells were taken from a 46-year-old man's pelvis and injected into arteries near his heart. The cells migrated to areas in the heart that had been damaged by a heart attack and turned into healthy muscle cells that began to beat. Using a person's own stem cells may be suitable as they will have the same DNA and will not be rejected. However, research into cloning will continue in spite of ethical problems that will need to be resolved, as there could be real benefits to disorders that affect nerves and muscles, such as Parkinson's Disease and Multiple Sclerosis.

Improvements in transplant surgery

As transplant surgery becomes more routine and acceptable, the demands for the service will continue to increase. However, the current shortage of donors could continue. Donors from black and minority ethnic groups are less likely to come forward. Research has shown that this is because of cultural and religious beliefs about the body needing to be maintained in its whole state after death. Transplant surgery is expensive, not just because of the procedure itself, but because of the medication that patients need to take for the rest of their lives to guard against tissue rejection. Demand for transplants will always out strip supply.

Genetic engineering

This is another controversial development in health care. Genetic screening is developing, especially when there is a family history of disease, such as breast cancer or ovarian cancer. In the field of cancer research inherited genetic factors seem to regulate some aspects of risk that an individual faces. Certain genes such as (BRCA–1) which increases some women's susceptibility to breast cancer, have been identified; others, such as hMSH2 on chromosome 2p, have been identified as a potential cause of colo-rectal cancer. "In genetic" screening, harmful genes such as these can be looked for in a person's DNA. There are ethical and practical considerations. The knowledge that a potential health risk is present could affect a person's chances of employment or insurance. It would also be a cause of anxiety, especially if there is no effective treatment to prevent the disease developing. Certain genetic conditions are more common among certain ethnic groups, for example, Ashkenazi Jews carry a higher incidence of genetic mutations associated with certain cancers. Genotypic prevention involves the diagnosis of a genetic disorder before birth, with the implication of offering the parents a choice of termination. Many disabled people have criticised this type of screening as they feel that people with genetic conditions are being discriminated against.

In October 2000 the Government announced that Britain will be the first country to allow insurers to use the results of genetic tests to identify people with hereditary illnesses. Approval would first be given for Huntingtons Chorea. Hereditary breast cancer and Alzheimer's disease are also expected to be approved. Critics of the decision feel that vulnerable groups would find it difficult to get life insurance or a mortgage as people would be asked to disclose the results of any genetic testing they had undergone. However, this is still under discussion and although insurance companies may request results of genetic testing in the future, clients may be allowed to refuse to divulge the information.

Activity

Mary is expecting her first baby. Her husband has achondroplasia (a condition that used to be called dwarfism). She has been told that male children are more likely to have this condition and she has been offered a pre-natal screening test to identify if the baby is a boy. If the baby is a boy, the foetus could be genetically screened to find out if it has the condition. Her husband, Brian, has mixed feelings about this. His father had the condition and had a successful career in paediatric medicine. He is a teacher. He feels that the condition has not affected his life chances and that by offering genetic screening it encourages a form of selection of the fittest, by assuming that people with disabilities are a drain on society. If you were the health worker involved in this case how would you approach this situation?

In this chapter we have covered a range of issues that affect workers in health and social care. We have seen how present-day social policy has its links with the past. If you wish to study social policy in more detail, you may find the following book useful: *Social Policy for Health and Social Care* by Tina Lovell and Claire Cordeaux (1999) Hodder and Stoughton.

References and resources

Community Care is a weekly publication that contains useful articles relevant to this area.

Brendon, V. (1994) *The Age of Reform 1820–1850*. Hodder and Stoughton

Holden, C. *et al.* (1996) *Further Studies for Social Care*, First Edition. Hodder and Stoughton.*

Lawson, T. and Garrod, J. (1996) *The Complete A–Z Sociology Handbook*. Hodder and Stoughton.*

Lovell, T. and Cordeaux, C. (1999) *Social Policy for Health and Social Care*. Hodder and Stoughton.*

Meggitt, C. (1997) *Special Needs Handbook for Health and Social Care*. Hodder and Stoughton.*

'Our Healthier Nation: Saving Lives' – White Paper (1999) HMSO.

Richards, J. (1999) The Complete *A–Z Health and Social Care Handbook*. Hodder and Stoughton.*

'Social Trends' (2001) HMSO.

'Tackling Health Inequalities' (2001) DOH.

Thomson, H. *et al* (2000) *Vocational A Level for Health and Social Care*. Hodder and Stoughton.*

Items marked with an asterisk are recommended reading for students.

Useful websites

Department of Health
www.doh.gov.uk

Department of Social Security
www.dss.gov.uk

Department of Trade and Industry
www.dti.gov.uk

Government Actuary Department
www.gad.gov.uk

Health Inequalities report
www.official-documents.co.uk/doh/ih/contents.htm

Immigration and Asylum Statistics
www.homeoffice.gov.uk/rds/index.htm

Institute for Social and Economic Affairs
www.iser.essex.ac.uk

National Assembly for Wales
www.wales.gov.uk

National Insurance Statistics and Research Agency
www.nisra.gov.uk

National Statistics
www.statistics.gov.uk

NHS in Scotland
www.show.nhs.uk/isd

NHS Plan
www.doh.gov.uk/nhsplan

'Our Healthier Nation' White Paper
www.doh.gov.uk./ohn.htm

Sure Start Programme
www.surestart.gov.uk

Teenage Pregnancy Unit
www.teenagepregnancyunit.go.uk

Glossary

Ageing population   A population in which the proportion of people over 65 is increasing.

Ageism   Negative feelings towards, and discriminatory behaviour against, a person on the basis of age.

Birth rate   The number of live births per 1000 of the population.

Black Report   A report on the inequalities of health, which shows there is a marked social class difference in health and health chances of the British population.

Care in the community   Policy of deinstitutionalisation introduced during the 1990s, when large-scale hospitals for the long-term care of people with mental health problems, learning disabilities, physical disabilities and older people, were closed and provision of care was placed in the community.

Census   Full-scale national survey taken every 10 years since 1801 (apart from 1941). Statistics from the census form the basis for planning welfare services.

Child Support Agency   Established 1993 by the Conservative government to reduce the cost to the taxpayer of financial support to one-parent families. Absent parents (usually fathers) were traced by the CSA and required to pay an appropriate amount of support.

Council housing   Homes built for, and rented out by, the local council as a low-cost alternative to buying. Public housing stocks have reduced following the selling-off of council homes to tenants.

Death rate   The crude death rate is expressed as the number of deaths per 1000 of the live population.

Demography   The study of population, with particular reference to its size and structure, and how and why it changes over time, through changes in the birth and death rates, marriage rates, patterns of migration and other factors.

Dependency Culture   New Right view that universal welfare provision has led people to expect the state to provide for them.

Direct taxation   Taxes – income tax or inheritance tax – directly levied on a person's income or wealth.

DNA (deoxyribonucleic acid)   A nucleic acid mainly found in the chromosomes of cells. It is the hereditary material of all organisms except for some viruses.

Epidemiology   The study of the nature, amount and spread of disease, in order to develop an appropriate approach to prevention and cure.

Family credit   A social benefit in the UK which tops up the income of low-paid workers with children.

Feminism   The ideological perspective that examines society and events within society from the viewpoint of women.

Genetics   The study of biological inheritance and the extent to which individuals are the product of their parental DNA.

Gross National Product (GNP)   A measure of the value of the productivity of a country, and therefore its wealth.

Ideology   A systematic set of beliefs which explains society and its policies.

Income support   A means tested benefit for unemployed people, single parents and disabled people whose income has been assessed as inadequate.

Indirect taxation   Taxes that are levied on goods and services (VAT). This form of taxation takes a greater proportion of the income of poorer groups.

Infant mortality rate   The number of deaths of infants under one year old per 1000 live births. It is an indicator of general prosperity.

Liberal Democratic Party   Formed from the amalgamation of the Liberal Party and the Social Democratic Party (SDP – a splinter group from the Labour Party).

Life expectancy   The average number of years a new-born baby can expect to live. Male babies born in 1994 in the UK can expect to live until about 74 years of age, and female babies until 79 years of age.

Local authorities   Local political bodies that control towns, cities and rural areas.

Marketisation   The process by which market principles and practices are introduced into areas that were not markets before, for example, health, schools and social services. In the view of the New Right, this approach is more likely to respond to service users' needs.

Means tested benefits   Social benefits that are delivered only when the claimant is able to show need. Many older people in need tend not to apply for these benefits.

Mixed economy   The public, private and voluntary sectors provide goods and services for service users, for example, day centres and nursing homes.

New Deal   Government programmes assisting unemployed people to enter work. Special advisors offer support to women, young people and people with disabilities.

New Right   Traditionally a Conservative approach, which has links to the *laissez-faire* policies of the nineteenth century, in which a free market with little intervention by the State is seen as effective, by encouraging competition and individual responsibility.

Official Statistics   Statistical data provided by central and local government and government agencies on unemployment rates, crime rates, etc.

Ofsted (Office of Standards in Education)   Set up by the Conservative government to inspect, monitor and report on the performance of schools.

Patriarchy   Term used by feminists to describe society as organised by men for the benefit of men and the oppression of women.

Poverty   A lack of sufficient resources to achieve a standard of living considered to be acceptable in a particular society. The benefit system in the UK is based on the idea of an absolute poverty line – if the person's income falls below that line they are said to be in poverty. In the European Union, the poverty line is usually drawn at 50% of the average income in that particular society.

Privatisation   Government policy in which the public sector influence is reduced and services are transferred to private agencies, for example, gas, water and electricity.

Progressive taxation   Direct taxation which increases depending on the amount of income received. This measure is to achieve a greater equality of distribution of income and wealth in a society.

Racism   Ideas about race are translated into negative feelings and discriminatory action against a particular racial group.

Recession   Deteriorating economic conditions when unemployment increases and productivity declines.

Redistribution   In which income and wealth are taken from the rich by progressive taxation and given to the poor in the form of benefits.

Social engineering   Planned social change brought about by the implementation of particular social policies, for example, the development of comprehensive schools.

Social Fund   Budget made available under the Department of Work and Pensions to provide loans to the recipients of social security benefits.

Social Security   The system of welfare support provided by the State for its citizens. Unemployment and sickness benefits and pensions are contributory through National Insurance contributions; non-contributory benefits provide a safety net for those most in need.

Social Trends   Annual digest of statistics produced by the Central Statistical Office.

Universalism   An approach to welfare that maintains that all citizens have an equal right to free and accessible services provided by the State.

Voluntary Sector   Non-profit making organisations that provide services and/or act as pressure groups.

Welfare pluralism   Provision of services from many different sources: private, public and voluntary.

Welfare state   Areas of service provision in which the government has a role in funding, planning and regulating. The key areas are health, education, income maintenance, housing and personal social services.

Chapter 2

Education for health and social well-being

This chapter describes:

- Definitions of health and social well-being
- Levels of health education
- Areas of health education:
  - 1 Promoting a healthy lifestyle: diet, hygiene, physical activity, mental health and positive personal relationships;
  - 2 Reducing the likelihood of ill-health: immunisation, heart disease, strokes, cancer, Sexually Transmitted Diseases (STDs), substance abuse;
  - 3 Promoting personal safety: safety in the home, road safety
- The origins of health education campaigns
- The roles of organisations and professionals involved in health education
- Planning for health education
- Evaluating health education campaigns

What is health?

The **World Health Organisation** (WHO) defines health as 'a state of complete physical, mental and social well-being and not merely the absence of disease or infirmity.' A more useful definition of health includes three other very important aspects of health: emotional, environmental and spiritual. Health is a resource for everyday life not the object of living. It is a positive concept emphasising social and personal resources as well as physical capabilities, and is regarded by WHO as a fundamental human right.

1 **Physical health** is the easiest aspect of health to measure. It involves the physical functioning of the body and includes the growth and physical development of the baby and child.

2 **Emotional health** involves how we express emotions such as joy, grief, frustration, hurt and fear. This ability to express our own emotions and to react to other people's emotions leads on to coping strategies for anxiety and stress.

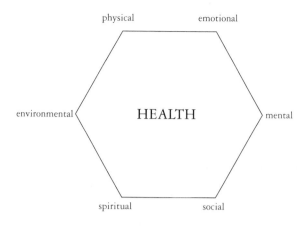

Figure 2.1 The six aspects of health

3 **Mental health** involves our ability to organise our thoughts logically, and is closely linked to emotional and social health.

4 **Social health** involves the way we relate to other people and form relationships.

5 **Spiritual health** involves personal and moral codes of conduct as well as religious beliefs and practices.

6 **Environmental health** refers to the general health of the society in which we live. In areas of famine – where the first priority for health is to obtain enough food – people may be denied access to health. Poverty and overcrowded living conditions are all negative aspects of environmental health.

What is health education?

Health education focuses on the individual and describes any activity that promotes health-related learning. It is also a means of **self-empowerment**. This means that by providing advice and information on health matters, people are able to take more control over their own health and the factors that affect their health. **Health promotion** is the umbrella term given to programmes of health education; it describes the process of enabling people to increase control over, and to improve their health.

It is now recognised that people's lifestyles and behaviour have a great effect on their health and social well-being.

Social influences on health and social well-being

- Ill health is not a matter of chance or bad luck. Some people have a greater or lesser chance of good health than others. There is now a mass of evidence detailing variations in health status according to socio-economic factors, gender, culture ethnicity and age.

- The existence of social inequalities in health is generally accepted. The new government health strategy 'Our Healthier Nation' recognises that there are inequalities in health across society:

  > The poorest in our society are hit harder than the well off by most of the major causes of death. In improving the health of the whole nation, a key priority will be better health for those who are worst off.
  >
  > *(From the summary of 'Our Healthier Nation', Department of Health 1998.)*

- Income is a key factor affecting health. An individual's income can determine access to resources such as a good diet and warmth. It also has an effect on people's psychological health, with those on a low income experiencing stress, depression and social isolation.

- Employment is a key factor affecting health. People who work live longer lives.

Unemployed men and women are more likely to die prematurely from heart disease, cancer (particularly lung cancer) or suicide.

- A social network can protect people against stress. Social exclusion that may arise from unemployment, a low income or isolation can significantly affect health. A social network that offers practical and emotional support has been shown to have a protective effect on health.

Behavioural influences on health and social well-being

- Many major causes of death are preventable and are the result of people's lifestyles:
  - smoking is deemed to be responsible for lung cancer in 90% of all cases;
  - a lack of fibre in the diet is responsible for stomach and colon cancer in up to 30% of all cases;
  - a lack of exercise is a contributory factor in hypertension (or high blood pressure).
- Individual responsibility for health. The government health strategy 'Our Healthier Nation' acknowledges a 'contract' for health between government, communities and individuals. The government and its lead agencies (including the Health Development Agency) have also set up media campaigns to persuade the population to change to healthier ways of living. The role of the health educator has thus been seen to give advice and information to encourage people to change and to equip people with the skills and confidence to make changes.
- Healthy behaviour is not evenly distributed across the population. There are differences in health across society and personal behaviour has a part to play in this. Damaging behaviours such as smoking are far more common in lower socio-economic groups. Forty per cent men in social classes IV and V smoke, compared with 21% in social class I. These groups are also less likely to take up healthier behaviours such as exercise.
- Lifestyles are partly determined by income: For example: a healthy diet has been shown to cost an average £5 more per 'shopping basket'; other factors over which people have little control, such as access to leisure facilities or shops selling fresh produce, may also be affected by income.
- People's behaviour can be a response to social circumstances. Smoking, drinking and illegal drug taking can all be seen as ways of coping with stressful lives.
- There is a danger of 'victim blaming'. If the focus is solely on changing behaviour, people may be blamed for ill health over which they have little control – 'victim blaming'.

Levels of health education

Table 2.1 Three levels of health education

Type of health education	Aim	For whom
Primary health education	Prevention of ill-health	Directed at reducing risks to the entire population in order to prevent ill-health from arising. **Examples:** Children in school learn about healthy eating, road safety and basic hygiene; immunisation.
Secondary health education	Reducing risk of ill-health	Directed at reducing risk factors for people already at risk, i.e., people with a health problem or a reversible condition. **Examples:** Encouraging overweight people to change their eating habits or a smoker to quit smoking; **screening** (routinely examining) apparently healthy people who are likely to develop a particular disease.
Tertiary health education	Promoting rehabilitation and adjustment	Directed at people whose ill-health or disabling condition has not been, or could not be, prevented and who cannot be cured completely. **Examples:** Rehabilitating a person who has undergone major heart surgery, to enable the individual to get the most out of life; educating parents and carers to help a child with brain damage to achieve their own potential.

Areas of health education advice

Table 2.2 Main areas of health education advice

Promoting a healthy lifestyle	Reducing the likelihood of ill-health	Promoting personal safety
Diet, hygiene, physical activity, mental health and positive personal relationships	Immunisation, heart disease, strokes, cancer, STDs (Sexually Transmitted Diseases), substance abuse	Safety in the home, road safety

Promoting a healthy lifestyle

A healthy lifestyle is a combination of a balanced diet, suitable physical activity or exercise and avoidance of harmful lifestyle practices such as smoking or substance misuse.

Healthy eating

No single food contains all the nutrients we need for health. The key to healthy eating, therefore is to enjoy a variety of foods without eating too much of any one kind. Food is energy that we burn constantly, even when we are sitting or sleeping. However, if we take in more energy than we need, the excess is stored as fat. Research shows that too much fat and oil in our diets may lead to obesity, heart disease and some cancers. The Government's 'Health of the Nation' programme recommends a balanced diet as a way of avoiding these problems and gives eight simple guidelines for a healthy diet:

- enjoy your food;
- eat a variety of different foods;
- eat the right amount to be a healthy weight;
- eat plenty of foods rich in starch and fibre;
- don't eat too many foods that contain a lot of fat;
- don't have too many sugary food and drinks;
- don't eat too much salt;
- if you drink alcohol, keep within sensible limits.

You should aim to eat foods from each of the main food groups every day.

The five main food groups are:

1 Starchy foods such as bread, cereals and potatoes.
2 Fruit and vegetables, including fresh, frozen and tinned.
3 Milk and dairy foods, including cheese, yoghurt and fromage frais.
4 Protein-rich foods, including meat, fish, nuts, beans and pulses.
5 Fatty and sugary foods.

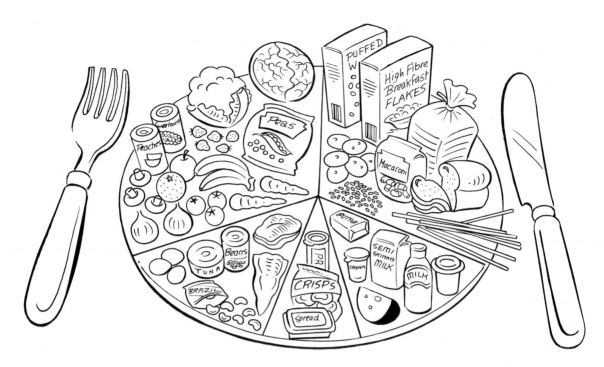

Figure 2.2 The balance of good health

Risks to health from poor diet

Risks from a poor diet include:

- **Cancer.** The risk of certain cancers is lower in people who eat diets rich in vegetables, fruit and starchy foods. The risk of certain cancers is higher in people who eat large amounts of red and processed meats, drink too much alcohol or become obese.

- **Heart disease.** Saturated fats are a major part of fat in foods such as milk and milk products (e.g., butter), and in meat and meat products. They are also found in some vegetable oils such as palm and coconut oil, and in some cooking fats, biscuits, cakes and pastries. Increasing intake of saturates increases levels of blood **cholesterol**. Having too high a level of cholesterol in the blood can increase the risk of having a **heart attack**, as it can be deposited on the walls of the blood vessels and cause damage.

Eating disorders

These include obesity, anorexia nervosa and bulimia nervosa. Boys, girls, men and women from all types of background and ethnic groups can suffer from eating disorders. Eating disorders are not just about food and weight, but about feelings. It may be difficult to face up to, and talk about, feelings such as anger, sadness, guilt, loss or fear. An eating disorder is often a sign that a person needs help in coping with life and sorting out personal problems.

Obesity

Obesity literally means fatness, but it is now recognised as an **eating disorder** that results in the person being overweight. Obesity is common in North America, Australasia and Europe. It also occurs, but is less common, in developing countries. In 1996, 45% of men and 34% of women in England were overweight. A further 16% and 18% respectively were obese. It is likely that the incidence is similar in other parts of the UK. Obesity tends to be more common among people aged 40–60 years and those from lower income groups. Today, more people are obese than ever before. Obesity in children is on the increase in the UK. Not only is this a health hazard while they are young, but it also sets a pattern for later life.

Obesity is caused by a mixture of factors, and each will contribute to obesity:

1 Lack of exercise.

- A more sedentary lifestyle: using the car has taken over from walking and using public transport, and watching TV is a popular leisure activity.
- Cycling or even walking to school is not as safe as it was. Parents are now more likely to run their children to school by car.
- Non-physical playing: television and computer games compete with games that involve physical activity.

2 Inappropriate diet.

- We live in a fast-food society: we eat more restaurant food, junk food, instant snacks and pre-cooked foods. These foods are usually very high in the two most fattening ingredients: fat and sugar.
- People eat more sweets and crisps and drink more fizzy drinks, partly because of advertising but also because they are more available.
- Poor fresh fruit consumption: despite it being more readily available, many people do not eat enough fresh fruit, preferring processed varieties that often contain extra sugar and fat products.

Being overweight can lead to problems such as:

- recurrent chest infections;
- diabetes;
- heart disease;
- high blood pressure (hypertension) and stroke;
- some cancers;
- arthritis and gout.

Obese people may also have poor self-esteem; they don't just have a struggle to contain and manage their *physical* problem, they also have to deal with people's *attitudes*. Those attitudes can range from disrespect, through mockery, to bullying and prejudice. Obese children are particularly vulnerable: it is not just other children who hold these attitudes – adults unwittingly pass on their ideas about 'fatness' and personality.

Anorexia nervosa

Anorexia is often, but wrongly, called the 'slimmer's disease'. It is most common in teenage girls, especially at about $14^{1}/_{2}$ years and again at 18. However, it has been diagnosed in children as young as five years of age. It is characterised by severe weight loss, the wilful avoidance of food and an intense fear of being fat. The following signs and symptoms are frequently experienced:

Physical	Psychological	Behavioural
• Severe weight loss • Periods stopping • Difficulty sleeping • Dizziness • Stomach pains • Feeling bloated • Growth of downy hair (lanugo) • Constipation • Feeling cold • Chilblains	• Believing they are fat when underweight • Being irritable • Setting high standards • Wanting to be left alone and losing friends • Increased interest in food, calories and cooking • Difficulty in concentrating	• Excessive exercising • Having ritual behaviours • Lying about eating meals • Lack of interest in normal activities • Cooking cakes and meals for the family

There is no single known cause for anorexia, but theories include:

- Those affected see it as a way of taking control over their lives.
- It may be a result of not wanting to grow up and change their body shape.
- Media obsession with the importance of achieving the 'perfect' (i.e. slim) body.
- It may be a physical illness caused in part by hormonal changes during adolescence.
- It may be caused by depression or a personality disorder.

Hospital treatment is often necessary to help the anorexic person return to a normal weight. Treatment is usually a combination of:

- a controlled re-feeding programme – in severe cases, a naso-gastric tube may be used;
- individual psychotherapy;
- family therapy.

Bulimia nervosa

Bulimia nervosa is characterised by episodes of compulsive overeating (bingeing) usually followed by self-induced vomiting. As with anorexia, those with bulimia nervosa are also obsessed with the fear of gaining weight. The foods eaten tend to be high in carbohydrate and fat. Sufferers may also use large quantities of laxatives, slimming pills or strenuous exercise to control their weight. Many bulimics have poor teeth due to regular vomiting (vomit is acidic and can erode teeth). The following symptoms are commonly experienced:

Physical	Psychological	Behavioural
• Sore throat and mouth infections	• Feeling emotional and depressed	• Eating large quantities of food
• Damaged teeth enamel – caused by the acid present in vomit	• Feeling out of control	
• Irregular periods	• Mood swings	• Being sick after meals
• Dry or poor skin condition	• Obsessions with dieting	• Taking laxatives
• Feeling tired		• Being timid and lying
• Difficulty sleeping		
• Swollen glands		

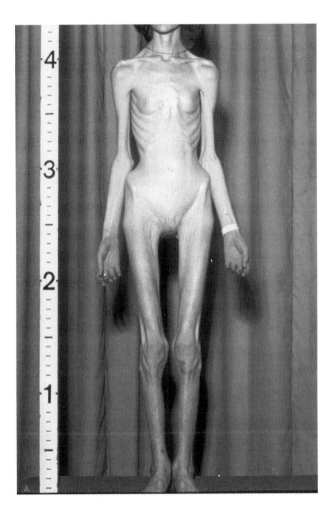

Figure 2.3 Anorexia

Media blamed for rise in eating disorders

Women on television, including news presenters and actresses, are 'abnormally thin' and are causing a rise in the number of young women suffering from eating disorders. A report by the British Medical Association shows that the position has reached an 'unacceptable level' with every family doctor in the country treating two patients suffering from anorexia and 18 with bulimia nervosa.

Doctors called for the media to show 'more realistic body shapes' to reduce the number of deaths caused by eating disorders. The research shows that the gap between the perceived ideal body shape and reality is widening, as women are generally getting larger while models, actresses and women who appear on television are getting smaller. The research showed that more female characters on television are thinner than average. It has been estimated that models and actresses in the 1990s have 10 to 15 per cent body fat, whereas a healthy woman has 22 to 26 per cent.

'We need more Sophie Dahls and fewer Kate Mosses,' said Professor Nathanson. 'Actresses on popular drama and television and news presenters tend to be thin. Whereas male news presenters are all different shapes and sizes, female news presenters are all thin. The pressure on these women to be thin and conform is enormous.'

There are an estimated 60,000 people in Britain with eating disorders. One in 10 is male but the majority are young women. Anorexia nervosa affects 1 to 2 per cent of women, aged 15 to 30 in the UK. Of those who develop the disorder, 15 to 20 per cent will die within 20 years. Dieting is a factor in the development of eating disorders and recent research showed that more young girls are expressing dissatisfaction with their body shapes; one in seven girls aged 11 is on a diet, rising to one in three by the age of 16.

Professor Sir William Asscher, the chairman of the board of science and education at the association, said that although there was no scientific proof of a direct causal link between media images of superthin women and eating disorders in young women, all the research pointed to a direct impact on teenage girls. 'In societies where there is no culture of thinness, eating disorders are very rare,' he said. 'Increasing Westernisation has led to an increase in eating disorders in several cultures.'

The BBC and ITV dismissed the notion that they only represented 'superthin' women on television. 'The BBC seeks to depict real life across the board and shows people of all shapes and sizes,' said a spokesman for the corporation. 'When we do specifically address the issue of body image through campaigns or programmes, we put the emphasis on health and fitness rather than body size.'

A spokesman for ITV said there were a lot of presenters on television, such as Dawn French, Gaby Roslin and Lisa Tarbuck, who were not 'superthin' but were among the most successful.

Rebecca Martin, editor in chief of *Jump*, a monthly magazine for teenage girls, said that it was very difficult to pin down the media as solely responsible for the increase in eating disorders in young girls. 'Editors can help by not putting people who look unhealthily thin in their magazines,' she said. 'We have girls of all shapes and sizes in *Jump* and try to portray normal women but this does not mean we are anti-thin, some girls are naturally thin.'

However, Premier agency, which represents the supermodels Naomi Campbell and Claudia Schiffer, said women who bought fashion magazines featuring thin models were as much to blame as the editors and advertisers. 'Statistics have repeatedly shown that if you stick a beautiful skinny girl on the cover of a magazine you sell more copies,' said a spokesman for the agency.

Adapted from an article in The Independent, *31 May 2000.*

Activity

1 Read the article 'Media blamed for rise in eating disorders'. Discuss the prevalence of slim role models on film and on television. Would it be 'healthier' if such media reflected society more honestly? (40% of adult women in the UK wear size 16 or more clothes).

2 Collect some magazines aimed at young women and young men. How prevalent is the image of the perfect (i.e. thin) body? Discuss the content of 'lifestyle' articles and specific reducing diets. Do you feel that these magazines encourage an unhealthy obsession with physical appearance?

Physical activity

Physical activity is necessary to stimulate the body's own natural maintenance and repair system. Whatever your age physical activity plays an important part in your health and social well-being. Some people think only sportsmen and women need to build physical activity into their lives. However, everyone needs to do some sort of physical activity in order to be healthy. Your bones, joints and muscles – especially your heart – will actually stay younger if you keep them busy. If you are not physically active you increase your health risks in many ways.

The three main components of being physically fit are **stamina**, **strength** and **suppleness**.

Stamina

You need a well-developed circulation to the heart and lungs to give you the ability to keep going without gasping for breath. With stamina you have a slower, more powerful, heartbeat, and are able to cope more easily with prolonged or heavy exercise.

Strength

You need well-toned muscles to give you the ability to do physical work. When your shoulder, trunk and thigh muscles are toned-up, they will work well and you will not experience strains and injuries as often.

Suppleness

Developing good mobility in your neck, spine and joints will prevent you spraining ligaments and pulling muscles and tendons. You will also be less likely to experience aches and pains from stiff joints.

Physical activity is now accepted as a major contributor to good health and an increasingly important focus for health promotion. Evidence from epidemiological studies clearly indicates that morbidity and mortality from a range of chronic diseases are lower in physically active groups compared to sedentary groups. Half-an-hour a day of physical activity, of at least a moderate intensity, helps to prevent and reduce risks to health.

The risks of not taking enough exercise include:

- coronary heart disease;
- non-insulin-dependent diabetes mellitus;
- mild depression;

- stroke;
- obesity;
- cancer of the colon;

- high blood pressure;
- osteoporosis;
- stiff joints.

Most people are aware that they feel better both physically and mentally when they have taken some physical activity. The report below describes the benefits of exercise to people with mental health problems, particularly depression.

Exercise 'helps mental health'

Many people say exercise helps them feel good. Many people with mental health problems use physical exercise to make them feel better, a survey has found. The survey by the charity Mind found that 83% of people with mental health problems looked to exercise to help lift their mood or to reduce stress. Two-thirds said exercise helped to relieve the symptoms of depression and more than half said it helped to reduce stress and anxiety. Some people even thought it had a beneficial effect on manic depression and schizophrenia. Six out of ten said that physical exercise helped to improve their motivation, 50% said it boosted their self-esteem and 24% said it improved their social skills. Mind found that people with mental health problems were more likely to get their exercise from everyday activities like walking, housework and gardening. However, 58% did not know that GPs can sometimes prescribe exercise sessions and activities.

The biggest barriers that prevented people from taking part in physical exercise were motivation problems, the cost of sport and lack of confidence.

One respondent to the survey said: 'I would not have recovered over the last few years without daily exercise, combined with alterations of diet.' Another said: 'I still suffer from depression, anxiety and stress, but doing exercise does give relief and greatly helps me through the days.'

Report author Sue Baker said: 'Our survey proves, beyond any doubt, that physical activity and exercise has a valid place in the "treatment" of mental health problems. As such it deserves far more recognition and should be made more widely available.'

However, she stressed that physical exercise could not prevent all mental health problems from developing, and should not be seen as a replacement for other 'treatments'. Mind is calling for:

- More information about the availability of exercise prescriptions from GPs.
- Greater access to leisure facilities for people with mental health problems.
- Subsidies to leisure centres for people on limited or low incomes.
- Increased provision of exercise in mental health services, for instance as part of care treatment plans.

Source Taken from a survey conducted by the mental health charity, Mind

Promoting positive social relationships

Mental health and social well-being

Mental health problems range from the stresses and worries that all of us experience at some times in our lives, to life-changing conditions which affect our whole personality and our general health and well-being.

The scale of the problem

- Between 7% and 12% of men will suffer diagnosable depression at some point in their lives; for women the figure is as high as 20–25%.
- One in 10 children between the ages of five and 15 have mental health problems.
- One person in 10 is likely to experience a 'disabling anxiety disorder' at some stage in their lives.
- One in 100 people will have schizophrenia at some point.
- Suicide is the second most common cause of death in young people in the UK under the age of 35.
- Since 1985 suicide attempts have risen by more than 170%.
- In Scotland, the number of young male suicides is more than double that of England.

Who has mental health problems?

Mental health problems can result from the range of adverse factors associated with **social exclusion** and can also be a *cause* of **social exclusion**. This is why they have such a profound effect on an individual's health and social well-being. For example:

- Unemployed people are twice as likely to have depression as people in work.
- Children in the poorest households are three times more likely to have mental health problems than children in well-off households.
- Half of all women and a quarter of all men will be affected by depression at some period during their lives.
- People who have been abused or been victims of domestic violence have higher rates of mental health problems.
- People with drug and alcohol problems have higher rates of mental health problems.
- Between a quarter and a half of people using night shelters or sleeping rough may have a serious mental disorder, and up to half may be alcohol dependent.
- Some black and minority ethnic communities are diagnosed as having higher rates of mental health problems than the general population – refugees are especially vulnerable.
- There is a high rate of mental health problems in the prison population.
- People with physical illnesses have twice the rate of mental health problems compared to the general population.

The most common mental health problems in the UK today are:

- depression;
- anxiety disorders;
- alzheimer's disease;
- schizophrenia
- eating disorders (see pages 53–7).

What is depression?

Depression is a common mental illness. It can strike at any age and the feelings of hopelessness and helplessness attached to it can make it difficult for people to carry out their normal activities. It can be more or less severe and symptoms are varied, making it often hard to diagnose. It is thought that some individuals may be more prone to depression, whether because of life experiences, their body chemistry or genetically inherited conditions. Anyone can suffer from depression. The most common symptoms include:

- feelings of helplessness and hopelessness;
- feeling useless, inadequate, bad;
- self hatred, constant questioning of thoughts and actions, a need for reassurance;
- feeling vulnerable and being oversensitive to criticism;
- feelings of guilt;
- loss of energy and the ability to concentrate and be motivated to do even the simplest tasks;
- harming oneself;
- sudden loss or gain in weight;
- sleep disruption or a need to sleep very long hours;
- agitation and restlessness;
- loss of libido;
- physical aches and pains.

Most people only suffer two or three of these symptoms at any one time. People with severe depression may also experience suicidal feelings, stop eating or drinking and suffer from delusions or hallucinations.

Different types of depression

There are many different types of depression, including

- **clinically diagnosed depression;**
- **bi-polar disorder** (or manic depression): marked by extreme mood swings, between highs when a person experiences excessive energy and optimism, and lows when they may feel total despair and lack of energy;
- **post-natal depression** can occur from about two weeks after the birth of a child to two years after and differs from the mood swings suffered by many in the first few days after the child is born (also called 'post-natal blues').

Other forms of depression include **Seasonal Affective Disorder** which is thought to be associated with the approach of winter and may be linked to lack of sunlight.

Causes of depression

Depression can be caused by a combination of factors:

- It often runs in families, suggesting a **genetic** component, but it may be triggered by stressful events.
- Major depressive illness is usually linked to some form of chemical imbalance in the brain.
- It is also thought that people with low self-esteem, a pessimistic outlook on life and difficulty coping with stress are more prone to depression.

- Life events that may trigger depression include bereavement, chronic illness, relationship problems and financial difficulties.

Treatment of depression

- **Anti-depressant drugs**, which include **Prozac** are thought to correct chemical imbalances in the brain.
- Other types of drugs may also be used to treat depression.
- **Psychotherapy**, which aims to uncover the reasons for depression and help the patient to find ways of overcoming them.
- **Self-help groups** may also offer people a forum for talking about their condition and sharing it with others so that they do not feel isolated and alone.

In extreme cases, a person with depression may need to be treated in hospital if, for example, they are threatening or have attempted to commit suicide – or if they pose a threat to others.

Anxiety disorders

Anxiety disorders are among the most common mental illnesses in the UK. They cover everything from **panic disorder, phobias** and **obsessive compulsive disorder** to **post-traumatic stress disorder**. Each has its own particular symptoms and differs greatly from normal feelings of nervousness.

Causes of anxiety disorders

There are several possible reasons for anxiety disorders; these include:

- genetic factors;
- biochemical changes in the brain;
- traumatic life events.

Symptoms of anxiety disorders

These vary from person to person but may include:

- panic, fear, apprehension;
- uncontrollable obsessive thoughts;
- repeated flashbacks of traumatic experiences;
- nightmares;
- ritualised behaviour such as repeated hand-washing;
- problems sleeping;
- cold or sweaty hands;
- palpitations;
- shortness of breath;
- inability to be still and calm;
- a dry mouth;
- numbness or tingling in the hands or feet;

- upset stomach;
- tense muscles.

Often there appears to be no particular reason why symptoms occur since the feelings of panic are dissociated from events which are happening or about to occur. People who suffer from anxiety disorders may also have other mental illnesses, such as depression.

Treatment of anxiety disorders

Anxiety disorders often respond well to treatment:

- behavioural therapy;
- counselling to find out the cause of the anxiety;
- relaxation techniques;
- drugs which control the symptoms or correct chemical imbalances.

Alzheimer's disease

Alzheimer's disease is a progressive, degenerative and irreversible brain disorder that causes intellectual impairment, disorientation and eventually death. It is linked to gradual formation of plaques in the brain, particularly in the hippocampus and adjoining cortex. As the disease develops, it destroys chemical messengers used by the cells of the brain to communicate with each other.

Causes of Alzheimer's disease

So far no one single factor has been identified as a cause for Alzheimer's disease. It is likely that a combination of factors is responsible, including:

- age;
- diet;
- overall general health;
- genetic inheritance;
- environmental factors.

Age continues to be the greatest risk factor for dementia. Dementia affects one in 20 over the age of 65 and one in five over the age of 80. But Alzheimer's is not restricted to elderly people: there are 18,500 people under the age of 65 with dementia in the UK.

Symptoms of Alzheimer's disease

- Poor or decreased judgement
- Difficulty in performing difficult tasks
- Problems with language
- Disorientation to time and place
- Problems with abstract thinking
- Problems with memory
- Change in mood and behaviour

- Change in personality
- Loss of initiative
- Listlessness and apathy

The disease is often associated with depression, anxiety and sleep disturbance. The rate of decline varies from person to person. The disease course runs anywhere from three to twenty years, with eight years being the average life span after diagnosis.

Treatment of Alzheimer's disease

- Drug treatment is often used, for example antioxidants designed to limit the impact of free radicals and Cholinesterase Inhibitors including tacrine and donepezil.
- Therapies: art therapy, music therapy, reminiscence therapy.
- Aromatherapy and massage may help alleviate agitation, anxiety, sleep disturbance and may relieve physical discomfort in people with dementia. Also for carers complementary treatments can offer natural ways to relax.

Those caring for a friend or relative with Alzheimer's disease need a great deal of practical help and emotional support.

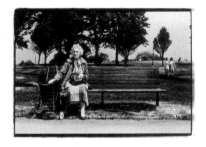

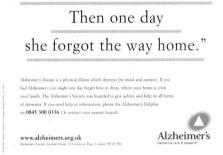

"Mum always loved shopping. Then one day she forgot the way home."

Alzheimer's disease is a physical illness which destroys the mind and memory. If you had Alzheimer's you might one day forget how to dress, where your home is, even your family. The Alzheimer's Society was founded to give advice and help on all forms of dementia. If you need help or information, phone the Alzheimer's Helpline on **0845 300 0336**. Or contact your nearest branch.

www.alzheimers.org.uk
Alzheimer's Society, Gordon House, 10 Greencoat Place, London SW1P 1PH

Alzheimer's
Dementia care & research

Figure 2.4 A poster from the Alzheimer's disease society

Schizophrenia

Schizophrenia is a severe mental illness that is characterised by changes in perception, thoughts and behaviour. The illness has been described in all cultures and its incidence (about 1 in 100) is much the same throughout the world. Schizophrenia can be confused with other mental disorders, such as bi-polar disorder (see page 61) and with physical illnesses. Schizophrenia affects males and females equally and typically starts between the ages of 15 and 30. There are some false ideas about schizophrenia:

- It isn't about having a 'split personality'.
- It doesn't mean a person will automatically be violent, ill, or in hospital for life.

Causes of schizophrenia

The cause of schizophrenia is unknown but it may have a genetic component. If a grand-parent had the illness, the risk rises to three per cent. If one parent was affected, the risk is as high as 10 per cent. This rises to 40 per cent if both parents have schizophrenia. Other predisposing factors include complications during pregnancy or childbirth and difficulties in childhood development. Factors which may trigger an episode of schizophrenia include stressful life events, and the use of illegal drugs such as cannabis. Schizophrenia is not caused by bad parenting.

Symptoms of schizophrenia

The symptoms and severity of schizophrenia vary widely from person to person. But in general, during an episode of schizophrenia, the way someone experiences and interprets the outside world becomes disrupted. A person may:

- Lose touch with reality: have difficulty organising their thoughts or difficulty concentrating.
- Have disturbances of thinking: see or hear things that aren't there, or feel as if thoughts are put into or taken out of their head, or are being broadcast to the world.
- Develop delusions (or 'false beliefs'): for example, that other people can read their thoughts; that somebody is trying to harm them or perhaps actually trying to kill them; that things they see or hear have a special message for them, for example, seeing a red car may mean the world is about to end.
- Experience hallucinations: that is, hearing, seeing or smelling things that are not seen, heard, or smelled by other people.
- Have difficulty expressing their emotions.

During an acute phase the person may deny that they are behaving unusually as their altered perception is very real to them. They will usually behave in unusual ways in response to their experiences. An episode of schizophrenia can last for several weeks, and can be frightening or disturbing for the person themselves and their friends or family. After this acute phase, people can go into a long-term period of 'negative' symptoms, including:

- lack of motivation;
- a feeling of flatness;
- social withdrawal.

Treatment of schizophrenia

- Antipsychotic drugs such as chlorpromazine and haloperidol are used to improve symptoms and to prevent relapse.
- Antipsychotic medication can also be given as an injection that lasts for days or weeks. This is known as a depot injection, and is often used for people with schizophrenia who have recovered from their acute illness and want to prevent a relapse, or who maybe find it easier to have an injection than to remember to take daily medication.
- Psychological and social therapies: Research shows that interventions with the families of people with schizophrenia can reduce relapse rates. These family interventions usually last several weeks and consist of education about the illness and help with problem solving.
- Cognitive behavioural therapy may help to reduce relapse rates.

A review of almost 2000 patients' life histories suggests that 25% of those with schizophrenia achieve full recovery; 50% recover at least partially; and 25% require long-term care.

Case study

Joanne's story

I had quite a wild time as a teenager – truanting, shoplifting, taking drugs – but somehow I still managed to get good marks at school. I went to university, to study sociology and ended up in a house with people who were quite restrained and middle class – very different from me. I don't know what brought it on but things started to feel strange when I became convinced my housemates were thinking bad thoughts about me and whispering all the time behind my back. Slowly I just got more paranoid, until I thought people could read my thoughts just walking down the street. I was hearing voices all the time but I didn't even realise I was ill. I thought maybe it was an after-effect of drugs I'd taken when I was younger.

My friends didn't really know how to treat me – I think friendships and social relationships can really suffer when you've got a mental health problem, either because people are scared, or they don't understand, or sometimes just because they're just thoughtless. I've had friends who have dropped me – they seem to have written me off as a worthwhile person. One friend used to go round 'warning' people about me before they met me, so of course they were pretty suspicious when they actually did meet me.

I became really depressed and even attempted suicide. It took about a year for me to get help, and I went to hospital as a voluntary patient. I was diagnosed with schizophrenia. Things got worse first but then with treatment they slowly got better. Eventually I managed to go back and complete my degree and now I work for a project that helps people with mental health problems get into employment. I feel much better about myself, just knowing that I have come through and that I can do a job that helps others in my situation – it's really rewarding.

I also think the media is very biased and this doesn't help people to understand what mental illness is all about. Schizophrenia only seems to exist in the media whenever a violent crime takes place. Otherwise we're the forgotten people and our stories are not told. People believe what they read in the papers, so what journalists write can have a real impact on the general public's view of schizophrenia and other mental health problems.

Activity

Exploring mental health

1 Find out about the support groups in the field of mental health, for example, the Alzheimer's Society, the Schizophrenia Fellowship, SANE, MIND, etc. How do these charities help those with mental health problems and their families?

2 Using material from the voluntary organisations, mount a display focusing on *one* mental health problem and provide the following information:

- what it is;

- who is likely to have the problem;

- help and support available.

3 Read Joanne's story above. What could have been done to help her when she first started experiencing problems? Find out about the different therapies available for those with schizophrenia.

Stress

Stress affects virtually everyone at some time in his or her life. Stress has physical effects on the body because it is part of the instinct we need to flee from danger quickly. Faced with pressure, challenge or danger, our bodies release hormones such as cortisol and adrenaline. These affect our metabolic rate, heart rate and blood pressure to prepare us for optimum performance. Unless we can compensate with physical activity, this natural reaction to stress reduces our ability to cope.

What causes stress and who is at risk?

Many events (or the anticipation of them) can lead to stress, including:

- pressure to perform at work, at school or in sports;

- threats of physical violence;

- money worries;

- arguments;

- family conflicts;

- divorce;

- bereavement;

- unemployment;

- moving house.

It is important to differentiate between temporary stress, which you know will soon go away, and long-term or **chronic stress**. Temporary stress can often be relieved by relaxing, by taking a walk or by a good night's sleep, but chronic stress is harder to deal with and can be damaging, both psychologically and emotionally.

Chronic stress can lead to:

- irritability or anger;
- apathy or depression;
- constant anxiety;
- irrational behaviour;
- loss of appetite;
- 'comfort eating';
- lack of concentration;
- increased smoking, drinking or drug-taking.

The physical effects can include:

- fatigue;
- skin problems;
- aches and pains resulting from tense muscles, including neckache, backache and tension headaches;
- increased pain from arthritis and other conditions;
- heart palpitations;
- in women, missed periods.

In moments of extreme stress, you may begin to shake uncontrollably, to hyperventilate (to breathe faster and deeper than normal) or even to vomit. If you suffer from asthma, stress can trigger an asthma attack.

Dealing with stress

Strategies to help deal with stress include:

- delegating or sharing your responsibilities at work;
- avoiding confrontation with difficult colleagues;
- learning to be more assertive;
- taking regular exercise;
- looking for humour or absurdity in stressful situations;
- never taking on more than you know you can complete;
- organising your time better to get as much done as possible;
- talking to friends or family, sharing your thoughts and fears;
- listening to music or relaxation tapes;
- breathing can help release tension and stress – learn to breathe deeply from your diaphragm and practise holding your breath for a few seconds before slowly exhaling.

Complementary therapy

There are many stress management techniques in the form of counselling, psychotherapy and hypnotherapy. Aromatherapy and reflexology may provide a quiet, relaxed environment in which to wind down. The Alexander technique may help to relieve muscle pains and help to control breathing in stressful situations.

Stress-related illnesses

As well as the emotional and psychological disruption it causes, **stress-related medical problems** are becoming increasingly common. Various illnesses may be said to be either caused or triggered by stress, including:

- **Stomach ulcers**, which may sometimes be caused by too much acid being produced in the stomach at a time of anxiety or worry.
- **Heart attacks**: it is thought that the fat released into the bloodstream when the body responds to demands gets trapped in the walls of the heart's own vessels. This gradually narrows these tubes, and when increased demand is placed on the heart, the narrowed tubes prevent the flow of oxygen, causing the heart muscle to die.
- **Skin disorders** such as eczema and psoriasis.
- **Myalgic encephalomyelitis (ME)**: the role of stress has been well documented in this very distressing condition.

ME is sometimes called **post-viral fatigue syndrome**. Studies have shown that people in the caring professions make up the largest group affected, with three times as many women as men suffering from ME.

No one definite cause is known, but theories have suggested the following:

- persistent viral infection;
- damage to the immune system following a viral infection;
- a neurotic disorder, for example, hyperventilation.

The main symptoms are:

- muscle fatigue;
- exhaustion;
- headaches;
- dizziness.

Other symptoms common to many people with ME are:

- muscular pains;
- fever;
- depression;
- bowel and digestive problems.

There is no diagnostic test, although entero-viruses can be traced in the colon of more than half of ME sufferers. Diagnosis is by process of elimination of other illnesses and diseases. The medical profession has little to offer in terms of scientific explanation or treatment of ME. The following treatments are among the more common:

- Anti-depressants: these are often prescribed, but the long-term use of these drugs is not recommended.
- A sugar and yeast-free diet: many sufferers follow this, in common with sufferers from *Candida Albicans* (Thrush) a yeast infection of the gut. It is thought that stress can lead to a weakening of the immune system, thus allowing this infection to flourish.
- Relaxation techniques such as meditation, the Alexander technique and yoga are often practised.
- Homeopathy.
- Acupuncture.
- Herbal treatments, for example with evening primrose.
- Counselling: this can enable a person to lead a less stressful lifestyle, thereby reducing his or her propensity to further bouts of ME.

 ## Case study

Holly's story

Before becoming ill with ME, Holly, aged 32, had led an active life both at work as a social worker and outside her job, having many interests which occupied most of her spare hours. She made little time for relaxation and her diet was high in sugar and carbohydrates. Her emotional history had been stressful. When she became ill, she suffered from most of the common symptoms of ME and was bedridden for three months. After numerous setbacks and relapses, she is now in the fifth year of her illness and has used diet, homeopathy, herbal treatments and counselling as her path to recovery. The most difficult experiences for Holly were the financial implications of being ill. She lost her job and has been living on state benefits; she has found her practical circumstances difficult to reconcile with her need for relaxation and a reduction in stress. After five years out of work it will be difficult for her to find a job, particularly with this history of ill-health. She says that counselling has empowered her to face the stresses and difficulties which the future might hold, without becoming ill again.

Activity

Stress-related illness

Study Holly's story, then answer the following questions:

1 What advice and recommendations should be made to a person with ME pre-disposing factors, to avoid contracting ME?

2 What support should be made available to people with ME by:

   a the NHS;

   b the DHSS;

   c the workplace;

   d friends and family?

3 Many ME sufferers feel isolated as there is still a lot of ignorance about the illness. How could this be combated?

Reducing the likelihood of ill-health

This area covers education programmes aimed at increasing awareness about the ways in which ill-health can be prevented. These programmes focus on:

- immunisation;
- heart disease;
- substance abuse: smoking, alcohol, drugs;
- sexually transmitted infections;
- cancer.

Immunisation

Immunisation is the use of vaccines to protect people from disease. As babies and children are particularly vulnerable to infection, they are offered immunisation, but parents or guardians must give their written consent. In the UK parents can choose whether to have their children immunised. The advantages of immunisation include:

- Children who are not immunised run a risk of catching diseases and having complications.
- Immunisation is the safest way to protect children from particular diseases that may have long-lasting effects.
- Having children immunised at an early age means they are well protected by the time they start playgroup or school where they are in contact with lots of children.
- Immunisation also protects those children who are unable to receive immunisation, by providing what is called **herd immunity**: this is a term used to describe partial uptake of immunisation, where enough people are immunised to prevent the spread of the disease.

Table 2.3 The current recommended immunisation schedules in the UK

Age	Disease	Vaccination method
2 months	Polio Hib* Diphtheria Tetanus Whooping cough	By mouth One injection
3 months	Polio Hib Diphtheria Tetanus Whooping cough	By mouth One injection
4 months	Polio Hib Diphtheria Tetanus Whooping cough	By mouth One injection
12 –15 months	MMR:† Measles Mumps Rubella	One injection
3–5 years	Measles Mumps Rubella Diphtheria Tetanus Polio Whooping cough	One injection By mouth
10–14 years School Leavers 13–18 years	BCG (tuberculosis) Diphtheria Tetanus Polio	Skin test followed by one injection; if required One injection By mouth

Meningitis C vaccine: The new immunisation will be given to children aged 2, 3 and 4 months and around 13 months with their routine immunisations. Extra appointments will be organised where necessary. Depending on their age, all other children will be invited through their GP, school or college to have the vaccine in a special catch up programme.

*Hib : Vaccination against the bacteria haemophilus influenzae, type B, which may cause meningitis (cerebrospinal meningitis) and infection of the epiglottis (back of the throat).

†MMR: Vaccination against measles, mumps and rubella (German measles).
The vaccinations at the ages of 2 months and 3–5 years are usually combined with routine children's medical examinations.

The Department of Health issues the following guidelines:

- Children should *not* be vaccinated if they have a fever. When children have a fever, the vaccination should be postponed. If the child just has an ordinary cold, but their temperature is normal, it is safe for them to be vaccinated.
- Side effects to the vaccines do occur, but **allergy** to the vaccines is **very** rare:
- The vaccines for diphtheria-tetanus-whooping cough, Hib and diphtheria-tetanus may cause a red area and swelling to occur on the vaccination spot. However, it will disappear within a few days. A fever may also be noticed on the day of the jabs and for 7–10 days later.
- The MMR vaccine may cause a brief reaction that may begin at any time from a few days to three weeks after the vaccination. The child may have symptoms like the diseases, which are being vaccinated against, but only in a mild form. That is, a cold, a skin reaction, a fever and perhaps swollen salivary glands. The child will not be contagious.

The meningitis C vaccine may have the following effects:

- **Babies**: Some swelling and redness where the injection is given.
- **Toddlers over 12 months**: Some swelling and redness where the injection is given. About one in four toddlers may have disturbed sleep. About one in 20 toddlers may have a mild fever.
- **Pre-school children**: About one in 20 may have some swelling at the injection site. About one in 50 may have a mild fever within a few days of the vaccination.
- **Children and young people**: About one in four may have some swelling and redness at the injection site. About one in 50 may have a mild fever. About one in 100 may have a very sore arm from the injection, which may last a day or so.
- On very rare occasions, vaccinations may cause serious complications.

Alternatives to immunisation

There is no proven, effective alternative to conventional immunisation. **Homeopathic medicine** has been tried as an alternative to the whooping cough vaccine but it was not effective. The Council of the Faculty of Homeopathy (the registered organisation for doctors qualified in homeopathy) advises parents to have their children immunised with conventional vaccines.

Activity

1. Find out how parents receive information about having their children immunised.
2. Do you think immunisation should be made compulsory (as it is in some countries) to eradicate childhood illnesses?

Drugs

A drug is any chemical substance that changes the function of one or more body organs or alters the process of a disease. Drugs may be:

- prescribed medicines, for example, antibiotics;
- over-the-counter remedies, for example, paracetamol or cough medicines;
- alcohol, nicotine (in tobacco) and caffeine (in coffee and other drinks).

When their use is considered harmful or socially unacceptable, this is termed **drug abuse**. Many more deaths and illnesses are caused through the use of legal drugs than through the use of illegal drugs.

Drug dependence

Drug dependence is the compulsion to continue taking a drug, either to produce the desired results, or to prevent the ill-effects that occur when it is withdrawn. There are two types of drug dependence:

1 **Physical dependence** is when someone has taken drugs in quantity for a time and comes to rely on the use of a drug in order to feel well and for their body to function 'normally'. It usually happens when the body has built up a tolerance to the drug and in its absence, physical withdrawal symptoms appear. It mainly occurs with **depressant drugs** such as **alcohol, barbiturates, heroin** or **tranquillisers**. However, the deep depressions and even suicidal feelings that can follow **cocaine** and **ecstasy** use could be counted as physical dependence, because users will take *more* of the drug to escape these feelings.

2 **Psychological dependence** is when the user experiences an overwhelming desire to continue with the drug experience. This can be because of the pleasurable effects and the desire to keep experiencing them. It can, however, also represent some sort of psychological prop. The drug experience can become a way of blocking out reality, making life bearable and a way of facing the world. Without the prop life seems worthless. It can happen with any drug or any activity which takes over a person's life including eating, sex, work, or jogging.

Drug tolerance refers to the way the body gets used to the repeated presence of a drug, meaning that higher doses are needed to maintain the same effect. The body learns to tolerate the drug in the system. Alcohol, barbiturates, heroin and **amphetamine** are all drugs to which the body can build up tolerance.

There are four main groups of drugs which are commonly abused:

- . stimulants
- depressants;
- hallucinogens or psychedelics;
- analgesic drugs.

1 A **stimulant** is a drug that speeds up the central nervous system to *increase* neural activity in the brain. They are rarely prescribed for any medical problem. Such drugs tend to make people feel more euphoric, alert and wide-awake, and are sometimes called 'uppers'. Examples are amphetamines, nicotine (in cigarettes), cocaine and crack, caffeine and ecstasy.

2 Depressants are drugs that slow down the central nervous system to *suppress* neural activity in the brain. Large quantities make people feel sleepy. They are sometimes called 'downers'. Very large doses can lead to fatal overdose as the vital systems of the body such as breathing are slowed to the point where they stop. Examples are alcohol, sleeping tablets, tranquillisers, solvents (as in glue-sniffing).

3 An **hallucinogen** is a drug which alters **perception**: the way you see, hear, feel, smell or touch the world. This can mean that the senses can get all mixed up or changed. People may see colours much more brightly or hear sounds differently, or say that they can 'hear' colours and 'see' sounds. They might also see things that aren't there, which some people find very frightening. Examples are LSD and magic mushrooms and the strongest types of cannabis are hallucinogenic; to a certain extent, ecstasy can also be hallucinogenic.

4 Analgesic drugs are used medically to treat moderate and severe pain. Abuse of analgesic drugs for their euphoric (or intoxicating) effects often causes tolerance and both physical and psychological dependence. Examples are heroin, morphine, methadone, pethidine, codeine and opium

Illegal drug abuse

Illegal drugs are those that are banned for any *non-medicinal* use by the **Misuse of Drugs Act**. Table 2.4 gives information on the most commonly used of these. Banned drugs are placed in different classes – Class A offences carry the highest penalties and Class C offences the lowest penalties.

Types of drug use

1 Experimentation. Some people take a drug because they are curious about what the effects feel like.

2 Recreational use. Most young people who take drugs take them in particular social settings – at a club or a party, for example. They may not suffer any major harmful effects to their health, although occasionally young people die from a strong adverse reaction.

3 Problem drug use. Some people may need to take a drug just to feel able to cope with everyday life. Their drug use is likely to affect their health and they may experience:

- mental health problems, such as anxiety, depression or inability to concentrate;
- loss of friends;
- money problems;
- trouble with the law.

Illegal drug taking is *not* a part of normal life, and most people who do try drugs do not continue using them. More young people experience problems caused by drinking too much alcohol than from drug use.

Why do people take drugs?

Surveys of young people in Britain suggest many are experimenting with illegal drugs. The misuse of drugs and solvents appears to be widespread in secondary schools. In the UK, drug use often starts at around the age of 13, yet drugs education may not start until the age of 14–16. Many adults think that young people use illegal drugs only if they are having problems. This is

A Guide to Illegal Drugs

Drug name	Alkyl Nitrates
Other names	• Poppers • Amyl nitrate, butyl nitrate, isobutyl nitrate • Product names include: Ram, Thrust, Rock Hard, Kix, TNT, Liquid Gold
What it looks like	• Clear or straw-coloured liquid in a small bottle • Vapour which is breathed in through the mouth or nose from a small bottle or tube.
Effects	• Brief but intense 'head rush' • Flushed face and neck • Effects fade after 2 to 5 minutes
Health risks	• Headache, feeling faint and sick • Regular use can cause skin problems around the mouth and nose • Dangerous for people with anaemia, glaucoma, and breathing or heart problems • If spilled can burn the skin • May be fatal if swallowed • Mixing Viagra with alkyl nitrates may increase risk of heart problems
Legal status	• Amyl nitrate is a prescription-only medicine • Possession is not illegal, but supply can be an offence

Drug name	Amphetamines
Other names	• Speed, whizz, uppers, amph, billy, sulphate
What it looks like	• Grey or white powder that is snorted, swallowed, smoked, injected, or dissolved in drink • Tablets which are swallowed
Effects	• Excitement – the mind races and users feel confident and energetic
Health risks	• While on the drug, some users become tense and anxious • Leaves users feeling tired and depressed for one or two days and sometimes longer • High doses repeated over a few days may cause panic and hallucinations • Long-term use puts a strain on the heart • Heavy, long term use can lead to mental illness • Mixing Viagra with amphetamines may increase the risk of heart problems
Legal status	• Class B (but Class A if prepared for injection)

Drug name	Cannabis
Other names	• Marijuana, draw, blow, weed, puff, shit, hash, ganja, spliff, wacky backy **Cannabis is the most commonly used drug among 11 to 25 year olds**
What it looks like	• A solid, dark lump known as 'resin' • Leaves, stalks ands seeds called 'grass' • A sticky, dark oil • Can be rolled (usually with tobacco) in a spliff or joint, smoked on its own in a special pie, or cooked and eaten in food
Effects	• Users feel relaxed and talkative • Cooking the drug then eating it makes the effects more intense and harder to control • May bring on a craving for food (this is often referred to as having the 'munchies')
Health risks	• Smoking it with tobacco may lead to users becoming hooked on cigarettes • Impairs the ability to learn and concentrate • Can leave people tired and lacking energy • Users may lack motivation and feel apathetic • Can make users paranoid and anxious, depending upon their mood and situation • Smoking joints over a long period of time can lead to respiratory disorders, including lung cancer
Legal status	• Class B (but Class A penalties can apply to cannabis oil). NB Proposed change to Class C is imminent

Drug name	Ecstasy
Other names	• E, doves, XTC, disco biscuits, hug drugs, burgers, fantasy • Chemical name:MDMA (currently many tablets contain MDEA,MDA, MBDB) **4% of 16 to 25s have used ecstasy in the last 3 months.**
What it looks like	• Tablets of different shapes, size and colour (but often white) which are swallowed
Effects	• Users feel alert and in tune with their surroundings • Sound, colour and emotions seem much more intense • Users may dance for hours • The effects last from 3 to 6 hours
Health risks	• Can leave users feeling tired and depressed for days • Risk of overheating and dehydration if users dance energetically without taking breaks or drinking enough fluids (users should sip about a pint of non-alcoholic fluid such as fruit juice, sports drinks or water every hour) • Use has been linked to liver and kidney problems • Some experts are concerned that use of ecstasy can lead to brain damage causing depression in later life • Mixing Viagra with ecstasy may increase the risk of heart problems
Legal status	• Class A • Other drugs similar to ecstasy are also illegal and Class A

Drug name	Gases, Glues, and Aerosols
Other names	• Products such as lighter gas refills, aerosols containing products such as hairspray, deodorants and air fresheners, tins or tubes of glue, some paints, thinners and correcting fluids
What it looks like	• Sniffed or breathed into the lungs from a cloth or sleeve • Gas products are sometimes squirted directly into the back of the throat
Effects	• Effects feel similar to being very drunk • Users feel thick-headed, dizzy, giggly and dreamy • Users may hallucinate • Effects don't last very long, but users can remain intoxicated all day by repeating the dose
Health risks	• Nausea, vomiting, black-outs and heart problems that can be fatal • Squirting gas products down the throat may cause body to produce fluid that floods the lungs and this can cause instant death • Risk of suffocation if the substance is inhaled from a plastic bag over the head • Accidents can happen when the user is high because their senses are affected • Long-term abuse of glue can damage the brain, liver and kidneys
Legal status	• It is illegal for shopkeepers to sell to under 18s, or to people acting for them, if they suspect the product is intended for abuse

Drug name	Heroin
Other names	• Smack, brown, horse, gear, junk, H, jack, scag
What it looks like	• Brownish-white powder which is smoked, snorted or dissolved and injected
Effects	• Small doses give the user a sense of warmth and well-being • Larger doses can make them drowsy and relaxed
Health risks	• Heroin is addictive (even when smoked) • Users who form a habit may end up taking the drug just to feel normal • Excessive amounts can result in overdose, coma, and in some cases death • Injecting can damage veins • Sharing injecting equipment puts users at risk of dangerous infections like hepatitis B or C and HIV/AIDS
Legal status	• Class A

Drug name	LSD
Other names	• Acid, trips, tabs, blotters, microdots, dots
What it looks like	• ¼ inch squares of paper, often with a picture on one side, which are swallowed. Microdots and dots are tiny tablets
Effects	• Effects are known as a 'trip' • Users will experience their surroundings in a very different way • Sense of movement and time may speed up or slow down • Objects, colours and sounds maybe distorted
Health risks	• Once a trip starts, it cannot be stopped • Users can have a 'bad trip' which can be terrifying • 'Flashbacks' may be experienced when parts of a trip are re-lived some time after the event • Can complicate mental health problems
Legal status	• Class A

Table 2.4 Facts about drugs

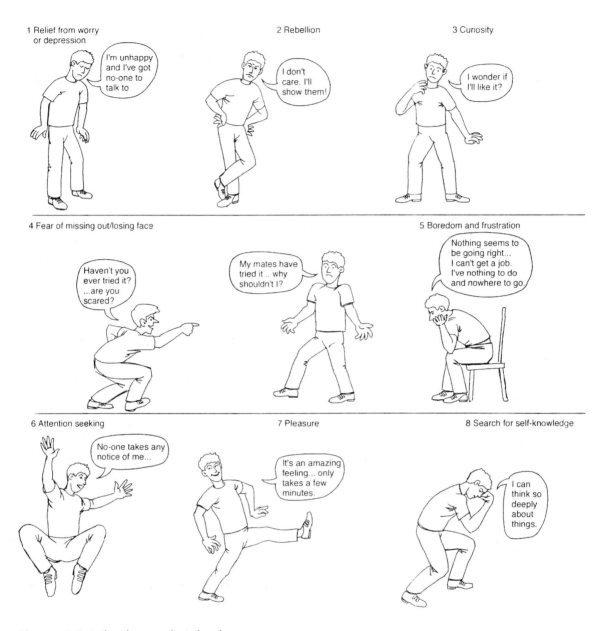

Figure 2.5 Why do people take drugs

not always true. They may be attracted to drugs for similar reasons as they are to alcohol (see Figure 2.5)

Risks of using illegal drugs

The following are risks involved in using *any* illegal drug:

- users can never be sure of exactly what they are taking;
- what is taken is unlikely to be pure, and users won't know what it has been mixed with;
- not knowing the strength of what has been bought could lead to an accidental overdose;

- users can't be sure of what effect a drug will have, even if they have taken it before;
- it is often very dangerous to mix different drugs, including drugs and alcohol;
- sharing needles or syringes carries a serious risk of dangerous infections being spread such as HIV and hepatitis B or C;
- a drugs conviction can cause problems obtaining a travel visa, and can affect job prospects.

Table 2.5 What to do in an emergency

Symptom	Response
tense and panicky	<ul><li>calm them and be reassuring</li><li>explain that the feelings will pass</li><li>settle them in a quiet, dimly lit room</li><li>if they start breathing very quickly, calm them down and tell them to take long, slow breaths</li></ul>
very drowsy	<ul><li>calm them and be reassuring</li><li>don't frighten or startle them, or let them exert themselves</li><li>never give coffee – or any other stimulant – to rouse them</li><li>if symptoms persist, place them in the recovery position</li><li>call an ambulance if necessary</li></ul>
unconsciousness	<ul><li>call an ambulance</li><li>place them in the recovery position so they won't choke if they vomit</li><li>check breathing – be prepared to do mouth-to-mouth resuscitation</li><li>keep them warm, but not too hot</li></ul>
For all symptoms	<ul><li>stay with them at all times</li><li>if you know what drug has been taken, tell the ambulance crew; if you have a sample of the drugs, give them to the ambulance crew</li></ul>

What to do in an emergency

Drugs affect everyone differently. It is not always possible to tell if someone has taken drugs. However, it is important to know what to do if you suspect that someone has reacted badly to a drug (see table 2.5).

Activity

1 Draw up a chart showing the 'pleasant' and 'unpleasant' effects of ecstasy, amphetamines and cocaine.

2 Choose one of the following drugs and research it:

• Alcohol

• Tobacco

• Cocaine

• Heroin

Include as much information as you can. Use your library's resources centre and internet sites such as the BBC sites and consumer support groups.

The project should be well illustrated and presented, and include the following information:

• What is the drug, how is it taken and what are its effects?

• Who uses the drug and why?

• How can health educators change the patterns of drug abuse?

Alcohol

Alcohol is probably the most commonly abused drug in the developed world. It is absorbed into the body through the stomach and intestines and distributed throughout the body by the bloodstream. In pregnant women, alcohol crosses the placental barrier to reach the developing baby.

Calculating the amount of alcohol

All alcoholic drinks contain pure alcohol (ethanol) in different amounts. You can compare the amount of alcohol in different types of drink using 'units'. All alcoholic drinks containers show the amount of alcohol they contain. By law they have to be labelled with the **alcohol by volume (%ABV)**. This number shows the percentage of the drink that is pure alcohol – the higher the number, the stronger the drink.

You can work out how many units are in a drink by multiplying the %ABV by the quantity in millilitres and dividing by 1000.

So a 330 ml bottle of lager at 5% abv can be worked out as:

$$330 \times 5 = 1650/1000 = 1.7 \text{ units of alcohol}$$

Many drinks now are also being labelled with the number of units of alcohol they contain – this makes it much easier to keep track of how strong certain drinks are.

Each of these drinks contains one unit:

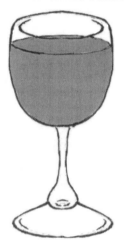 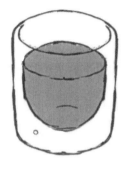 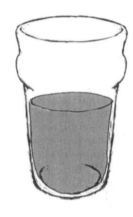

A small glass of wine = 1 unit   A 25ml pub measure of spirit = 1 unit   Half pint of ordinary strength lager/beer/cider = 1 unit

(NB A 330 ml bottle of alcopops (5% ABV) = 1.7 units)

Figure 2.6 Measuring alcohol as units

How does alcohol affect physical and mental behaviour?

The short-term effects of alcohol are almost immediate as it enters the bloodstream within minutes of taking a drink. It is carried to all parts of the body including the brain. The effects can take hours to wear off and the time it takes depends on:

- how much has been drunk and how quickly;
- what sort of drink (stronger drinks such as spirits and fizzy drinks such as sparkling cider are absorbed more quickly);
- how used people are to drinking alcohol;
- size and weight of the drinker.

Even in small amounts, alcohol affects:

- physical co-ordination;
- reaction times;
- judgement.

It takes about an hour for an adult body to get rid of one unit of alcohol. This may be slower in young people, and depends on drug tolerance and body weight.

The long-term effects are shown in Figure 2.7.

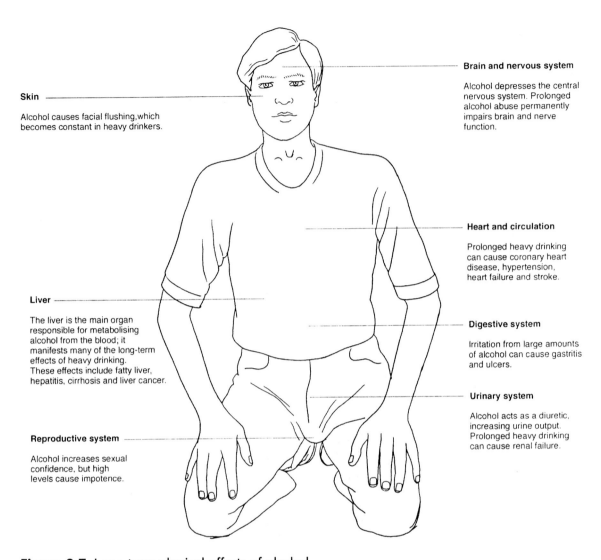

Skin

Alcohol causes facial flushing,which becomes constant in heavy drinkers.

Brain and nervous system

Alcohol depresses the central nervous system. Prolonged alcohol abuse permanently impairs brain and nerve function.

Heart and circulation

Prolonged heavy drinking can cause coronary heart disease, hypertension, heart failure and stroke.

Liver

The liver is the main organ responsible for metabolising alcohol from the blood; it manifests many of the long-term effects of heavy drinking. These effects include fatty liver, hepatitis, cirrhosis and liver cancer.

Digestive system

Irritation from large amounts of alcohol can cause gastritis and ulcers.

Urinary system

Alcohol acts as a diuretic, increasing urine output. Prolonged heavy drinking can cause renal failure.

Reproductive system

Alcohol increases sexual confidence, but high levels cause impotence.

Figure 2.7 Long-term physical effects of alcohol

Alcohol abuse

Alcohol-related problems occur at all educational and social levels and in every age group. There are several signs that a person is having difficulty controlling their alcohol intake:

- drinking for relief from pain and stress;
- pattern drinking (drinking every day or every week at a certain time, particularly in the morning);
- making alcohol the centre of life or of all pleasurable leisure activities.

Some quick alcohol facts

- The heaviest drinkers are 18–25 year olds, of both sexes on a Friday or Saturday night.
- 78% of all assaults are alcohol related.
- Drink plays a part in 50% of all murders.

- Alcohol is involved in 40% of all domestic violence incidents.
- One third of divorce petitions cite alcohol as a contributory factor.
- One in 3 drivers killed in road accidents were over the limit
- 1000 children under the age of 15 are admitted to hospital each year with acute alcohol poisoning
- Being drunk is no excuse if you end up in court on a charge of criminal damage or violence.

Warning

If you are going to drive you shouldn't drink. Even small amounts of alcohol increase the risk of an accident. Anyone caught driving above the legal limit will lose their driving licence for at least a year, face a stiff fine and may end up in prison.

Recommended guidelines on alcohol intake

The daily benchmarks (below) for adult men and women are a guide to how much you can drink without risking your health. These benchmarks are not appropriate for young people, pregnant women and specific circumstances, for example driving.

- Men: 3–4 units daily
- Women: 2–3 units daily

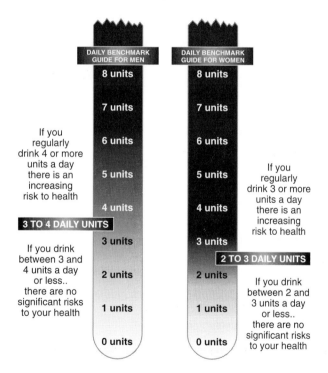

Figure 2.8 Daily benchmark guide for safe drinking

Activity

Researching alcohol abuse

1 Describe some of the ways in which people who drink excessive amounts of alcohol endanger

 a themselves

 b other people.

2 Find out why women are more sensitive to comparable doses of alcohol than are men.

3 Collect advertisements for drink from magazines, and also the posters and ads put out by bodies such as Alcohol Concern, Drinkwise and the Health Development Agency, which warn of the dangers of heavy drinking. In groups, discuss which posters are more effective – and why?

4 Research the condition known as Foetal Alcohol Syndrome. How many babies are affected each year in the UK and what problems does it present?

5 Find out what treatment or therapy is available for people with a drinking problem (alcoholism) in your area? What does the self-help group Alcoholics Anonymous offer?

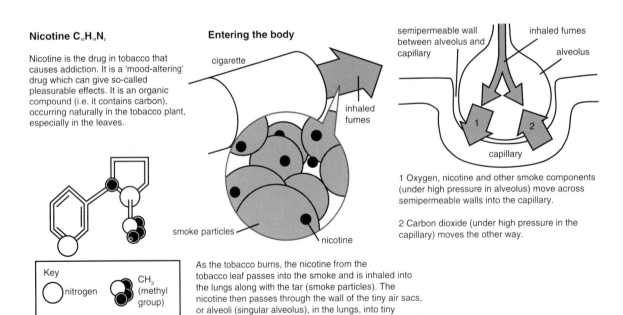

Nicotine $C_{10}H_{14}N_2$

Nicotine is the drug in tobacco that causes addiction. It is a 'mood-altering' drug which can give so-called pleasurable effects. It is an organic compound (i.e. it contains carbon), occurring naturally in the tobacco plant, especially in the leaves.

Key

nitrogen

hydrogen

CH_3 (methyl group)

Entering the body

cigarette

inhaled fumes

smoke particles

nicotine

As the tobacco burns, the nicotine from the tobacco leaf passes into the smoke and is inhaled into the lungs along with the tar (smoke particles). The nicotine then passes through the wall of the tiny air sacs, or alveoli (singular alveolus), in the lungs, into tiny blood vessels (capillaries). It enters the bloodstream and is carried around the body.

semipermeable wall between alveolus and capillary

inhaled fumes

alveolus

capillary

1 Oxygen, nicotine and other smoke components (under high pressure in alveolus) move across semipermeable walls into the capillary.

2 Carbon dioxide (under high pressure in the capillary) moves the other way.

Figure 2.9 How smoking affects your body

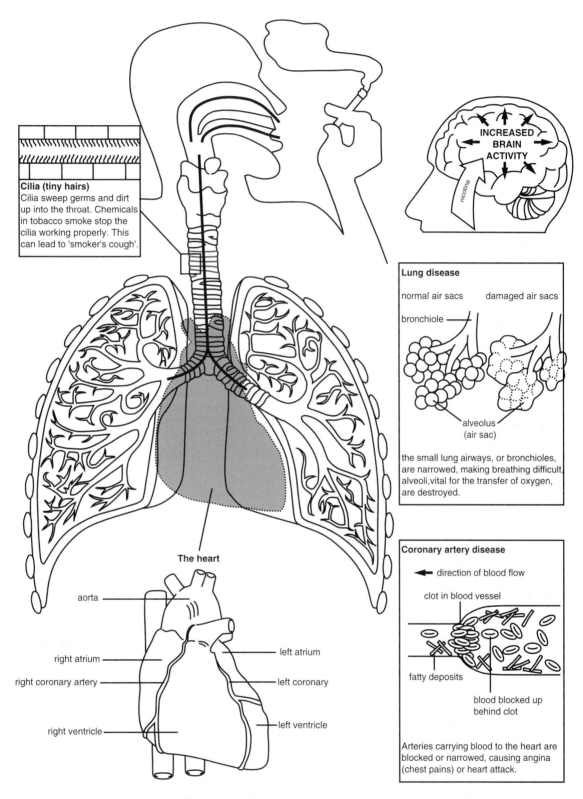

Cilia (tiny hairs)
Cilia sweep germs and dirt up into the throat. Chemicals in tobacco smoke stop the cilia working properly. This can lead to 'smoker's cough'.

INCREASED BRAIN ACTIVITY

nicotine

Lung disease

normal air sacs   damaged air sacs

bronchiole

alveolus (air sac)

the small lung airways, or bronchioles, are narrowed, making breathing difficult. alveoli, vital for the transfer of oxygen, are destroyed.

The heart

aorta

right atrium

right coronary artery

right ventricle

left atrium

left coronary

left ventricle

Coronary artery disease

◄— direction of blood flow

clot in blood vessel

fatty deposits

blood blocked up behind clot

Arteries carrying blood to the heart are blocked or narrowed, causing angina (chest pains) or heart attack.

Figure 2.10 How smoking affects your body

Smoking

Smoking is the largest single cause of preventable disease and premature death.

How smoking affects your body

Figures 2.9 and 2.10 show the physical effects of smoking. Many diseases and health problems are caused or complicated by smoking; these include:

- cancer: of the mouth, lip, larynx, oesophagus, lung, pancreas, cervix, stomach, bladder and kidney. NB The direct evidence that cigarette smoking causes cancer of the lung is clear – fewer than 10% of lung cancers occur in non-smokers
- chronic lung disease: bronchitis and COLD, Chronic Obstructive Lung Disease
- leukaemia
- emphysema
- fertility problems
- early menopause
- cataracts of the eye
- stroke
- sickle-cell anaemia
- stomach ulcers

Some quick smoking facts

- Smoking causes 31,820 deaths from lung cancer every year in the UK, and overall results in approximately 120,000 deaths each year.
- If you regularly smoke and drink, you are more likely to get cancer of the throat than someone who doesn't. If you do contract it you have a high chance of dying within five years.
- It is not only smoking cigarettes that is dangerous and puts your health at risk, cigars and pipes also increase your chances of getting cancer.
- Although lung cancer caused by smoking is the most common cancer in men and the second most common in women, smoking can also cause cancer of the throat, mouth, gullet, larynx, bladder, kidney, pancreas and stomach.
- Apart from the serious risk of cancer that you undertake when you smoke there are also other negative health implications: tar builds up on your lungs and your lung capacity is reduced, which can lead to a difficulty when breathing, and your chances of a heart attack are increased.
- On average, babies whose mothers smoke throughout pregnancy weigh 200g less at birth than babies of non-smokers.
- Giving up smoking reduces the risk of premature death; the risks return to those of a non-smoker within five to ten years.
- The best way to reduce the risk of getting cancer whilst simultaneously improving your general health and appearance is to stop smoking.

Why do people start smoking?

Smoking usually begins in adolescence. Various factors combine to make it more likely that a young person will smoke; these include:

- Availability: if cigarettes are readily available at home.
- Role models: if role models, e.g. parents, teachers and friends smoke.
- Peer pressure: there is a strong need to conform to the norms of one's peer group.
- Confidence: smoking is a social habit which gives confidence.
- Rebellion: as a gesture of defiance against authority.

Studies have shown that a teenager who smokes just two or three cigarettes has a 70% chance of becoming addicted.

Passive smoking

Breathing other people's smoke is called passive, involuntary or second-hand smoking. The non-smoker breathes **sidestream** smoke from the burning tip of the cigarette, and **mainstream** smoke that has been inhaled and then exhaled by the smoker. The smoke emitted from the end of a burning cigarette has *double* the concentration of nicotine and tar when compared to the smoke actually inhaled by the smoker (through a filter). It also contains three times the amount of benzopyrene (a known carcinogen) and five times the amount of carbon monoxide (a poisonous gas). The risks to non-smokers of passive smoking include:

- **Cot death.** World Health Organization figures indicate that babies are at five times greater risk of cot death if their mothers smoke.
- **Asthma.** Children also have a 20–40% increased risk of asthma if they are exposed to tobacco smoke, and a 70% increased risk of respiratory problems if their mother smokes. People whose partners smoke are nearly five times more likely to develop asthma in adulthood than those who are not exposed to passive smoking, according to new research.
- **Heart disease.** Short term exposure to tobacco smoke also has a measurable effect on the heart in non-smokers. Just 30 minutes' exposure is enough to reduce coronary blood flow. A study published in 1997 by the American Heart Association found that the risk of heart attack and subsequent death is 91% higher (i.e. almost double) for women who were regularly exposed to second-hand smoke and 58% higher for those who were only occasionally exposed.
- **Respiratory problems.** In the UK, long term exposure to second hand cigarette smoke has been shown to increase the risk of **lung cancer** by 20–30%. Those who are exposed to second hand smoke at work are more than twice as likely to develop respiratory problems.

Giving up smoking

The Health Education Council gives the following advice to those who wish to give up smoking:

- Cut out the first cigarette of the day to start with, then the second, and so on.
- Start by cutting out the most 'enjoyable' cigarette of the day, such as the one after a big meal.
- Give up with a friend.
- Tell everyone you are giving up smoking.

Activity

> ## Campaign against smoking
>
> Set up a 'No Smoking' campaign in your school or college.
>
> - Obtain posters from any organisation committed to helping smokers to give up, for example, the NHS site or ASH (Action on smoking and health). Or make your own using the quick facts section on page 86.
>
> - Choose a prominent site to display posters and fact sheets – don't forget to ask permission.
>
> - Obtain several **peak flow meters**. (A peak flow meter is a small device that measures how well air moves out of the airways). Health clinic and GP practices might be willing to loan them out. Learn how to use them and to instruct others in their use. (**NB** Follow the rules of hygiene.)
>
> - Ask each volunteer if he or she smokes and offer them the chance to test their own peak flow rate.
>
> - Record results from smokers and non-smokers on separate charts.
>
> - At the end of the session, analyse the results and present them on a poster.

Lung diseases

Lung diseases, which include conditions ranging from asthma to lung cancer, are now the biggest killers in the UK, accounting for one in four deaths. Respiratory conditions are now the most common long-term illness among children. They are also responsible for most emergency hospital admissions in the UK. It is also the most common reason patients give for visiting their GP and is estimated to cost the NHS £2.5bn each year – more than any other disease.

Cancer

What is cancer?

There are over 200 different cancers, yet each starts in the same way – with a change in the normal make-up of a cell. Normal cells grow in a controlled way. But cancer cells are different from normal cells:

- They go on and on growing. One cell becomes cancerous. This grows into two, then four, then eight and so on. By the time a cancer is big enough to see on a scan, or to feel as a lump, there are billions of cells in the tumour.

- Cancer cells may not stick together well, and are able to spread around the body.

- Cancers start because some of the information that is carried in the cell's DNA has become altered. For example, this altered information might tell the cell to carry on growing instead of stopping.

- There are many different types of cells in the body and any of these can become cancerous. This is why there are so many different types of cancer.

- Cancer cells use the blood stream and the circulation of tissue fluid (in the lymphatic system) to spread around the body. In order to grow, a cancer needs a good blood supply, just like any other growing body tissue. The fact that cancers grow is harmful to the body because they damage the tissues around them.

- Cancers are also harmful because they can spread. Doctors use a system called **staging** to describe the size of a tumour and gauge whether it has spread. Many people will have their cancer diagnosed and successfully treated before it has spread. Some cancers are more likely to spread than others. Certain cancers are more likely to spread to particular parts of the body.

- The **immune system** may have a role to play in fighting the cancer. Cancer treatments such as chemotherapy and radiotherapy can weaken the immune system for a time. Some people have genes that make it more likely that they will get cancer, some have genes that protect them. Things around us can also damage our genes and make a cell cancerous. This includes poisons in **cigarette smoke** and **radiation**. The older a person gets, the more likely it is that they will get cancer.

- Cancers can cause different symptoms in different people because of where they are. A cancer may press on a nerve, or another body organ that is nearby. The place where the cancer starts also affects what treatment can be used because doctors have to take into account the risk of damaging neighbouring organs.

Cancer is the cause of a quarter of all deaths in the UK. Experts have estimated that more than 80% of cancers may be avoidable by changing lifestyles or the environment. In 1996 there were 156,000 deaths from cancer – nearly a quarter of these were from lung cancer and a further quarter were caused by cancers of the large bowel, breast and prostate. Cigarette smoking has been identified as the single most important cause of preventable disease and premature death in the UK.

Some quick cancer facts

- 30% of all cancer deaths are caused by smoking.
- Every year smoking causes over 30,000 deaths from lung cancer.
- 3% of all cancers are related to excess alcohol consumption.
- Heavy drinkers are at risk of cirrhosis of the liver, which can lead to cancer in later life
- About 35 % of cancers may be related to diet.
- Diets containing a variety of fruits and vegetables seem to protect against certain cancers.
- Too much sun can lead to skin cancer.
- Skin cancer is the second most common cancer in the UK.
- Britain has the highest death rate from breast cancer in the world.
- 16,000 women die each year from breast cancer in the UK.
- About 2,000 women in the UK die each year from cervical cancer (cancer of the cervix or neck of the womb).

- Testicular cancer is the commonest cancer in the UK in men aged 20–34, with 1000 new cases reported each year.

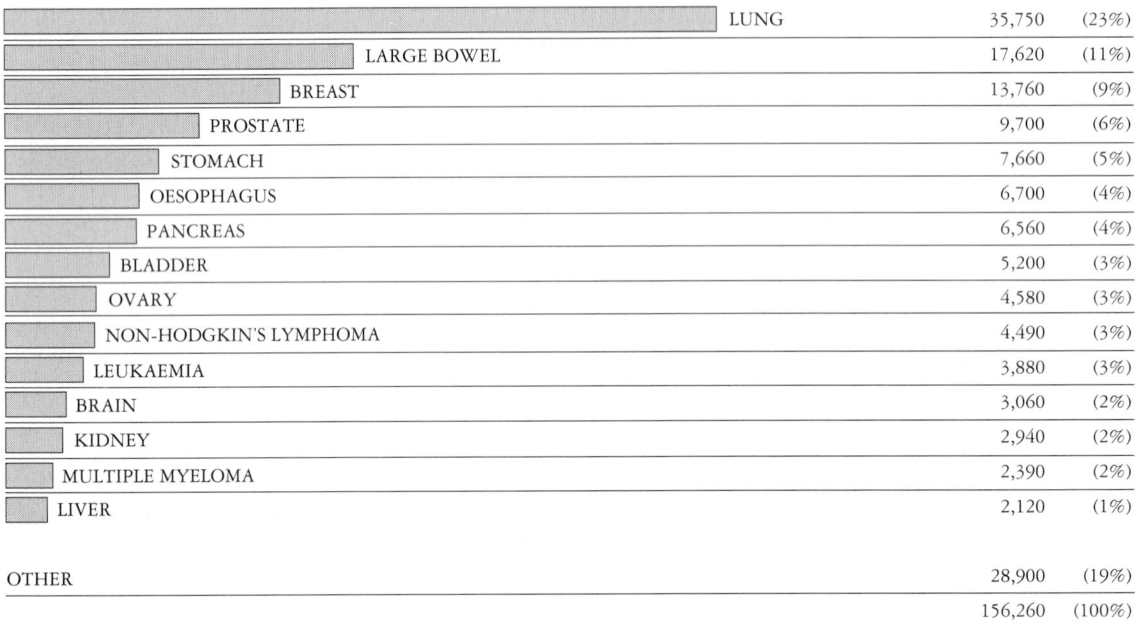

LUNG	35,750	(23%)
LARGE BOWEL	17,620	(11%)
BREAST	13,760	(9%)
PROSTATE	9,700	(6%)
STOMACH	7,660	(5%)
OESOPHAGUS	6,700	(4%)
PANCREAS	6,560	(4%)
BLADDER	5,200	(3%)
OVARY	4,580	(3%)
NON-HODGKIN'S LYMPHOMA	4,490	(3%)
LEUKAEMIA	3,880	(3%)
BRAIN	3,060	(2%)
KIDNEY	2,940	(2%)
MULTIPLE MYELOMA	2,390	(2%)
LIVER	2,120	(1%)
OTHER	28,900	(19%)
	156,260	(100%)

Figure 2.11 Deaths from different types of cancer

The risks of radiation

Radiation is used therapeutically to treat various forms of cancer, but it can also cause cancer. Everyone is exposed to that which comes naturally from the earth and the sky; other sources of radiation need to be fully monitored:

- X-ray examinations and treatment, including dental X-rays.
- Houses found on certain types of ground in some counties in England, Scotland and Wales are more likely to have high levels of radon, which is produced in granite and other rocks.

Reducing the risks of cancer

- Stop smoking, or better still don't start; after ten years your risk of lung cancer is about half that of a continuing smoker.
- Try to avoid places where you will be exposed to passive smoking.
- Know the limits of sensible drinking and keep within them.
- Eat more fruit and vegetables.
- Eat more starchy and fibre-rich foods.
- Eat less fatty foods.
- If you want to tan, do it gradually and protect against sunburn by using a sun lotion with the correct sun protection factor (SPF).
- Women aged between 50 and 64 should attend a breast screening centre every three years for mammography (X-rays) of both breasts; early detection gives a better chance of successful treatment.

- To reduce the risk of cervical cancer, use a barrier contraceptive (cap, condom, female condom or diaphragm) during intercourse; women aged 20–64 should attend a clinic for a free cervical smear test every 3 years.
- A good way of detecting testicular cancer in its early stages is for men to examine their own testicles.
- If you work with radiation, make sure that the safety regulations are fully observed.
- The radon level in your home can be measured by writing to NRPB.

 # Activity

Cancer risks

Prepare a fact file detailing the links between certain lifestyle practices and different types of cancer. Include information about cancer support groups.

Heart disease and stroke

There are two *main* types of coronary heart disease: angina and heart attack.

1 **Angina pectoris** is characterised by a crushing pain in the chest because of insufficient oxygen being carried to the heart muscles. It is often brought on by exercise or stress. The patient will usually have special tablets (glyceryl trinitrate or Trinitrin) that dissolve under the tongue and bring rapid relief

2 **Heart attack** is caused by either:
- myocardial infarction, when part of the heart muscle has died as a result of blood starvation;
- coronary thrombosis, when the blood supply to the heart muscles is stopped by a blood clot.

Both kinds of heart attack are usually caused by **atherosclerosis** – the build-up of fatty deposits, called atheroma, in the blood vessels.

Stroke

Stroke or cerebral vascular accident (CVA), occurs when an area of the brain is deprived of its blood supply for 24 hours or more – usually because of a blockage or burst blood vessel – causing vital brain tissue to die. It is caused by:

- atherosclerosis;
- weakening in an artery wall (aneurysm);
- atrial fibrillation – a kind of irregular heartbeat (arrhythmia); this can cause a blood clot to form in the heart which can shear off and travel to the brain.

Some quick heart disease facts

- One fatal **heart attack** occurs in Britain every three minutes. In about one-third of all heart attacks the patient dies before reaching hospital.
- An estimated 20% of deaths from heart disease in men and 17% in women are due to **smoking**.
- It is estimated that in the UK about 36% of deaths from heart disease in men and 38% of deaths from heart disease in women are related to **lack of physical activity**.
- Heart disease causes nearly one-third of all deaths in the UK in people under the age of 75.
- The UK has one of the highest levels of heart disease in the world.
- One reason why heart disease rates are high in the UK is because the average **diet** is so unhealthy. In particular, fat intake – especially of saturated fat – in the UK is too high, and fruit and vegetable consumption is too low.
- **Moderate alcohol consumption** (one or two drinks per day) is associated with a reduced risk of heart disease. At high levels of intake – particularly in 'binges' – the risk of heart disease is increased.

Reducing the risks of heart disease and stroke

- Don't smoke.
- Take regular exercise – a brisk walk for 20 minutes each day will improve circulation.
- Drink alcohol sensibly – think of a pint of beer or two glasses of wine as the maximum for one day.
- Eat healthily.
- Try to avoid stress.

 Activity

Lifestyles and health

Arrange a debate around a specific lifestyle issue, for example, diet, smoking or alcohol use. Suggested topics:

- Should overweight (obese) people or smokers be refused a heart transplant by the NHS?
- Should smokers pay compensation directly to those damaged by passive smoking?
- Should health professionals prescribe courses to change health-damaging behaviour (for example, a strictly monitored diet or an exercise programme at a leisure centre?

Sexually transmitted infections (STIs)

There are several different types of sexually transmitted infections (infection you can only catch through having sex with a partner). They cannot always be recognised because some do not have any signs or symptoms. Using a condom is not a 100% guarantee of not catching a STI but it does offer very good protection. STIs will not go away unless treated and some of them are easy to treat.

Table 2.6 describes the different infections, and how they may be recognised and treated.

Top tips if you've got an STI

- Make sure your partner is checked out and cleared of infection before you have sex again.
- Avoid sex until the STI has been treated and has gone away.
- Always use condoms if you have sex.
- If you are at all worried about having an STI, make sure you visit a GUM clinic.
- Once you become sexually active it is important to look after your sexual health by visiting a GUM clinic if you have had unprotected sex.
- If you're having sex, avoid catching a love bug... use a condom, it's the only way! You can't tell by looking – don't leave it to chance.

Remember – you can catch an STI the first time you have sex with someone!

Most sexually transmitted infections are treatable...just go to your local GUM clinic. A GUM clinic is one of the most confidential places you can visit. It's also free and totally non-judgmental. Even though these clinics are often found in hospitals, your medical records can never be passed on to your GP or other parts of the hospital. All you have to do for a test is turn up, and wait your turn.

(Material adapted from the family planning charity Marie Stopes International website: www.likeitis.org.uk)

Promoting personal safety

Many people believe that as individuals they have little control over risks to their health because of large-scale environmental problems – such as global warming or industrial pollution. While it is true that many environmental issues require global policies to be managed effectively, risks to one's immediate environment *can* be controlled.

Some quick accident facts

- Two-thirds of all fatal accidents involving school-aged children are the result of **road accidents.**
- In 1998, over 40,000 children were killed or injured on our roads.
- The severity of injury is closely linked to speed. Hit at 20mph, one in 20 pedestrians is killed, while at 40mph only one in ten survives. Drivers can make the biggest contribution to reducing road accidents by slowing down, especially when children are around.
- About 4000 people are killed in **home and garden** accidents in the UK each year and almost 3 million people seek medical attention in hospitals as a result of accidents at home.

Table 2.6 Sexually transmitted infections (STIs)

Infection	What is it?	How can I tell if I've got it?	What will clear it up?
AIDS and HIV	**HIV (Human Immunodeficiency Virus)** is a virus which damages the body's immune system. When someone has **AIDS (Acquired Immune Deficiency Syndrome)**, it means they are HIV+ and have gone on to get a series of serious illnesses. HIV can be passed on by having sex without a condom with someone who has HIV. HIV is only passed on through bodily fluids and blood, for example through sex, injecting drugs or from mothers to their unborn children.	You can't. The only way to tell if you have HIV is to have a blood test.	At present there is no cure for HIV or AIDS but new combination therapies mean improved management of the illness.
Chlamydia	This is the most common STI amongst young women and men. It's caused by a bacteria, which, if left untreated, can cause pelvic inflammatory disease (a disease that infects your pelvic region and can lead to infertility in women and men).	In 15–20% of cases there will be symptoms 5–10 days after infection (look for a discharge and pain). However, *most people do not get any symptoms.*	Antibiotics after a simple chlamydia test at a genito-urinary medicine (GUM) clinic.
Genital warts	Genital warts are small fleshy lumps (like the warts you can get on your hands). They appear around your genitals and are caused by a virus called human papilloma virus (HPV).	The big problem with warts is that there are often no symptoms, or the warts develop inside the vagina (usually on the cervix) so you can't see them. If they do appear they may itch but are usually painless.	If you have been infected the good news is that in many cases the body's immune system will cause most warts to disappear without treatment after six months. Large visible warts need to be treated. You will be given a special lotion that you will be asked to apply to the warts. If this doesn't clear the warts, or the warts are in a tricky place, stronger lotions may be used. Occasionally, warts may be frozen or burned off, but usually this is not painful.

Infection	What is it?	How can I tell if I've got it?	What will clear it up?
Herpes	There are two types of herpes that cause small, painful blisters. Herpes Simplex Virus (HSV) Type 1, which usually causes cold sores, and HSV Type II, which causes genital sores. Herpes Type 1 is passed by kissing and herpes Type II is passed through sex. Type 1 can become Type II, through oral sex.	Look for small, painful clusters of sores. It can be diagnosed from a sample taken for testing, or a doctor may know just by looking. Remember, herpes is highly infectious and during an outbreak you should avoid sex and kissing (if you have cold sores). Outbreaks are treated with salt baths and/or medication.	There is no cure for herpes.
Gonorrhoea	Gonorrhoea is a disease caused by bacteria. The danger of this is, if left undiagnosed, it can cause pelvic inflammatory disease and infertility.	In five out of every six cases, there are no symptoms. Symptoms to look for are a discharge and a burning sensation when going for a wee.	Antibiotics.
Syphilis	An infection caused by a bacteria, which, if left untreated, can have very serious consequences.	A sore on your genitals, and a rash. If left untreated, the symptoms become severe.	Syphilis can be cured with one course of antibiotics.
Pubic lice	Also known as crabs, pubic lice are small insects that are spread through sex and intimate contact (bedding, towels etc.).	You'll have severe itching throughout your pubic region.	Usually a doctor will be able to tell if you have pubic lice and will prescribe a lotion to kill them off.
Trichomoniasis	This is an infection that affects the vagina, cervix, urethra and bladder.	Look for a greenish-yellow discharge with a strong and offensive smell, itching of the vagina and a burning when going for a pee. Boys/men have no symptoms.	A swab will be taken and antibacterial drugs prescribed.
Hepatitis B	This is a serious condition that causes inflammation of the liver caused by a virus passed on through vaginal or anal intercourse.	Usually there are no symptoms but look for unusual tiredness.	There is no effective cure, but in some cases your body fights off the virus and the infection goes away.

- There were 656 deaths associated with **work activities** in Great Britain during 1997–8.
- Nearly one-third of home fire victims are killed in fires that are related to cigarette smoking.
- Around half of pedestrians aged between 16 and 60 killed in road accidents have **blood alcohol levels** above the legal drink drive limit.

Many deaths can be avoided if simple precautions are taken.

Table 2.7

Fire safety	Home safety	Road safety
• Install a smoke alarm in your home, a least one per floor, and check regularly that it is working correctly. Replace the batteries as soon as they are low.	• Make sure pan handles are turned to the back of the hob while cooking.	• Infants and children should always ride in approved child car safety seats that are correctly adjusted and installed. Look for car seats with a British Standard kitemark. Other passengers should wear car seat belts.
• Extinguish all cigarettes carefully, especially before retiring for the night. Never smoke in bed.	• Store sharp objects such as scissors, razors and knives in a drawer.	• Never fit a rear-facing child safety seat in a passenger seat fitted with an airbag.
• Don't overload electrical sockets.	• Keep medicines and vitamins in a cupboard out of children's reach.	• If you are cycling, wear a helmet that meets a recognised safety standard. When riding in the dark, use front and rear lights (and have a rear reflector fitted) as required by law. Try to wear something fluorescent and reflective so that you can be seen more easily by other road users.
• Keep a fire extinguisher in the kitchen and learn how to use it properly.	• Store cleaning chemicals in a cupboard with a safety catch or in a high cupboard.	• Teach children how to cross roads safely and wherever possible cross at a zebra or pelican crossing.
	• Keep the stairs clear of toys and other items that could trip you up.	• Do not drink and drive and, even if you are not driving, don't put yourself at risk of road accidents by drinking too much. Alcohol affects physical coordination and reaction times so people who are drunk are more likely to be involved in accidents. Half of all pedestrians aged between 16 and 60 killed in road accidents are over the legal drink drive limit.
	• Fit locks on children's bedroom windows and keep furniture away from the window to prevent them climbing up to the window sill.	• Do not use mobile phones while driving. They distract you from driving safely.
	• Remove any potentially poisonous house plants.	• Observe speed limits, particularly in built-up areas and when children are about.
	• Never leave babies and small children unattended in the bath or near other sources of water, even for a short time.	
	• Avoid trailing wires and clutter in walking areas.	
	• Remove or repair frayed carpet edges.	

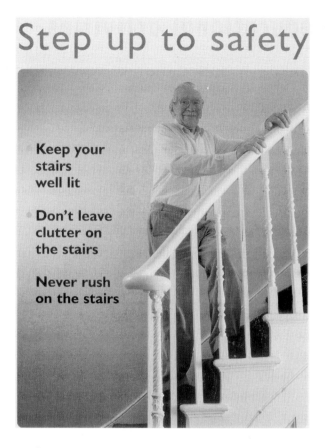

Figure 2.12 Step up to Safety: health promotion leaflet for elderly people

The Department of Education and Employment are developing the following pieces of software aimed at making the journey to school safer:

- Mapping software that will enable pupils to map safer, healthier and more sustainable routes to school
- Car-sharing database that will allow schools to develop a car-sharing scheme aimed at reducing the health and safety risks of the 'school run'.

 Activity

Road safety

Find out about recent campaigns to improve road safety awareness, for example, TV and poster adverts that focus on using seat belts, crossing the road safely and not drinking when driving. How effective and memorable are these ads? Can you think of a more effective way of getting the message across?

Origins of educational activities

Educational promotions for health and social well-being may be launched for many reasons, including the following:

- to meet international targets for health and social well-being;
- to meet national targets for health and social well-being;
- to address local/regional issues for informing social policy.

International targets

The World Health Organisation (WHO)

The WHO Regional Committee for Europe outlined 21 targets for health – called **HEALTH 21**. These targets are much less specific in their aims than the national targets set by Government Departments. Examples include:

- **Healthy start in life.** By the year 2020, all newborn babies, infants and pre-school children in the region should have better health, ensuring a healthy start in life.
- **Health of young people.** By the year 2020, young people in the region should be healthier and better able to fulfil their roles in society.
- **Healthy ageing.** By the year 2020, people over 65 years should have the opportunity of enjoying their full health potential and playing an active social role.
- **Improving mental health.** By the year 2020, people's psycho-social well-being should be improved, and better comprehensive services should be available to, and accessible by, people with mental health problems.

National targets

'Saving Lives: Our Healthier Nation'

This is a government national action plan to tackle the problem of poor health. It proposed a three-way partnership – between individuals, communities and government agencies to combat the 'four big killers' faced by people in the UK today:

- Every year **cancer** kills 127,000 people;
- Every year **heart disease and stroke** kill 214,000 people;
- Every year 10,000 people are killed by **accidents**;
- Every year **suicide** kills 4,500 people.

NB: Since the setting up of the **national action plan**, lung disease has been identified as a major health problem in the UK.

Tackling inequalities in health and social care

While overall life expectancy in England has been improving, the health gap between the rich and the poor has been widening. The stark fact is that a poor person is more likely to be ill and to die younger. Health inequalities are also evident for factors such as gender and ethnicity where differences in health can be similarly striking. The reasons for health inequalities are

Table 2.8 NHS Plan for tackling inequalities: (Access to NHS services; Children: ensuring a healthy start in life; Reducing smoking)

Access to NHS services	Children: ensuring a healthy start in life	Reducing smoking
• Allocating NHS resources to different parts of the country. • Fairer distribution of GPs. There will be a new way of distributing resources to address inequities in primary care services. • 200 new Personal Medical Services schemes principally in disadvantaged communities by 2004. • Health centres in the most deprived areas will be modernised. • The development of a new Health Poverty Index. • Health inequalities and equitable access to healthcare will for the first time be performance managed using the Performance Assessment Framework. • Free translation and interpretation service from every NHS premises by 2003.	By 2004 there will be: • An expansion of Sure Start to cover a third of all children under four living in poverty. • A new children's fund worth £450 million over three years. • A reform of welfare foods, with increased support for breastfeeding and parenting. • Full implementation of the Teenage Pregnancy Strategy. • Effective and appropriate screening programmes for women and children. • A new sexual health and HIV strategy. • Access to the Connexions Service, either through a Connexions Personal Advisor, drop-in centre, telephone or Internet-enabled support for every young person aged 13 to 19. • An additional 6,000 severely disabled children will receive a co-ordinated care package from health and social care services.	• Make Nicotine Replacement Therapy (NRT) available on prescription, to complement buproprion (Zyban) in 2001. • Ask the National Institute for Clinical Excellence to advise GPs on the most appropriate and cost-effective prescribing regimes for NRT and buproprion. • Ask the Committee on Safety of Medicines to consider whether more NRT can be made available for general sale. • Focus the efforts of specialist smoking cessation services on heavily dependant smokers needing intensive support and on pregnant smokers as part of ante-natal care. • If successful, this programme will mean that by 2010, approximately 55,000 fewer women will be smoking in pregnancy and at least 1.5 million smokers will have given up smoking. • In addition to the **Smoking Kills** target of reducing smoking in adults from 28% to 24% by 2010, the Cancer Plan (September 2000) announced new national and local targets to address the gap between socio-economic groups in smoking rates and the resulting risks of cancer and heart disease: • Smoking rates among manual groups will be reduced from 32% in 1998 to 26% by 2010. • Local targets will be set making explicit what this means for the 20 health authorities with the highest smoking rates. • Funding for smoking cessation work with black and minority ethnic groups has been increased to £1 million. • There will be new pilots in 10 deprived areas to reduce smoking prevalence in communities where there are particular opportunities for focused support, such as prisons and hospitals.

Table 2.9 NHS Plan for tackling inequalities: (Teenage pregnancy; nutrition; drugs and alcohol-related crime)

Teenage pregnancy	Improving diet and nutrition	Tackling drugs and alcohol-related crime
• The appointment of a local teenage pregnancy co-ordinator in every social services area supported by eight regional co-ordinators. • Local reduction targets which seek the largest reductions in areas with the highest rates. By 2010 we are seeking a 60% reduction in under 18 conceptions in the worst fifth of wards, thereby reducing the level of inequality between the worst fifth of wards and the average by at least a quarter. • A national media campaign with adverts in teenage magazines and in local radio. • The production of new guidance on sex and relationship education. • The production of new guidance for local co-ordinators on effective youth contraceptive services.	Action by 2004 includes: • A national five-a-day programme to increase fruit and vegetable consumption: • The National School Fruit Scheme which entitles school children aged four to six to a free piece of fruit each school day. • Five-a-day Community Projects have been set up to test the feasibility and practicalities of evidence-based community approaches to improving access to and increasing awareness of fruit and vegetables. National roll out begins in 2002. • Work with industry – producers, caterers, retailers – to increase provision of, and access to, fruit and vegetables. • A communications programme to increase awareness of fruit and vegetable consumption, particularly targeting those groups with the lowest intakes. • Evaluation and monitoring of the implementation and impact of the five-a-day programme. • A reform of the welfare foods programme to use the resources more effectively to ensure children in poverty have access to a healthy diet. • Increased support for breast feeding – inequalities in breast feeding exist, for example, over 90% of mothers in social class I breast feed their babies initially, compared to only 50% of mothers in social class V. • Reduce salt, sugar and fat in the diet: work with the Food Standards Agency and the food industry to improve overall balance of the diet. • Local action to tackle obesity and physical inactivity informed by advice from the Health Development Agency. The recent National Audit Office report on 'Tackling Obesity in England' highlighted that most adults are now overweight, and one in five is obese. • Hospital nutrition policy to improve the outcome of care for patients.	The new National Treatment Agency (NTA) came into being on 1 April 2001, and will have a budget that pools resources spent on services from health and other agencies. • The main purpose of the Agency will be to ensure that those requiring treatment are able to access quality services regardless of their route of referral. • Ministers have decided to set up the National Treatment Agency as a Special Health Authority. • The NTA will deliver the three key quality improvement elements of clear quality standards, effective local delivery and strong monitoring mechanisms. • The NTA will make a difference by setting standards of treatment provisions and commission, performance monitoring and development and tackling variations in treatment standards and availability. • The Agency will put in place new structures and mechanisms to ensure that every drug treatment programme is aimed at the outcomes of the best.

complex and tackling them is a tough challenge that requires concerted action at all levels. Tackling wider influences (or determinants) such as: poverty, education, social exclusion, employment, housing, and the environment will be key, and will involve contributions and partnership working from all Government departments as well as at a local level within individual communities. **The NHS Plan (2001)** gave a number of commitments on health inequalities – see tables 2.8 and 2.9.

The NHS cancer plan

This promises action on:

- preventive work to reduce risk;
- earlier detection;
- improved community support for sufferers;
- faster access to treatment;
- national standards of treatment;
- improved palliative care;
- a strengthened research base.

Performance targets

These include a maximum one-month wait:

- from urgent GP referral to treatment for children's and testicular cancers and acute leukaemia by 2001;
- from diagnosis to treatment for breast cancer by 2001;
- from diagnosis to treatment for all cancers by 2005.

There will be a maximum two-month wait:

- from urgent GP referral to treatment for breast cancer by 2002;
- from urgent GP referral to treatment for all cancers by 2005.

Other new measures include:

- a target to reduce smoking rates among manual workers from 32% in 1998 to 26% by 2010;
- £50m more investment and additional Lottery cash for palliative care and hospices.

Local and regional issues for informing social policy

Local **health promotion units** have a role in ensuring that national targets are achieved. The government has also set up **Health Improvement Programmes (HimPs)**, and **Health Action Zones (HAZs)**

Health Improvement Programmes (HimPs)

These are a partnership between:

- Health Authorities (including Primary Care Groups), Primary Care Trusts, NHS Trusts, to develop the aims and the objectives of the NHS;
- NHS bodies and local authorities to promote the health and well-being of the local populations.

Current Health Improvement Programmes aim to:

- improve health and tackle inequalities;
- modernise and improve local services;
- provide a more comprehensive and effective planning process within the local health care system;
- support the development of partnerships with local authorities, the voluntary sector and other organisations.

HImPs will involve:

1 Those who use local services – either as patients or carers – the voluntary sector, local communities etc. need to input into the current HImPs so they feel ownership of its objectives and are committed to its implementation. Here it is important to involve those groups (children, black and minority ethnic groups and older people) who are under-represented or hard to reach under the NHS's traditional consultation methods.

2 Others with an interest or contribution to offer: trade unions, TECS, local schools, employers, including their occupational health services, the Health and Safety Executive, relevant colleges and universities etc.

Health Action Zones (HAZs)

These are partnerships between:

- The NHS;
- local authorities;
- community groups;
- the voluntary and business sectors located in deprived areas with poor health status and significant service pressures.

The function of HAZs is to:

- trigger health action programmes;
- develop and implement a health strategy to deliver within their area measurable improvements in public health and in the outcomes and quality of treatment and care.

Educational programmes and activities for health and social well-being

The focus of health promotion activities

The main aims of health education programmes are to:

- raise individual and population awareness about health issues;
- provide information and advice;
- develop personal strengths and abilities;
- support people to make changes.

Whether health and ill health is seen as the consequence of individual lifestyles or as a response to the social environment will affect the focus of health promotion activities. Health promotion activities can have a variety of objectives:

- to prevent disease;
- to ensure that people are well informed and able to make choices;
- to change behaviour;
- to help people acquire skills and confidence to take greater control over the factors influencing their health;
- to change policies and environments to facilitate healthy choices.

Health promotion involves working with individuals, communities and society

The new health strategy, 'Our Healthier Nation', recognises the role of individuals in determining their own health but also sees a role for communities and government in tackling the root causes of ill health. Individual practitioners may be engaged in:

- advice and information giving;
- education and training;
- policy work and lobbying;
- community development;
- interagency collaboration;
- research, profiling and monitoring;
- media development and campaigns.

Significant educators of health and social well-being

Organisations

Table 2.10 Organisations involved in health education

World Health Organisation (WHO)
For detailed information (see Chapter 5, page 266)

HealthPromis: the national database for health promotion for England, containing references and links to a range of sources.

Health Development Agency (HDA) for England: The HDA aims to improve the health of the people of England through research, capacity-building, monitoring and setting standards. (This used to be known as the Health Education Authority.)

Health Education Board for Scotland

Health Promotion Wales

The Health Promotion Agency for Northern Ireland

Government departments
The Department of Health, (DOH), The Department of Health and Social Security, (DHSS); Department for Education and Employment (DfEE); Ministry of Agriculture, Fisheries and Food (MAFF); Department of the Environment (DofE); Department of Transport; Central Office of Information etc.

UK Public Health Association
The United Kingdom Public Health Association (UKPHA) is an independent UK wide voluntary association, bringing together individuals and organisations from all sectors, who share a commitment to promoting the public's health. It is a membership based organisation that aims to promote the development of healthy public policy at all levels of government and across all sectors, and to support those working in public health either professionally or in a voluntary capacity. The UKPHA is a registered charity.

National Health Service (NHS)
Health Improvement Programmes (HiPs).
NHS Direct.
For detailed information, see Chapter 1.

Health and Safety Executive (HSE)
For detailed information, see Chapter 5 (pages 273–4).

Local Education Authorities
Schools, colleges, school and college nurses.

Social Services
Parenting skills programmes and child protection.

Voluntary Agencies
Most voluntary organisations offer information and advice on health education specific to their interest, for example, RNIB, Age Concern, ROSPA, NCH etc. They are available online and usually have telephone helplines.

Local police forces
Citizenship programmes, road safety, home safety and personal safety.

Commercial organisations
Private preventive medical companies, for example BUPA, PPP. Manufacturers and retailers of 'healthy' products, such as Flora, Benecol etc.

Community groups
Local groups e.g. neighbourhood Watch, Friends of the Earth, Community centres.

The mass media
Newspapers, magazines, TV and radio.

People who work in health education

- **Health and social care professionals:** nurses, doctors, midwives, health visitors, health promotion officers, occupational health nurses (see Chapter 5 for information).
- **Environmental health officers**
- **Health and safety officers**
- **Housing officers**

  (see Chapter 5, pages 281–2)
- **Youth workers and social workers** (see Chapter 5, page 282).
- **Community liaison police officers:** specialist police officers visit schools to advise and teach children about healthy living practices, such as road safety, personal safety and substance abuse
- **Teachers and lecturers**
- **Family and friends**

Professionals work with individuals and with communities; each area requires different skills and strategies:

Supporting individual change

Health education with individuals involves:

- Helping individuals identify risks to their health and to assess the costs and benefits of change.
- Providing information.
- Developing a relationship of trust and mutual respect with a client.
- Being aware of other factors, such as the views of significant people in the client's life and the individual's own self esteem, that could influence the situation.
- Knowledge of health psychology: Naidoo and Wills (1994) suggest that before change can take place, six conditions must be met:

1 **The change must be self-initiated.** Some clients resist pressure from others to change their behaviour.

2 **The behaviour must become important.** Many behaviours, for example, smoking, have become a habitual part of the client's life. Something must happen to draw the individual's attention to the behaviour and prompt a reappraisal.

3 **The importance of the behaviour must emerge over a period of time.** The new behaviour (i.e. not smoking) must become a normal and accepted part of the individual's life. This process takes time.

4 **The behaviour is not part of the individual's coping strategies.** It is more difficult to change if the risky behaviour helps the individual to cope with other difficulties (for example smoking helps the person to feel less stressed). In some circumstances, it is possible to suggest alternative coping strategies.

5 **The individual's life should not be problematic or uncertain.** People who are already experiencing stress, perhaps because of poverty or significant life events, may find it more difficult to change their health behaviour.

6 Social support is available. The presence of other people who are interested in the behaviour change can be of immense help to the individual

Working with communities

There are many different kinds of communities. A community can be made up of individuals:

- living in the same geographic area;
- belonging to the same ethnic group;
- of the same age;
- working for the same organisation;
- sharing the same culture or sexual orientation.

Most people belong to several communities.

Health education with communities or groups of people involves:

- involving the group or community in planning their own health care – leading to empowerment;
- helping people to understand the influence of social factors on their health (see pages 49–50);
- initiating or facilitating support groups;
- working with other agencies;
- profiling health needs of local people;
- lobbying and campaigning.

Health educators must be good communicators. Whether communicating with an individual or with a group, the message conveyed must be clear, unambiguous and relevant.

Objectives of educational activities

Various sources of information or data are used to identify the aims and objectives of health education campaigns. These include:

Epidemiology

This is the study of the distribution and determinants (or decisive factors) of disease in communities; epidemiological data indicates how:

- How many people are affected by a health problem (**morbidity** statistics).
- How many people die from a particular health problem – if potentially fatal (**mortality** statistics).
- Who are most at risk, for example which age groups, men or women; which occupation; which geographical area; smokers or non-smokers; active or sedentary people etc.

Descriptive studies

These describe the situation, for example, describing the distribution of a certain disease in relation to the age of a given population.

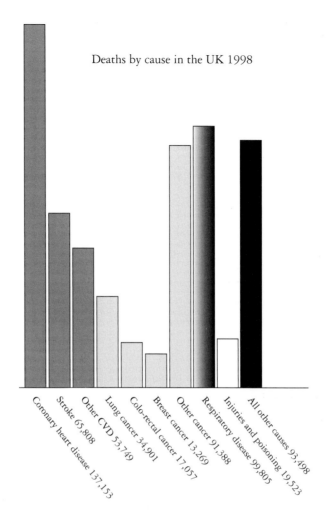

Figure 2.13 Mortality statistics: deaths by cause in the UK 1998

Analytical studies

These try to explain the situation by formulating and testing **hypotheses**, for example, trying to explain why a certain disease affects predominately males over the age of 60 in a given population.

Different study designs can be used in different situations and can use a mixture of **descriptive** and **analytical** approaches. Study designs can also be categorised as:

- **non-experimental**, where there is no **intervention** by the researcher, for example, case studies and surveys. Most surveys are **cross-sectional** (based on a random cross section of the population of interest, carried out at one point in time). **Longitudinal** surveys are carried out at more than one point in time, and aim to analyse cause and effect relationships. Most longitudinal studies follow-up the same population over time (for example, to measure the incidence of disease, and cause-effect relationships).

- **experimental** (intervention study), where the researcher *does* intervene, designed to test a cause- and-effect **hypothesis**. However, they can be carried out only if it is feasible and ethically justified to manipulate the postulated cause, for example, fluoridate the water supply of some towns, but not others, then compare the level of dental caries in children.

Table 2.11 Models and approaches in educating for health and social well-being

	Medical, preventive interventionist	Behaviourist	Empowerment	Educational	Social change
Aims	• medical interventions • disease reduction • compliance • scientific (e.g. epidemiology) • expert-led (top-down)	• encourage individuals to adopt healthy behaviours – key to improved health • health belongs to the individual – is their choice	• help people identify own health concerns – gain skills, ability, confidence to deal with them. • health educator facilitates (bottom-up) • self-empowerment, community empowerment	• provision of knowledge and skills to enable informed choice about behaviour. • does not aim to persuade or motivate in particular direction – *but* intended to lead to voluntary choice	• policy and environmental changes • to make the healthier choice the easier choice
Methods	primary preventive services (e.g. immunisation)	• mass media (e.g. HDA) • expert-led (top-down) but adaptable – could be client-led (bottom-up)	• developing plan with patient or client (e.g. nurses – care-plan) • client identifies areas for change • community development – identify shared concerns – plan action	3 aspects of learning: • cognitive (information and understanding) • affective (attitudes and feelings) • behavioural (skills) • teacher/facilitator • counselling, group discussion, role play	• targeting groups – organisational level (top-down) • public health legislation • support of groups or populations • lobbying, policy planning
Evaluation	**short-term:** uptake of preventive services **long-term:** morbidity and mortality rates	• is the result a change in behaviour? – problems with measuring behaviour	• extent to which specified aims met (outcome evaluation) • how group has been empowered (process evaluation)	• increased knowledge	• effectiveness of policy change
Disadvantages	• does not promote positive health • ignores social/environmental aspects of health • dependent on expert medical knowledge • removes health decisions • reinforces the medical model and medical hierarchy	• ignores social/economic factors • can lead to victim blaming (i.e. passive smoking issue) • expert-led • social engineering • targeting certain groups – can be manipulative	• evaluation problematic – long-term – difficult to decide the causes of change. • community development time-consuming and expensive • relinquishing control difficult for many professionals	• ignores social/economic factors • information alone insufficient to change behaviour	• long term and expensive • politically sensitive, e.g. no smoking policy in all public places, advertising and sponsorship of smoking

A **randomised controlled trial (RCT)** is the experimental approach of choice when assessing the effect of any type of health care **intervention**. The intervention could be:

- a new drug treatment compared to an existing medication;
- a new service, for example, practice nurse-led clinics for diabetes compared to routine general practice care.

These clinical trials must be carefully designed and conducted. The strength of an RCT lies in the *randomisation* of individuals from a defined sample population into either an 'experimental' group or a 'control' group.

Models and approaches

Models and approaches in educating for health and social well-being

The main models or approaches to health education are described briefly in Table 2.11. Professionals in the field of health education need to adapt and combine different approaches, or models, to suit the desired outcome of the programme.

Planning health education campaigns

All health education programmes need to be carefully planned. This planning process can be broken down into the following stages:

The eight stages of a health education programme

Stage 1: Identify the health issue

Examples are heart disease and the role of stress; exercise; nutrition; substance abuse; sexually transmitted infections; personal safety; road safety; immunisation, etc.

Stage 2: Identify the target group

Examples are middle-aged men who are at particular risk from heart disease; young people who have just started or may be tempted to start smoking. The age of the target group – that is, whether they are children, adolescents or adults – will affect the way health education advice is presented to them. It is important to be aware of the different needs of the audience to ensure that appropriate information and resources are used.

Stage 3: Identify the aims and objectives of the campaign

Aims

The aims or goals of the campaign are broad statements of what you are trying to achieve from a single session or event, or from the whole campaign. Examples are

to examine the issue of sexually transmitted infections; to increase knowledge of healthy eating.

Objectives

The objectives are more specific aims. They help you to pinpoint the most realistic method of presenting health advice and information and to evaluate your success in achieving them. Examples are

to provide parents with up-to-date information on immunisation so that they can make an informed decision regarding their own children; to prepare a display on 'Safe Sex' – outlining the risks of contracting a sexually transmitted infection; to devise a questionnaire for adolescents to assess their knowledge about the effects of alcohol on behaviour.

Stage 4: Planning to achieve the aims and objectives

Having identified your objectives, you now need to decide on the method of presentation. This will depend on such factors as cost, size of target group, ease of delivery, availability of material and/or equipment, and appropriateness for the target group. Suitable methods may include:

- display, perhaps tying in with a national awareness day or week, for example, AIDS awareness week or National No Smoking Day;
- video programme;
- leaflets;
- group workshops;
- formal lecture with slides or OHP transparencies.

Stage 5: Identify resources and equipment

The choice of resources and equipment will depend on several factors:

- availability of resources, for example, size of room, video rental, access to display boards and materials;
- cost of equipment;
- time available for activity;
- knowing how to operate equipment, for example, the use of a slide machine or OHP;
- relevance to the target audience.

Stage 6: Planning the content and method of the programme

This is where you work out *exactly* how to present the information, using the resources available. The objectives and the target group will guide your choice of method, but it must be one with which you feel confident. The more effort you put in at this stage, the greater the chance of success.

Guidelines for a presentation

- Produce a detailed time plan.
- Allow time to introduce yourselves and the topic.
- Do a timed test run to ensure that you have enough material.
- Check the room for seating arrangements and equipment.
- Rehearse the delivery of the talk – try to use prompt cards which emphasise *key points* even if you have written out the whole talk. Remember to maintain eye contact with your audience – this is difficult to do if you are reading large amounts of text.

- Sum up the main points.

- Discussion time – let your audience know that there will be time for any questions or debate at the end. You may need to initiate this by asking a question yourself – have a few ideas ready or split the audience into smaller groups for the discussion of key points and arrange for these groups to give feedback to the whole group.

- Empowering the audience – individuals need to make choices themselves. Your task is to present them with clear, relevant and above all *accurate* information. If you don't know the answer to any question, admit it and apologise!

Stage 7: Implementation

Carry out the plan and remember to evaluate the programme as you go along.

Stage 8: Evaluation

Evaluation is an important part of any health education activity; it allows you to **assess** and **review** all aspects of the programme. Always refer to the original aims and objectives and ask if these have been achieved. Before ending your presentation, ask the audience to complete an (anonymous) evaluation form so that you can review the outcome of the session.

Questionnaire on presentation on
SMOKING AND HEALTH

We would be very grateful if you could spare a few minutes to complete this form. Any information received is confidential and will help us to improve our technique.

On a scale of 1–5 (1 = poor; 5 = good):

a) How would you rank the information on smoking and risks to health?

   1   2   3   4   5

b) How useful was the information on ways to stop smoking!

   1   2   3   4   5

c) How would you rank the OHP charts and diagrams as a learning tool?

   1   2   3   4   5

d) How would you rank the display on 'Smoking: the facts'?

   1   2   3   4   5

e) Did the session cover all you expected?   Yes/No

Any other comments: ....
....
....
....

Thank you very much for your cooperation.

Figure 2.14 Sample evaluation form

Methods of educating for health and social well-being

Presenting the facts

The media have an important role to play in providing individuals with the information necessary to make decisions which may affect their health and that of their families. People are often confused by the sheer amount of sometimes conflicting advice they receive on health issues, for example, red wine is claimed to help protect against heart disease and cancer, but it is not always clear how much wine is beneficial and how much would be harmful in other ways. Most newspapers rely on interviews with 'experts' to present information about health issues, but there can be disagreement. For example:

- The link between BSE (Bovine Spongiform Encephalopathy) in animals and CJD (Jacob Kreutzfeld Disease) in humans.

- Repetitive strain injury – is this an occupational hazard? Experts disagree.

- Seasonal Affective Disorder (SAD) – often dismissed as a new neurosis.

Analogy

The most common analogy used in health education is that of the body as an *engine*. If it is looked after properly, given the right fuel and exercise, then it should give years of trouble-free service. Unfortunately this analogy does not take into account the inherited (genetic) dispositions we all have to certain disorders.

Shock/scare stories

Every decade has its share of shock stories. There is usually a 'knee-jerk' reaction by the public, but the adoption of avoidance strategies is sustained only if the initial scare is substantiated by informed debate and interest by health professionals. Examples include:

- The risk of listeria contamination of foods that have been cooked and then rapidly chilled.
- The role of toxins in cot mattresses as a contributory factor in cot deaths.
- The significance of aluminium-coated saucepans as a cancer risk.

Role models

Sports personalities and their lifestyles are very influential, particularly on young people, for example, the recent case of a footballer being treated for drug addiction received a lot of publicity and raised health awareness. Supermodels are often accused of promoting an unrealistic role model for adolescent girls – see page 57. Film stars and other people in the public eye advertise products and take part in health campaigns.

TV and radio

Programmes such as *Eastenders* and *The Archers* promote discussion on health issues, such as:

- child abuse;
- alcoholism and violence in the home;
- HIV/AIDS.

The role of the mass media in educating for health and social well-being

The mass media are the channels of communication to large numbers of people: they include: television, radio, magazines and newspapers, books and displays and exhibitions.

Health messages are conveyed through the mass media in various ways; these include:

- Planned deliberate health promotion, for example, displays and exhibitions on health themes, NHS or Health Development Agency adverts on television and in newspapers, Open University community education programmes on health.
- Books, documentaries and articles about health issues, for example, television programmes and magazine articles about diet, pollution or fitness.
- Health promotion by advertisers and manufacturers of 'healthy' products, for example, adverts for wholemeal bread or for low fat spreads, educational leaflets on 'feeding your baby' or 'slimming' which also promote the manufacturer's products.
- Discussion of health issues as a by-product of news items or entertainment programmes, particularly in 'soaps' where a character has a health problem.
- Health messages conveyed secretly, for example, well-known personalities or fictional characters refusing cigarettes or, conversely, chain-smoking.

Activity

TV and radio and health messages

1 In small groups, discuss a 'soap' on TV or radio. List all the health issues you can remember within the storylines:

- Do you think that TV or radio fiction is a good way of getting the message across? For example, have you learnt anything new?

- Does the inclusion of a telephone helpline detract from or enhance the impact of a health problem?

- Does the programme mirror real life or is it viewed as escapism?

2 Look at the TV listings for the next week. Make a list of all the programmes scheduled which have a health or social care focus. Arrange for each individual in your group to watch and analyse the message conveyed in the different formats, for example, documentary, soap, chat show, drama, film, etc. Discuss the impact of each format and its success in getting the message across.

The advantages and disadvantages of the different methods of health education are shown in Table 2.12

Ethical aspects of educating for health and social well-being

Any professional activity or campaign which 'interferes' in the lives of others will run into ethical problems. For example:

- Do health promotion agencies have a *right* to persuade or even coerce others into adopting a healthier lifestyle?

- Is there a risk that the individuals they target may suffer guilt and stress? Could they feel that they are being somehow blamed for their ill-health?

- Why should the general public take any notice of health 'experts' whose views often change over time or conflict with one another? (see page 111)

- How much should health professionals interfere in the legal pursuit of profits by a company which markets 'unhealthy' products such as cigarettes or fatty foods?

There have been many successful health campaigns over the last decades:

- **Grab 5:** The recent campaign led by Sustain (the alliance for better food and farming) to encourage primary school pupils to eat more fruit and vegetables (i.e. at least five portions per day.

- **Don't drink and drive campaigns:** These are run periodically on advertisement hoardings and on TV, but most frequently around Christmas and the New Year.

Table 2.12 The advantages and disadvantages of the different methods of health education

Resource method	Advantages	Disadvantages
Handouts and leaflets	• easy to produce • reduces need to take notes • information can be re-read as often as required	• not always read • can glance at information rather than read it carefully • difficult to obtain feedback
Display	• can be very attractive and eye-catching – especially when using a wide variety of interactive resources	• no captive audience
Posters	• can be very eye-catching when displayed in a prominent place	• often only glanced at – the overall message needs to be visually arresting
Videos	• can be useful as a trigger for discussion • useful for small to medium groups • can present information in a lively way	• danger of losing attention of audience if too long • must be previewed for relevance to target audience
Role play	• can be a lively way to encourage audience to think in depth about a health issue	• some people find role play threatening • may spend more time worrying about their 'acting' and not enough on the health issue
Presentations and workshops	• audience is captive – can't switch off or turn the page • information can be geared to the needs of the target audience • people have the opportunity to ask questions and to give feedback	• much depends on the skill of the presenter – to maintain audience attention • audience may be too shy to participate fully
TV and Radio	• can reach large numbers of people • can have a powerful instant impact through striking visual images • can raise awareness of a health issue which then stimulates group discussion	• difficult to obtain feedback • information or message may not be at the right level for a wide audience • audience can switch off if they don't like what is on
Newspapers & magazines	• can reach large numbers of people • information can be re-read whenever required • specialist magazines – such as *Top Sante* can target information at a particular audience	• difficult to obtain feedback • newspapers have a wide audience, so hard to target information • expensive to buy space in national newspapers and magazines • readers can ignore certain pages

- **Avoiding the risks of cot death:** This campaign took the form of TV documentaries and leaflets in clinics and hospitals.

- **Immunisation campaigns:** These are very successful and have done much to reduce the incidence of infectious diseases. However recent controversies over possible side-effects of the combined MMR vaccine have raised an ethical dilemma for both health professionals and parents.

- **Safety in the sun:** the increased public awareness of the depletion of the ozone layer and the risk of skin cancer

Many other campaigns have had more limited success, for example, those which have focused on secondary health education such as persuading women to attend for breast cancer screening.

Example of a national health campaign

National campaign: Smoking kills

The White Paper **Smoking Kills** is the first ever, comprehensive, government strategy to tackle smoking. Overall the government aims to persuade more smokers to give up, to aid them in doing so and to persuade non-smokers, particularly children, not to start.

The targets are:
- To reduce the number of 11–15 year-olds who smoke from 13 % in 1996 to 9% in 2010, with a fall to 11% by 2005.
- To help adults, especially the disadvantaged, to stop smoking. The target is to reduce the overall smoking rate in all social classes from 28% in 1996 to 24% in 2010, with a fall to 26% by 2005.
- To give special support to pregnant smokers and reduce the percentage of women who smoke in pregnancy from 23% in 1995 to 15% by 2010, with a fall to 18% by 2005.

(*All these targets apply to England only.*)

Target audiences

The key target audiences are:
- adult smokers aged 25–45;
- young people aged 11–16;
- pregnant women;
- ethnic minorities.

This campaign emphasises that:

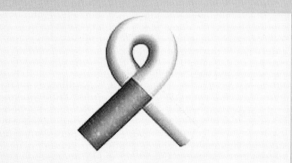

- giving up is a *process*, and that relapsing is a natural part of that process;
- most smokers don't give up for good the first time they try – it often takes five or six attempts;
- lapses are ok – what is not ok is giving up on giving up.
- becoming a non-smoker can be hard, and 'giver-uppers' need to persevere.

This campaign aims to offer these people support and encouragement.

NHS Smoking Helpline – 0800 169 0 169

This helpline provides information and support for smokers who want to give up. People can also order written material via the phone line. Details of smoking cessation services in local districts are available from the NHS Smoking Helpline, and callers can be referred to face-to-face support via this route.

Figure 2.15 Don't give up giving up

NHS Pregnancy Smoking Helpline – 0800 169 9 169

This was launched in September 2000, and is particularly aimed at younger pregnant women in low-income groups who are more likely to continue to smoke during pregnancy. Some of the less well known problems associated with smoking during pregnancy are highlighted along with a supportive message encouraging women to call the NHS Pregnancy Smoking Helpline.

Promotional material

There are a number of leaflets, posters and stickers available through the website and the telephone lines. The campaign leaflet, 'Don't give up giving up', is available to order in a large range of languages, on audio cassette and in large print, Braille and learning disability versions.

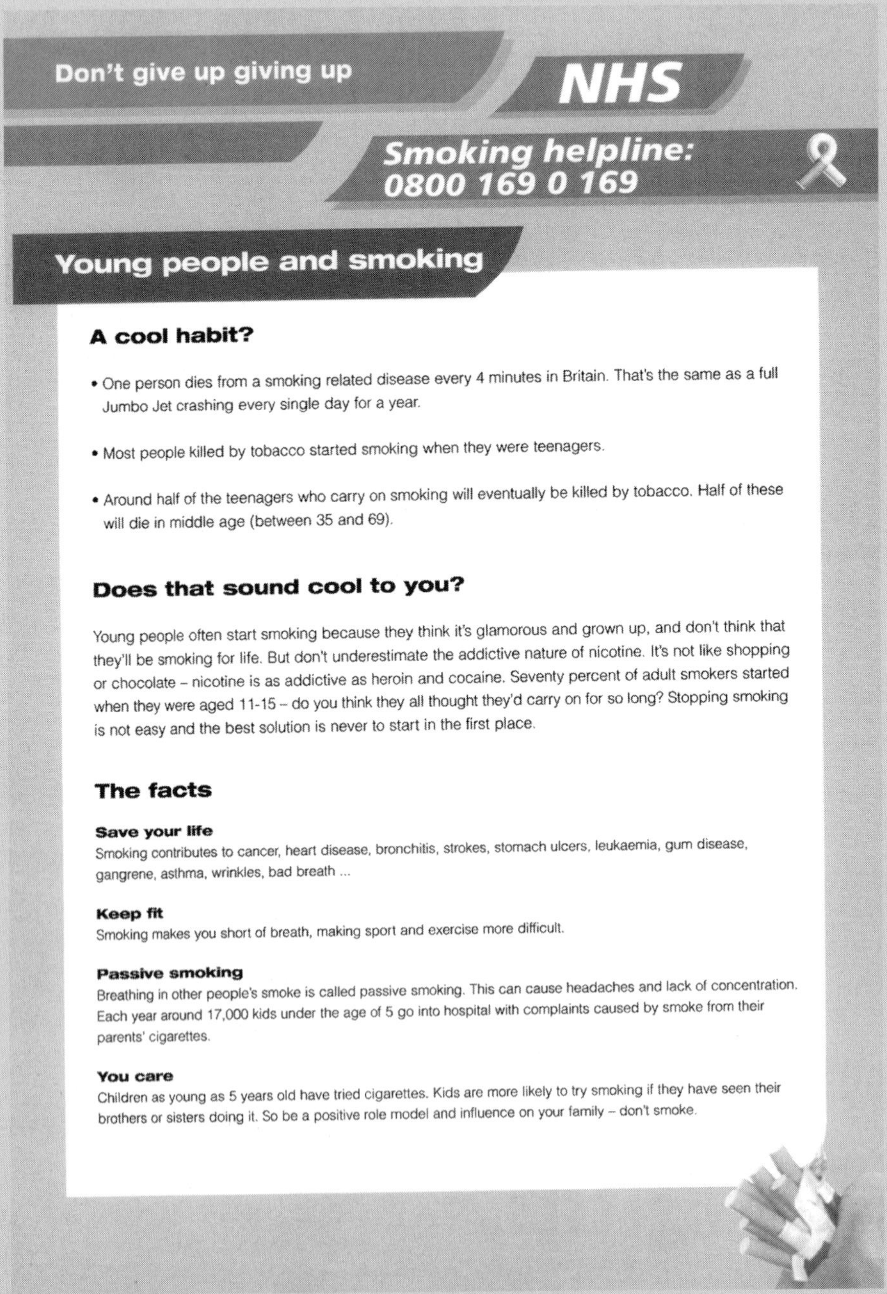

Don't give up giving up

NHS

Smoking helpline: 0800 169 0 169

Young people and smoking

A cool habit?

- One person dies from a smoking related disease every 4 minutes in Britain. That's the same as a full Jumbo Jet crashing every single day for a year.

- Most people killed by tobacco started smoking when they were teenagers.

- Around half of the teenagers who carry on smoking will eventually be killed by tobacco. Half of these will die in middle age (between 35 and 69).

Does that sound cool to you?

Young people often start smoking because they think it's glamorous and grown up, and don't think that they'll be smoking for life. But don't underestimate the addictive nature of nicotine. It's not like shopping or chocolate – nicotine is as addictive as heroin and cocaine. Seventy percent of adult smokers started when they were aged 11-15 – do you think they all thought they'd carry on for so long? Stopping smoking is not easy and the best solution is never to start in the first place.

The facts

Save your life
Smoking contributes to cancer, heart disease, bronchitis, strokes, stomach ulcers, leukaemia, gum disease, gangrene, asthma, wrinkles, bad breath ...

Keep fit
Smoking makes you short of breath, making sport and exercise more difficult.

Passive smoking
Breathing in other people's smoke is called passive smoking. This can cause headaches and lack of concentration. Each year around 17,000 kids under the age of 5 go into hospital with complaints caused by smoke from their parents' cigarettes.

You care
Children as young as 5 years old have tried cigarettes. Kids are more likely to try smoking if they have seen their brothers or sisters doing it. So be a positive role model and influence on your family – don't smoke.

Figure 2.16 Young people and smoking leaflet

Activity

1 Select a recent health education campaign that you found memorable (such as the NHS anti-smoking campaign). Evaluate the success of the campaign, with particular emphasis on the following:

  • A description of the aim of the campaign, for example, a new Government report may have highlighted an increase in alcohol-related road traffic accidents, which the campaign aims to address.

  • A description of the methods used, for example, newspaper coverage, use of famous personalities, use of shock/scare tactics, and how these methods relate to the target population of the campaign.

2 Interview at least six individuals from the target group of the campaign, using a structured interview format (see main textbook for guidance).

3 Use the results of these interviews to draw conclusions and to make recommendations about the effectiveness of the campaign.

Evaluating promotional activities

Evaluation involves identifying and grading the criteria, values and aims of a project and collecting information to assess if they have all been met. Overall, the main aim of evaluating a health education campaign is to see whether it has achieved its **objectives**. The objectives of any campaign should be SMART:

S Specific

M Measurable

A Agreed

R Realistic

T Timebound

The success of medical treatments is relatively easy to measure or evaluate – for example, the rapid recovery of servicemen with infections during the Second World War was certainly helped by the use of antibiotics, particularly penicillin. More recently, the use of drugs to treat and to prevent asthma has been successful. Most health education campaigns aim to increase public awareness and to affect lifestyle and behaviour; they are usually very difficult to evaluate. There are many reasons for this:

1 It is difficult to ensure strict comparability between the target group and a control group.

2 Any trial that aims to compare a target group with a control group must span a long period of time and cover a large population.

3 Primary prevention methods are usually matters of public policy, concerning healthy

individuals who are not actively seeking help or care. How do we decide whether their continuing good health is directly influenced by a campaign?

4   The mass media plays a large part in raising public awareness of health issues, but messages received via TV, radio and the press are often not acknowledged as being part of health education.

There are some issues which have not been the focus of recent health campaigns:

- Chlamydia: the most common sexually transmitted infection in the UK today and yet most people have never heard of it (see page 94).
- Dental decay: one of the most costly avoidable health problems.
- Head lice: the subject of infrequent campaigns, but a common problem in nurseries and schools
- Back pain: a very common reason for absence from work.
- Heart disease: experts disagree on the exact causes of heart disease, but it is the major killer of those over 75 in the UK.

 # Activity

Health campaign: group presentations

These could be arranged as a video or as an oral presentation, depending on the resources available. Discuss with your tutor how and when you are going to make your presentation. Draw up an *individual action plan*, following the advice on pages 109–11 to include:

1   Choice of health promotion area. Choose from:

- smoking;
- alcohol;
- drug abuse;
- safe sexual practices;
- stress and mental illness.

2   Detailed planning – delegate different responsibility for different tasks to each group member. The presentation should:

- only contain accurate information;
- outline your target group;
- include recommendations on ways in which the audience can contribute to their own health;
- provide a question-and-answer session at the end;

- ensure that all feedback made to the target audience is both constructive and non-judgemental.

After the presentation, write an individual evaluation of the exercise, commenting on:

- your own contribution;

- the audience response to your presentation;

- recommendations for the future (i.e. ways of improving the session).

Chapter 3

Physiological disorders

This chapter focuses on the abnormal physiology and dysfunction of body systems. You will be investigating disorder and disease, and increasing your knowledge of diagnosis and treatment. The unit provides a valuable knowledge base for those who might consider future careers in medical physics, laboratory work, nursing or medicine. A knowledge of diagnosis and treatment can be of value to anyone entering the caring professions to help them support clients who may require medical intervention. This unit utilises the knowledge of body systems you will have gained from Chapter 3, Physical aspects of health in Vocational A level Health and Social Care.

This chapter describes:

- signs, symptoms, diagnosis and treatment of disorders within the respiratory, cardiovascular, digestive, renal, nervous and endocrine systems;
- physiological measurements involved in diagnosis and treatment;
- care delivery;
- safe practice.

Throughout the chapter there are activities to help you reinforce your learning. Where appropriate, there are answers to questions at the end of the book. The chapter concludes with a Glossary and List of Resources.

Signs, symptoms, and treatment of physiological disorders

To make a diagnosis of a disease it is necessary to:

- have a knowledge of normal physiological function;
- understand the symptoms a client presents with;
- use information from a variety of physiological measurements.

A description of disorders of the six body systems are given below. For your AVCE unit you need to know about each disorder, and then select **three** disorders to learn about in depth, including signs, symptoms, diagnostic tests, causes, disease progression and epidemiology, treatments and prognosis. Before you start reading about each disease, you will need to refer back to an account of the relevant body system and physiological measurement techniques (Chapter 3, 'Physical aspects of health' in *Vocational A Level Health and Social Care*, Thomson, H. *et al.*). Once you have familiarised yourself with each body system, read through the accounts below of each disease before making your choice of which three disorders to select.

The respiratory system

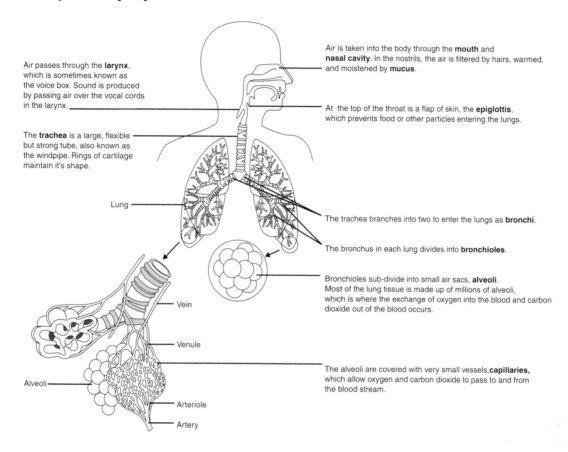

Air passes through the **larynx**, which is sometimes known as the voice box. Sound is produced by passing air over the vocal cords in the larynx.

Air is taken into the body through the **mouth** and **nasal cavity**. In the nostrils, the air is filtered by hairs, warmed, and moistened by **mucus**.

At the top of the throat is a flap of skin, the **epiglottis**, which prevents food or other particles entering the lungs.

The **trachea** is a large, flexible but strong tube, also known as the windpipe. Rings of cartilage maintain it's shape.

Lung

The trachea branches into two to enter the lungs as **bronchi**.

The bronchus in each lung divides into **bronchioles**.

Bronchioles sub-divide into small air sacs, **alveoli**. Most of the lung tissue is made up of millions of alveoli, which is where the exchange of oxygen into the blood and carbon dioxide out of the blood occurs.

Vein

Venule

The alveoli are covered with very small vessels, **capillaries**, which allow oxygen and carbon dioxide to pass to and from the blood stream.

Alveoli

Arteriole

Artery

Figure 3.1 The respiratory system

You need to be familiar with the following physiological detail:

- the structure of the respiratory system;
- the microscopic structure of the air passages and respiratory surface;
- the mechanism of gas exchange at the respiratory surface;
- the mechanism of breathing.

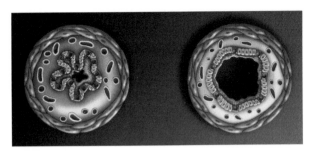

Figure 3.2 The difference between a normal bronchiole and a narrowed bronchiole

Bronchitis

Causes

The inflammation and swelling results in the bronchioles becoming narrower or closing (Figure 3.2). Bronchitis may be caused by infection and just last for a few days (**acute**), or it may be a serious long term disorder (**chronic**). Bronchitis is considered to be chronic if the sufferer has a persistent cough which lasts for at least three months of the year for more than two consecutive years.

In **acute bronchitis** 90% of cases are caused by viruses. In the other 10% of cases it is bacteria which cause the infection.

Chronic bronchitis can be caused by a number of different factors. For example:

- repeated attacks of acute bronchitis;
- industrial pollution such as coal or grain dust;
- atmospheric pollution;
- smoking (the most common cause).

Signs and symptoms: acute bronchitis

- hacking cough;
- the accumulation of thick phlegm (a mixture of mucus, bacteria and white blood cells);
- fever and chills;
- soreness and tightness of the chest;
- some shortness of breath;
- increased breathing (respiratory) rate.

Signs and symptoms: chronic bronchitis

- persistent coughing;
- wheezing and breathlessness.

Diagnosis: acute bronchitis

A stethoscope can be used to listen for the 'rattling' sound which is found in this condition.

Treatment: acute bronchitis

- inhaled bronchodilator (widens the bronchioles);
- inhaled or oral steroids to reduce inflammation (in severe cases);

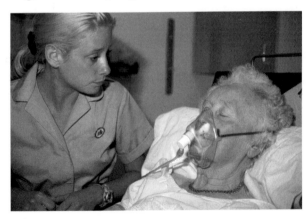

Figure 3.3 Oxygen is used in severe cases of bronchitis

- rest, drinking plenty of fluids and avoiding cigarette smoke.

Diagnosis: chronic bronchitis

- a stethoscope is used to listen for wheezing;
- a chest X-ray can be made to check for damage to the lungs;
- a spirometer can be used to measure lung volumes and respiratory rate (see page 141, below).

Treatment: chronic bronchitis

- smokers will be encouraged to stop;
- overweight patients will be encouraged to diet;
- inhaled bronchodilator;
- steroids;
- oxygen may be necessary in severe cases (Figure 3.3).

Asthma

Causes

Asthma is a chronic respiratory disease but the symptoms are not always present. The symptoms may be triggered by a variety of factors, for example, pollution, smoke, pollen, animals, exercise, respiratory infection and stress. The number and severity of asthma attacks vary from one sufferer to another. During an asthma attack the muscles of the airways are contracted. If mucus builds up, there will be coughing, and in severe cases the alveoli become damaged and scar tissue develops. Gases cannot diffuse through this scar tissue, so this reduces the effectiveness of the lungs.

Signs and symptoms

- tightening of the chest;
- difficulty in breathing;
- wheezing;
- coughing.

Diagnosis

A measurement of **peak flow** will be made (see pages 142–3). This is the maximum rate at which air can be exhaled. Asthma sufferers have a low peak flow reading; the more severe the attack, the lower their reading. Patients can monitor their peak flow at home.

Treatment

Asthma can be serious if not treated and controlled properly.

- bronchodilators relax the muscles of the airways;
- in severe cases steroids are prescribed.

Activity

Asthma is a common condition. Talk to a number of sufferers and find out what factors tend to trigger their attacks.

The cardiovascular system

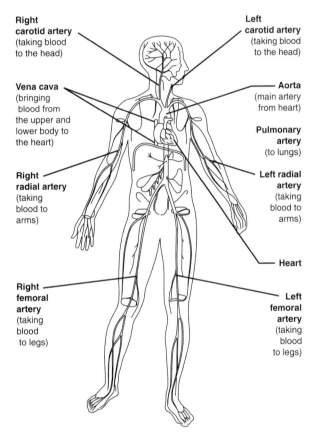

Right carotid artery (taking blood to the head)

Left carotid artery (taking blood to the head)

Vena cava (bringing blood from the upper and lower body to the heart)

Aorta (main artery from heart)

Pulmonary artery (to lungs)

Right radial artery (taking blood to arms)

Left radial artery (taking blood to arms)

Right femoral artery (taking blood to legs)

Heart

Left femoral artery (taking blood to legs)

Figure 3.4 The cardiovascular system, showing major arteries

You need to be familiar with the following physiological detail:

- the microscopic structure of cardiac muscle;
- cardiac cycle;
- cardiac rhythm;
- sino-atrial node, atrio-ventricular node, Purkinje fibres;
- innervation of the heart by the sympathetic and vagal nerves;
- the roles of arteries, veins and capillaries.

Hypertension (high blood pressure)

Causes

Blood pressure is a measure of the pressure of blood against the artery walls. It is given as two numbers: the higher number is the pressure during the contraction of the heart (systole), and the lower reading is the pressure during relaxation of the heart (diastole). It is measured with a sphygmomanometer (see pages 143–5). An individual's blood pressure will vary over time and blood pressure will vary from one individual to another. The following are considered to have a higher than normal risk of hypertension:

- members of families with a history of high blood pressure, heart disease or diabetes;
- pregnant women;
- women who take birth control pills;
- people who are older than 60;
- people who are overweight;

- people who do not exercise;
- smokers;
- people who drink a lot of alcohol;
- people who have high fat diets;
- people who have high salt diets:
- people who are stressed.

Signs and symptoms

High blood pressure is sometimes known as the 'silent killer' because there are rarely any symptoms of high blood pressure. If blood pressure is very high, a person may suffer:

- headaches;
- nosebleeds;
- numbness and tingling.

If hypertension is not treated it can lead to:

- vision problems;
- heart attack (see below);
- stroke;
- kidney failure (see pages 130–1).

Diagnosis

Because of the widespread harm that high blood pressure can cause to the body, it is important that blood pressure is regularly checked, particularly in people who are in a high risk group (see above). A healthy heart will give a reading of approximately 120 systolic and 80 diastolic (120/80). A blood pressure of more than (140/90) is considered abnormal. If it is as high as 200/120 immediate treatment will be required.

Treatment

When hypertension is diagnosed, a patient will generally be given advice about necessary **life style changes** which will help to lower blood pressure, for example, weight loss diets, exercise, relaxation techniques, drinking less, or giving up smoking could be recommended. **Medication** will be prescribed if blood pressure is particularly high or remains high after lifestyle changes.

Activity

What recommendations about diet would you make to a person with high blood pressure?

(See page 162 for answers).

Myocardial infarction (heart attack)

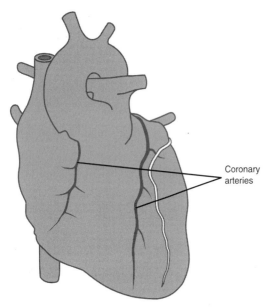

Figure 3.5 The coronary arteries

Coronary arteries

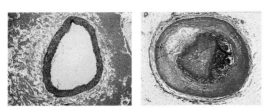

Figure 3.6 Cross-sections of a normal and blocked coronary artery

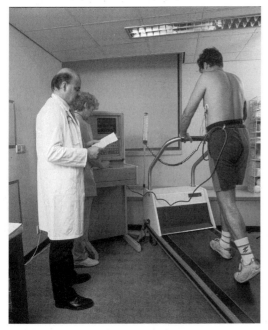

Figure 3.7 Producing an ECG

Causes

The muscle of the heart receives its blood supply through two coronary arteries (Figure 3.5). If a branch of one of these becomes blocked, some of the muscle cells will be starved of oxygen and die. A blockage can be caused by the build-up of fatty materials in the artery walls (**atherosclerosis**). **Plaques** (Figure 3.6) which are made of cholesterol, fibres, dead muscle cells and platelets can form. These build up in the artery wall and restrict the flow of blood. If they break through the lining of the wall, they create a rough surface which makes blood clot. The clot formed, known as a **thrombus**, restricts the blood flow further, leading to a heart attack. Table 3.1 shows factors which increase a person's risk of suffering a heart attack.

Signs and symptoms

- sudden and severe chest pain;
- pain or tingling in the left arm;
- breathlessness;
- lips become blue.

Diagnosis

An electrocardiogram (ECG or EKG) is used to monitor the nature of the heart beat. Electrodes are placed on the skin over the heart and the electrical excitation associated with each heartbeat is recorded over time (Figures 3.7 and 3.8).

Treatment

Drugs can be administered within the first 12 hours after a heart attack, which help to remove the blockage in the blood vessel and prevent any permanent damage to the heart. To reduce the chances of a heart attack reoccurring, a patient will be advised to:

- take gentle exercise;
- eat a healthy, low fat diet;
- keep stress levels to a minimum;
- if necessary, to take medication to reduce cholesterol, blood pressure and the risk of clotting.

Table 3.1 Factors which affect the risk of suffering a heart attack

Factor	Risk
Family history	If there is a history of heart disease in the family, there is an increased risk of a heart attack
Gender	Heart attacks are more frequent in males than females
Age	The risk of having a heart attack increases with age
Weight	Obese people are more likely to have a heart attack than people of normal body weight
Smoking	Smokers are more likely to have a heart attack than non-smokers
Alcohol consumption	Heavy drinkers are more likely to have a heart attack than moderate drinkers or non-drinkers
Diet	People with high fat diets are more likely to have high levels of cholesterol in the blood which increases the risk of a heart attack
Stress	Continued stress increases the risk of having a heart attack
Exercise	Inactivity increases the risk of having a heart attack
Blood pressure	High blood pressure (hypertension) increases the risk of a heart attack
Diabetes	People with diabetes have an increased risk of suffering a heart attack

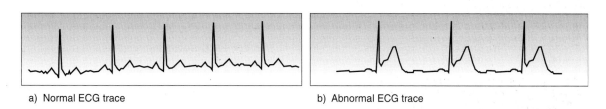

a) Normal ECG trace   b) Abnormal ECG trace

Figure 3.8 Compare the difference between a normal and an abnormal ECG trace

 Activity

1   Look at Table 3.1 and identify the factors over which a person has some control. From this, write a list of lifestyle choices young people can make to reduce their chances of suffering a heart attack in later life.

The digestive system

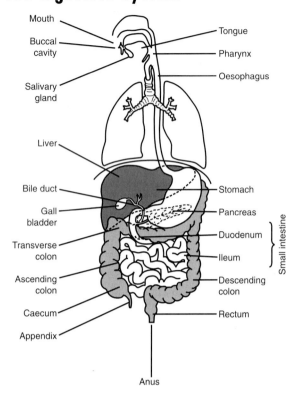

Figure 3.9 The digestive system

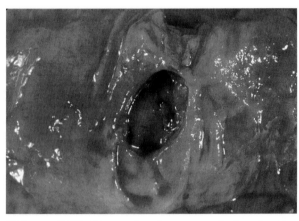

Figure 3.10 Stomach ulcers are holes in the lining of the stomach

You need to be familiar with the following physiological detail:

- the structure of the alimentary canal;
- the process of digestion;
- the process of absorption.

Stomach ulcers

Causes

- Stomach ulcers, also known as peptic ulcers, are holes in the protective lining of the stomach (Figure 3.10).
- Until recently, it was believed that they were caused by factors such as stress and poor diet, which led to excessive acid in the stomach. It is now thought that ulcers may be caused by an infection by the bacterium *Helicobacter pylori*.
- People are more susceptible to ulcers if they use over-the-counter painkillers, for example, aspirin, very frequently.
- A high level of alcohol consumption can lead to ulcers.
- Smokers are more likely to develop ulcers than non-smokers.
- Elderly people are more likely to develop stomach ulcers, possibly because of pain killers taken to treat arthritis.

Signs and symptoms

- a burning, gnawing abdominal pain particularly between meals or early in the morning;
- black or bloody stools;
- bloating;
- heartburn;
- nausea or vomiting;
- weight loss

Stomach ulcers can lead to more serious conditions, so it is important that they are diagnosed and treated.

Diagnosis

The symptoms listed above will help doctors to diagnose ulcers. To find out in which part of the gut the ulcers are, a patient will usually be given a **barium meal** before being **X-rayed**. The patient drinks the barium meal, a chalky liquid, and then has X-rays of the digestive gut taken from various angles. In some cases doctors may carry out a **gastroscopy** which allows them to see the stomach lining and to test for bacterial infections.

Treatment

Medications such as antibiotics, which kill bacteria, and antacids, which reduce the amount of acid produced by the stomach, are effective. In emergency situations surgery may be necessary.

Irritable bowel syndrome

Causes

Irritable bowel syndrome (IBS) is the most common disorder of the digestive system. It occurs when the normal contractions of the muscles of the gut, which move the contents through the digestive tract (**peristalsis**), are disrupted. It is not known why this happens, although the following have been suggested as triggers of the condition:

- stress;
- food allergies;
- overeating;
- high fat diet;
- various medications that affect the natural bacteria in the gut or cause constipation.

Signs and symptoms

Different people often experience different symptoms and these may vary over time. Some of the common symptoms are:

- abdominal pain or cramps;
- diarrhoea;
- constipation;
- bloating.

Symptoms of IBS may last for several weeks or longer.

Diagnosis

There are no specific tests to diagnose IBS, but doctors are likely to do tests to rule out other more serious conditions:

- a stool sample is sent to a laboratory;
- a barium enema is administered followed by an X-ray.

Treatment

Because there is no known specific cause of IBS, treatment is only given to relieve the symptoms of the disease:

- a patient may be given recommendations to change their diet, for example, to increase fibre and decrease fat;

- medication may be given to slow the movement of food through the gut and to relieve stomach cramps.

Activity

What recommendations would you make to a patient in order for them to reduce the level of fat in their diet and to increase the amount of fibre?

(See page 162 for answers).

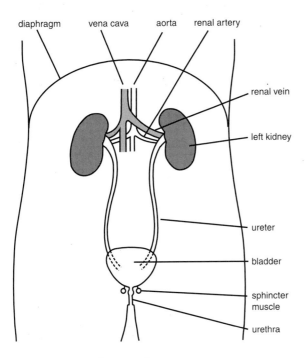

Figure 3.11 The renal system

The renal system

You need to be familiar with the following physiological detail:

- structure of a nephron;

- the histology of the nephron related to its function;

- ultra-filtration;

- selective reabsorption of water and solutes;

- role of osmoreceptors in the hypothalamus;

- the production and action of anti-diuretic hormone.

Renal (kidney) failure

Causes

Kidney failure can be either acute (function is lost suddenly) or chronic (function is lost gradually, possibly over a period of years). There are a variety of possible causes. Acute kidney failure may be caused by infection, poisons or a physical injury. Chronic kidney failure may be caused by factors such as diabetes, high blood pressure or a kidney disease. The elderly have a higher risk of developing kidney failure, and males are at higher risk than females.

Signs and symptoms

Because the kidneys stop working efficiently, toxins such as urea and creatinine build up in the blood. The build up of toxins may take place without the development of any symptoms. Alternatively, the following symptoms may be experienced:

- an increase or decrease in the amount of urine produced;

- swelling of tissues;

- nausea;
- vomiting;
- poor appetite;
- metallic taste;
- weight loss;
- fatigue;
- confusion;
- spasms;
- pale skin;
- dry, itchy skin;
- higher blood pressure.

In the long term, chronic kidney failure can lead to heart disease and an increased susceptibility to infections.

Diagnosis

Any of the above symptoms may be seen. Urinalysis (see page 148) may show abnormalities such as protein or red blood cells. A blood sample may show high levels of urea and creatinine or anaemia (low levels of red blood cells). If diagnosis is not possible from urine or blood samples, a kidney biopsy will be carried out. This involves using a special needle to take a small sample of kidney tissue to examine with a microscope.

Treatment

There are a variety of treatments such as:

- a protein restricted diet;
- limiting fluids;
- using drugs to control blood pressure;
- diuretics can be used to control salt-water balance;
- bicarbonate can be used to help control blood pH.

In cases of complete kidney failure:

- Haemodialysis may be regularly carried out. In this process blood is taken out of the body, passed through an artificial kidney to filter out impurities, and returned to the body (Fig. 3.12.).
- If a suitable donor can be found, a kidney transplant may be carried out. In this process a diseased kidney is replaced with a healthy kidney.

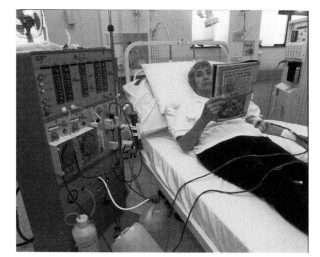

Figure 3.12 Patient undergoing dialysis

Activity

Find out more about an alternative to haemodialysis, peritoneal dialysis, in which the lining of the abdomen, the peritoneal membrane, is used to clean the blood.

Polycystic disease

Causes

A person suffering from polycystic kidney disease has many fluid filled cysts on the kidneys. These cysts reduce the amount of healthy kidney tissue, so kidney function is reduced and eventually, in about half of all sufferers, this may lead to total kidney failure. The condition may also lead to the formation of cysts in other organs such as the liver, heart and brain.

The most common form of polycystic kidney disease is inherited and symptoms usually develop between the ages of 30–40 years. There is a much rarer inherited form in which the symptoms are present in the first few months of a baby's life. Occasionally people who already have kidney failure will develop cysts on the kidney. This is not inherited and tends to affect older people.

Signs and symptoms

- pain in the back and sides (between the ribs and hips);
- urinary tract infection;
- blood in the urine;
- high blood pressure;
- kidney stones.

Diagnosis

Ultrasound imaging can be used to detect cysts in the kidney and perhaps in other organs. Because the condition is usually inherited, a patient will be asked about their family history. In the future DNA testing will be able to confirm the condition before the cysts develop.

Treatment

There is no cure available but treatment can reduce the symptoms and extend life expectancy. For example, drugs can be used to relieve pain and surgery can be used to temporarily reduce the cysts. If kidney failure develops, the patient will require dialysis or a kidney transplant (see renal failure, pages 130–1).

The endocrine system

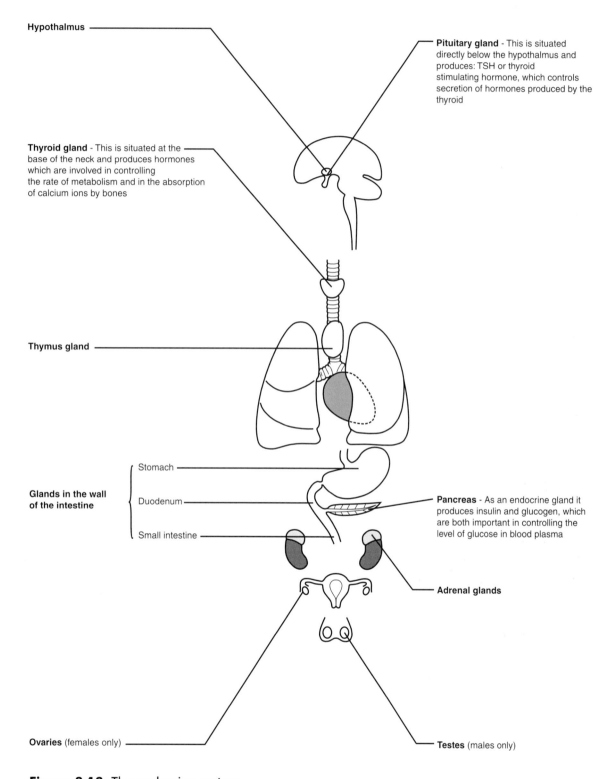

Hypothalmus

Pituitary gland - This is situated directly below the hypothalmus and produces: TSH or thyroid stimulating hormone, which controls secretion of hormones produced by the thyroid

Thyroid gland - This is situated at the base of the neck and produces hormones which are involved in controlling the rate of metabolism and in the absorption of calcium ions by bones

Thymus gland

Glands in the wall of the intestine

Stomach

Duodenum

Small intestine

Pancreas - As an endocrine gland it produces insulin and glucogen, which are both important in controlling the level of glucose in blood plasma

Adrenal glands

Ovaries (females only)

Testes (males only)

Figure 3.13 The endocrine system

You need to be familiar with the following physiological detail:

- the nature of hormones;
- the role of endocrine glands and target organs;
- homeostasis and negative feedback.

Thyrotoxicosis

Causes

This condition, which is sometimes known as hyperthyroidism, is caused by the thyroid gland (Figure 3.14) producing too much of the hormone. This hormone controls the rate of metabolism in the body. If there is too much thyroxine the rate of metabolism will be too fast.

There are a variety of reasons why the thyroid gland may not function correctly. Most commonly, thyrotoxicosis occurs when antibodies produced by the immune system attack the thyroid gland. This is a type of **auto-immune disease**. It is not known why this happens but there appears to be some genetic basis. The antibodies attack the TSH receptors on the thyroid gland, which has the effect of 'switching on' the continuous production of thyroid hormones.

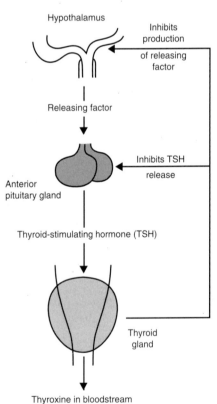

The hypothalamus is sensitive to the level of thyroxine in the blood. If the level falls below a certain level, the hypothalamus produces more releasing factor. This stimulates the anterior lobe of the pituitary to release more thyroid stimulating hormone, which in turn stimulates the thyroid gland to produce thyroxine. Thyroxine has an effect on both the anterior lobe of the pituitary and the hypothalamus, which leads to a reduction in the production of more thyroxine. This is an example of a negative feedback loop, which is so common in control systems.

Figure 3.14 Functioning of the thyroid gland

Signs and symptoms

The common symptoms of thyrotoxicosis are caused by a rapid metabolic rate and include:

- weight loss despite increased appetite;
- palpitations, fast or irregular heartbeat;
- higher blood pressure;
- tremor (shakiness);
- anxiety;
- tiredness or weakness;
- sweating;
- sore eyes;
- itching;
- thirst and diarrhoea;
- intolerance of heat.

There may be a swelling in the throat (goitre) from an increase in the size of the thyroid gland. In some cases the eyes appear swollen or prominent.

Diagnosis

Thyroid function tests (see pages 148–9), can be carried out to test for high levels of thyroid hormones in the blood. The results of these tests should be considered alongside the patient's signs and symptoms.

Treatment

- A number of **drugs** are available which can be used to help return the levels of thyroid hormones to normal.
- In a few cases it may be necessary to surgically remove most of the thyroid gland (**thyroidectomy**).
- **Radioactive iodine** can be taken as a capsule or drink to stop the thyroid gland working. Subsequently, the patients would need to take thyroxine tablets for the rest of their life.

Diabetes mellitus

Causes

This is the most common disorder of the endocrine system. People who suffer from this condition do not have sufficient insulin, the hormone which lowers blood sugar level. There are two distinct forms of diabetes mellitus – type 1 and type 2.

Signs and symptoms

Untreated diabetes can lead to the following symptoms:

- urine production increases;
- intense thirst;
- weight loss or weight gain;

- fatigue;
- breath smells of pear drops;
- the pH of the blood can drop (become more acidic) which could lead to nausea, rapid deep breathing, coma and death.

Diagnosis

Without treatment, diabetics accumulate high levels of sugar (glucose) in their blood. The high level of glucose in the blood means that glucose starts to appear in the urine. This can be detected by chemical tests, which are described on page 148.

Treatment

Diabetes can lead to serious long-term complications if it is not carefully controlled. The eyes, nervous system, kidneys, and cardiovascular system could be damaged. As shown in Table 3.2, type 1 diabetes is treated with insulin injections and controlled diet, and type 2 diabetes is treated with controlled diet alone. Regular exercise and the maintenance of an ideal body weight are both important to diabetics.

Table 3.2

	Type 1	Type 2
Age of people affected	Mainly young people under the age of 20.	Affects much older people.
Cause	Loss of some or all of the cells in the pancreas which make insulin. This is thought to be either because of destruction by the body's own antibodies, or because of a viral infection.	In some cases the level of insulin production drops; in other cases the cells that are affected by insulin become less sensitive to the hormone.
Treatment	Insulin injections (insulin would be digested if taken orally) and controlled diet.	Controlled diet (low sugar).
Onset	Sudden onset.	Develops gradually.

Word check

Insulin injections

Insulin is a protein so if it was taken orally it would be broken down in the digestive system. It therefore has to be injected under the skin. People with type 1 diabetes will need to have injections at least twice a day, and if necessary children can learn to do this themselves from an early age.

Diet

Both the content and the timing of meals is important to prevent fluctuations in blood sugar levels:

* three meals a day, and three or four snacks are usually recommended;

* carbohydrates should make up 50–60% of the total energy content of the diet, proteins 20–25%, fats 20–30%;

* carbohydrates in the diet should be in the form of starch rather than sugars. (This is because starch is broken down in the gut to slowly release a steady supply of sugar into the blood, whereas sugar in the diet will immediately enter the blood leading to a rapid increase in blood sugar level.);

* a carbohydrate snack should be eaten half an hour before exercise;

* if a diabetic starts to feel symptoms of **hypoglycaemia** (low blood sugar level) they should have a snack or drink which contains carbohydrates.

 Activity

1 If you know a person with diabetes who would be willing to talk to you about their condition, ask how they feel when they are hypoglycaemic.

2 Find out about implants of pancreatic tissue.

The nervous system

You need to be familiar with the following physiological detail:

* the structure and functions of the central and peripheral nervous systems;
* the structure of a nerve cell;
* a reflex arc;
* the autonomic nervous system.

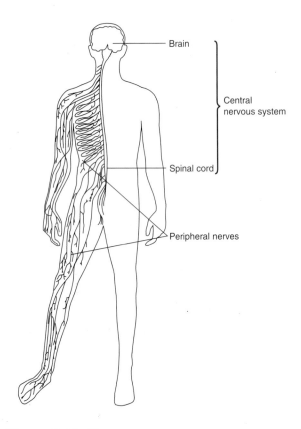

Figure 3.15 The nervous system

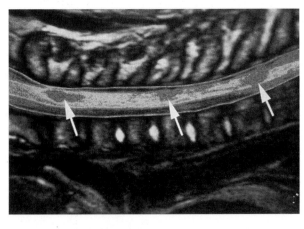

Figure 3.16 MRI scan showing damage (arrowed) done to spinal cord by MS

Multiple sclerosis

Causes

Most of the nerves in the body are covered with an insulating myelin fatty sheath, which allows nerve impulses to be transmitted efficiently. In multiple sclerosis (MS) sufferers the myelin sheath becomes inflamed and eventually becomes scarred, and even disappears in places (Figure 3.16). This affects the flow of nerve impulses. It is not known why the myelin sheath is affected but it is thought that there is some disruption to the immune system. Some researchers suggest that diet or pollution may be possible causes. It is not known why women are more susceptible to the condition than men.

Signs and symptoms

The symptoms of the disease depend on which nerves are affected, but they may include:

- weakness, stiffness or numbness of one or more limbs;
- sensations of tingling, pins and needles or tightness around one or more limbs or the body;
- shaking (tremors) or loss of balance;
- loss of muscular co-ordination;
- impaired vision;
- bowel or bladder incontinence;
- fatigue.

An initial attack may occur in teenage years but often the symptoms are so brief and mild that it goes undiagnosed. Attacks that last for weeks or months will then start to reoccur at some time between the ages of 20 and 40. The pattern of attacks has been divided into three categories of MS:

- **Relapse-remitting** (25% of MS cases): sudden and severe attacks occur at intervals. Between the attacks are periods of almost total remission.
- **Relapse-progressive** (40% of MS cases): less severe attacks occur, but the recovery in the periods between the attacks is less complete. It gradually causes a degree of disability.
- **Chronic-progressive** (15% of MS cases): there are no periods of remission and it rapidly causes disability.

Diagnosis

A person who is suffering from MS will be given a thorough neurological examination (see pages 149–51, below). Their nervous system may also be examined using magnetic resonance imaging (MRI) (Figure 3.17).

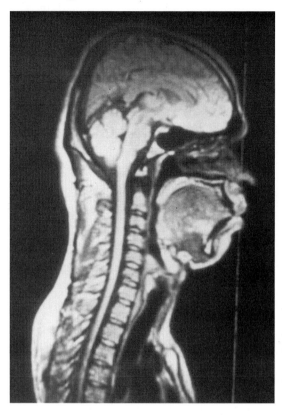

Figure 3.17 MRI scan of the head

Treatment

It is difficult to treat MS, partly because the symptoms vary from person to person and, within one person, from time to time. There is no cure but the following medications can be used in an effort to relieve symptoms:

- interferon beta to reduce the frequency and severity of attacks;
- corticosteroids to reduce inflammation and shorten attacks;
- muscle relaxants to reduce stiffness and pain.

Physiotherapy is important to maintain mobility.

Epilepsy

Causes

People with epilepsy have recurrent seizures. The nature of these seizures varies, as described below in 'Signs and symptoms'. It is not known what causes epilepsy, but it is thought that, in some cases, there may be a genetic basis. There are a number of factors which may trigger a seizure and these vary from person to person. Examples include stress, lack of sleep, certain foods or drugs and flashing lights.

Signs and symptoms

The first signs of epilepsy are usually seen in childhood. As mentioned above, the nature of the seizures vary:

- **Absence (petit mal) seizures:** staring straight ahead; a few seconds of complete immobility; repetitive swallowing. These may occur several times a day.
- **Tonic/clonic(grand mal) seizures:** loss of consciousness; rigidity; jerking movements; bladder incontinence. This may be followed by a period of confusion or deep sleep. Before the attack the person may experience an 'aura' or warning, for example, a particular taste or smell.
- **Temporal lobe seizures:** repetitive movements such as lip smacking and aimless fiddling; a sense of detachment from the surroundings.

- **Motor seizures:** rhythmic twitching of muscles in a hand foot or face which spreads to the whole body. After the seizure there may be a period of weakness or paralysis.

Diagnosis

A doctor will ask for details of any history of seizures within the family and will need a description of the symptoms shown by the person before, during and after a seizure. The structure of the brain may be examined using MRI (magnetic resonance imaging) (see Figure 3.17) or a CAT scan (computer axial tomography) (Figure 3.18). An electroencephalogram (EEG) may be made, which gives information about a person's brain activity.

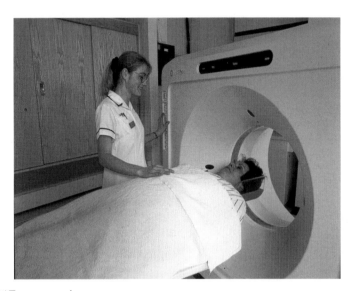

Figure 3.18 A CAT scanner in use

Treatment

- Medication can be used to control seizures.
- Brain surgery can be carried out if medication has no effect.
- Possible triggers of attacks can be avoided, for example, stress or particular foods.
- Family and friends need to be educated on how to help a person fall and then put them in a safe recovery period.

Activity

Find out what action you should take if someone you are with suffers a grand mal seizure.

(See pages 162–3 for answers)

Physiological measurements and observations

You will need to know about the particular physiological measurements which are used to diagnose and investigate your three chosen disorders.

Respiratory rate (used to diagnose bronchitis)

Respiratory rate is the number of breaths taken per minute. At rest this is usually about 8–18 breaths per minute. However, a person suffering from bronchitis will have a higher than normal breathing rate.

It is often difficult for a subject to breathe at their normal rate if they know they are being monitored. It is therefore useful, if circumstances permit, to observe the chest movements associated with breathing without the subject being aware that their breathing rate is being monitored. For example, a nurse can take the pulse and then count the number of breaths in a timed period without the patient noticing.

If necessary, a **spirometer** can be used to measure breathing rate (Figure 3.19). The apparatus is usually filled with oxygen. The lid of the apparatus is pivoted at one end and moves up and down in a water tank as the subject breathes in and out. These readings can be recorded on graph paper on a revolving drum (**kymograph**). The mouthpiece contains a one-way valve to ensure that the same air is not rebreathed. The subject wears a nose clip while using the apparatus. Figure 3.20 shows a spirometer trace of a person suffering from bronchitis compared with a normal spirometer trace.

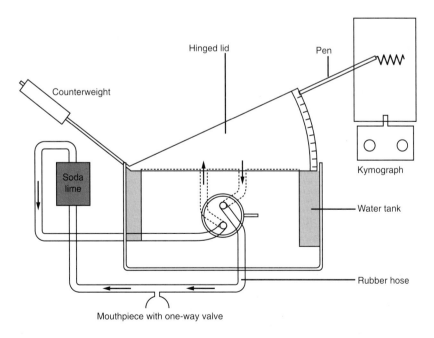

Figure 3.19 A spirometer is used to measure a person's breathing rate

A spirometer showing

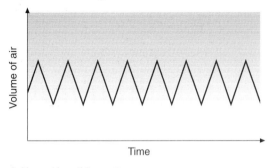

a) Normal breathing pattern

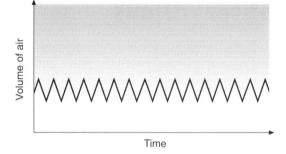

b) Breathing pattern of a bronchitis sufferer

Figure 3.20 Spirometer traces showing normal and abnormal patterns

Peak flow measurements (used to diagnose asthma)

Peak flow estimation is the commonest test of lung function. This can be carried out with a simple piece of equipment known as a **peak flow meter**. The person is asked to blow into it as quickly as they can. The rate at which air is expelled fastest (peak expiratory flow) is recorded on a scale.

It is important that the subject is encouraged to blow as hard and fast as possible. Three readings should be taken and the highest of the three readings used.

A normal peak flow reading is between 400 and 600 dm^3 per minute. Peak flow readings vary according to sex, age, height and even the time of day the measurement is taken.

* Peak flow readings are usually higher in men than in women.
* The highest peak flow usually occurs between the ages of 30 to 40 years.
* The taller a person is, the higher their peak flow is likely to be.
* Peak flow is often higher in the morning than in the evening.

Peak flow measurements are often used to diagnose and monitor the severity of asthma (see page 123).

Asthma sufferers will have a low peak flow reading; the more severe their asthma, the lower their reading. Because peak flow may vary tremendously from time to time, a one-off reading at a clinic may not give a doctor or nurse sufficient information. The asthma sufferer will therefore be asked to take their own readings, morning and evening, over a period of time and plot them on a chart (Fig. 3.21).

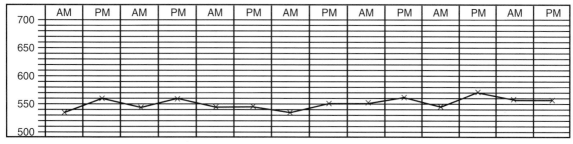

a) peak flow chart of a person without asthma or a person whose asthma is well controlled

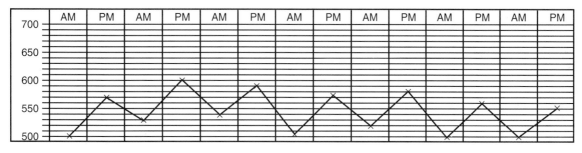

b) peak flow chart of a person whose asthma is not well controlled

Figure 3.21 Peak flow charts

Blood pressure (used to diagnose hypertension)

See also 'Recording blood pressure' in the 'Safe practice' section on page 159, below.

As explained in the section on Hypertension on pages 124–5, the pressure at which blood flows through the circulatory system can be measured using a **sphygmomanometer** ('**sphgymo**' for short). Traditionally a mercury column sphygmomanometer has been used for measuring blood pressure. However, there are a number of drawbacks associated with these:

- Most importantly, European legislation requires the phasing out of all equipment containing mercury.
- Using such models is a skilled operation involving the use of a stethoscope.
- There are no audible or visual indicators of pressure measurements for a group of people (for example, in a classroom situation) to experience.

Table 3.3 Sources of error when taking blood pressure

The observer

- Observer bias – prior recording viewed by the nurse or a preference for a specific figure

- Lack of understanding of the correct procedure, e.g. incorrect positioning of the patient sitting/standing, support of the arm, positioning of the cuff bladder over the centre of the brachial artery, the equipment not level with the heart

- Lack of concentration

- Hearing problems/deficit

- Sight problems

The equipment

- Cuff bladder size

- Maintenance – BP (Blood Pressure) machines should be recalibrated and assessed every 6–12 months

- Defective control valves caused by leakage, making control of the pressure release difficult

- Leaks from cracked or perished tubing

- If used, the stethoscope should be in good condition and have clean and well-fitted ear pieces

The patient

- The patient may be suffering from excessive heat, cold, be wearing constrictive clothing, have a full bladder, recently exercised, been smoking, just had a meal or there may be a distraction, all of which will serve to either increase or decrease the BP

- Older patients have calcified/rigid arteries or anaemia which can all influence the BP reading

- A patient suffering from a high temperature may have a low BP due to vasodilation, causing BP to fall

- In conditions where BP is low it is common to underestimate the BP

- In some patients the white coat syndrome (caused when doctors appear at the bedside) affects BP, giving an inaccurately high BP reading

- Patient BP does vary during the day – higher systolic in the evening and a low recording in the morning

- Fear, anxiety, apprehension, pain can all raise the BP and these can be apparent on admission. It is recommended in this instance to wait at least 1 hour following admission to take the BP

(from 'Adv. voc. H&SC' Thomson *et al* 2000 publ H&S. Page 193)

It is therefore better that, where possible, an electronic model should be used. A cuff is inflated around the upper arm. The high pressure compresses the brachial artery and so prevents blood flow to the lower arm. The cuff is then slowly deflated and as the blood flow resumes the sounds are detected by the transducer or microphone which is built into the cuff. (A transducer is any device which changes a physiological variable into an electronic signal.) Measurements are read from a gauge or digital display.

In a hospital ward the measurements will be recorded on the patient's chart. If blood pressure has been measured in less than optimum conditions, for example, if the patient is very anxious, this should also be recorded.

Table 3.3 shows the main sources of error associated with measuring blood pressure.

Weight (used to diagnose digestive disorders)

Height and weight

A person's weight can be an important guide to their physical health. Someone who is very overweight or underweight gives cause for concern. However, as the example below shows, a measurement of weight alone will not give sufficient information to allow conclusions to be reached.

Activity

Paul is an 18-year-old student who weighs 77kg. Can you make any comments on the state of his physical health?

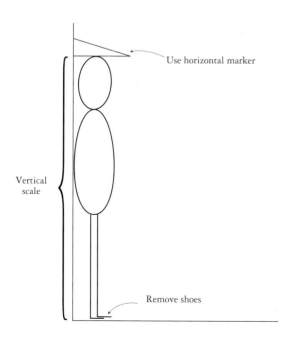

Use horizontal marker

Vertical scale

Remove shoes

To allow any conclusions to be drawn about physical health from the weight of a person, we obviously need to have an idea of their **height**, too. In the example above, you would have formed a different opinion of Paul's physical health if you had been told that he was 1.83m or 1.60m. Height should be measured as shown in Figure 3.22.

Figure 3.22 The correct way to measure height

Activity

Figure 3.23 shows the relationship between weights and heights.

a Take a straight line across from your height and a line up from your weight. (When you weigh yourself take 2 kg off to allow for your clothes.) Check which category you fit into. Do you need to alter your diet/exercise regime?

If so, how?

b Looking at Figure 3.23, what advice would you give to the following people about their diet/exercise based on their weight and height?

Palin: 65 kg   1.55 m

Kate: 47 kg   1.68 m

Peter: 70 kg   1.75 m

See page 163 for answers.

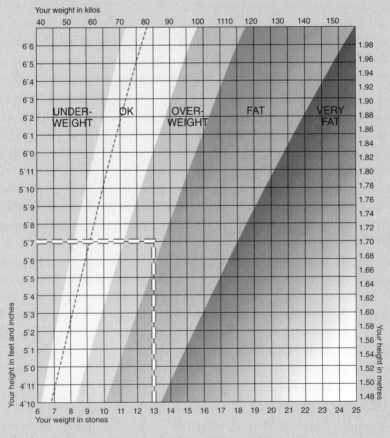

Figure 3.23 The relationship between height and weight

Body mass index

Body mass index (BMI) is a measure which takes into account both height and weight. It can, therefore, be used to indicate whether a person's weight is healthy for their height. BMI is given by the equation:

$$\text{BMI} = \frac{\text{body mass (kg)}}{(\text{height/m})^2}$$

To calculate your BMI you should:

1 Use your calculator to find the square of your height in metres.

For example, a height of 1.63m will have a squared value of $1.63 \times 1.63 = 2.82\text{m}^2$.

2 Divide your mass in kg by the value calculated in step (1). This gives you your BMI.

3 Compare your calculated BMI with the values given below:

Body mass index	Interpretation
Below 20	Underweight
20–25	Ideal weight
25.1–30	Overweight
Above 30	Obese

Activity

Table 3.4	Height (m)	Mass (kg)
Guy	1.60	74
Heather	1.50	54
Rachel	1.75	77

1 Table 3.4 shows the height and weight of three patients. For each patient calculate their BMI and say which are overweight.

2 Read the article from *The Times* (15 February 2001). What would be:

a the main advantage,

b the main disadvantage of using waist measurement to diagnose obesity?

See page 163 for answers.

The heart bears the ultimate burden

By Thomas Stuttaford

The cost to the State of the medical ill-effects stemming from obesity is not confined to those resulting from heart disease, high blood pressure, strokes, cardiovascular disease and type 2 diabetes.

People who are obese are more likely to suffer from gall bladder disease, osteoarthritis and chest troubles as well as cancer of the breast, uterus, prostate and colon.

Doctors, if not their patients, classify obesity as preventable. The medical way of deciding whether patients are overweight is to work out their body mass index, which is the weight in kilograms divided by the patient's height in metres squared. If the answer is more than 25 a person is overweight, if it is more than 30 he or she is clinically obese.

A simpler way is to measure the waist. Any waist measurement of over 40in (102cm) in men, or 35in (88cm) in women, is a warning of obesity and medical troubles ahead.

Urinalysis (used to diagnose renal failure)

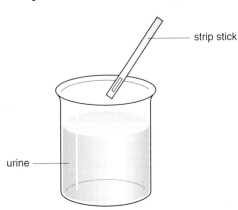

Figure 3.24 Strip-stick chemical analysis of urine

Urine can be analysed to diagnose kidney failure or urinary-tract infections. Urinalysis is usually carried out by a laboratory technician, nurse or doctor but there are home self-tests available (see 'Testing urine' on page 158). Any abnormal appearance (colour, cloudiness) should be noted. The chemical tests only take a few minutes. Strip-sticks (Figure 3.24) are used to test for:

- protein;
- sugar;
- ketones.

Thyroid function tests (used to diagnose under- and over-secretion of the thyroid gland

It is very difficult to diagnose under- or over-secretion of the thyroid gland from signs and symptoms alone. The symptoms are non-specific and can be caused by other conditions. Because of this there has been a huge increase in the number of thyroid function tests carried out. These are biochemical tests in which the concentration of thyroid stimulating hormone and/or thyroxine (T3) in the blood serum is measured. In the UK it is estimated that there are currently 9–10 million tests carried out each year. Some professionals argue that a diagnosis of hypothyroidism (under-secretion of the thyroid gland) or hyperthyroidism (over-secretion of the thyroid gland) can be made on the basis of the biochemical tests alone. Others argue that the biochemical tests are misleading and that diagnosis should be made on the basis of signs and symptoms alone.

When thyroid function tests are carried out it is important to remember that:

- Many factors can affect the levels of thyroid stimulating hormone in the blood.
- Changes in the level of the hormone are poorly understood in patients with illnesses that affect the whole body.
- It is possible to obtain false positive and false negatives (i.e. readings which indicate there is no over- or under- secretion when in reality there is, or readings which indicate there is over- or under-secretion when in reality there is not).

Blood glucose measurement (used to diagnose diabetes mellitus)

It is important that people with type 1 diabetes regularly check their blood sugar (glucose) level. This will indicate whether extra insulin needs to be taken to reduce the blood sugar level. Maintaining a constant blood sugar level will both keep a person feeling well and reduce the chances of long term complications. A blood test can be done very quickly and easily with very little discomfort. A finger-stick test using a blood glucose meter measures the level of sugar in the blood.

Recently a laboratory test (haemoglobin A1c test) has been developed, which shows the average content of a person's blood over the last three months. This is the best test for showing if the person's blood sugar level is well controlled. It is based on analysing the amount of sugar attached to the red blood cells.

When doctors are first diagnosing diabetes, a blood test will be done after an overnight fast. An **oral glucose tolerance test** may also be carried out. The patient starts off by fasting (drinking only water) for at least 10 hours. The blood sugar level is tested and then a drink with a high level of glucose is given. The blood sugar level is then tested again five times at intervals for the next three hours. In a person without diabetes, the blood glucose level will increase rapidly after the drink, and then, as insulin is produced, the level rapidly returns to normal. However, in people with diabetes the blood glucose will rise higher and return to normal more slowly.

Neurological examination (used to diagnose disorders of the central nervous system, such as multiple sclerosis)

There are no tests that are specific to multiple sclerosis. It is usually diagnosed by eliminating other conditions. Because of this, several tests and procedures are needed, for example, MRI (see page 139). The tests will include a full neurological examination by a neurologist. The following may be examined.

Mental status

Patients are observed as they are asked a number of questions so that their personality and emotional state can be assessed. Attention, memory and cognitive function are tested.

Cranial nerves

To find out if there is any damage to the cranial nerves, the patient is given tests to check:

- their ability to smell;

- their ability to distinguish visual symbols;
- their field of view;
- the reaction of their pupils to variations in light intensity;
- their eyelid movements;
- their eye movements;
- their jaw movements;
- their facial movements;
- their hearing;
- movement of their palate and gag reflexes;
- movement of the neck muscles;
- control of the tongue.

Motor skills

Tests are carried out to detect abnormalities of movements and muscle tone. Abnormal spontaneous movements such as muscle twitches and tremors are looked for. The patient's strength will be tested to check that it is normal. Table 3.5 shows a scale which is often used by neurologists.

Table 3.5 Scale used by neurologists for rating strength

Grade	Indicates
0	No muscle movement
1	Visible muscle movement, but no movement at the joint
2	Movement at the joint, but not against gravity
3	Movement against gravity, but not against added resistance
3.5	Moves against gravity, plus slight additional resistance (severly weak)
4	Moves against moderate resistance
4.5	Slightly weak
5	Normal strength

Co-ordination and gait

The following tests may be carried out to test **co-ordination**:

Finger-to-nose: the tester holds out their finger and the patient alternately touches their nose and the tester's finger. The tester moves their finger between touches.

Heel-to-shin: the patient lies on their back, places the heel of one leg on the other knee and then slowly slides the heel down the shin bone to the ankle.

In the above two tests, the neurologist will be looking for jerky, uncoordinated movements.

Rapid alternating movements: the patient is asked to slap one palm with the other hand using, alternately, the palm and the back of the hand. This should be repeated as rapidly as possible. To test **gait**, the patient's walking should be observed. Their **tandem gait** may also be observed. To check this, the patient will be asked to walk by placing the heel of one foot immediately in front of the toe of the other foot. If the patient is unstable, help must be available to provide support should it be necessary.

Reflexes

A reflex is an automatic or involuntary response to a stimulus. Examining reflexes gives an objective way of assessing neurological function. A number of reflexes can be tested. A well-known reflex is the knee jerk reflex. The patient is seated with their legs dangling. The tendon below the kneecap is then struck. A normal reflex is for the quadriceps muscle at the front of the upper leg to contract, which extends the knee.

Sensory responses

A number of stimuli can be applied to the patient, and their ability to detect these stimuli should be recorded. Examples of such stimuli include:

- pressure with a sharp point (but not sharp enough to draw blood);
- temperature (cold and warm objects placed against the skin);
- touch (stroking skin with a finger);
- position (the index finger or big toe is moved gently and the patient has to identify if it is moving and in which direction);
- vibration (a vibrating tuning fork is applied to a finger or toe).

Treatment and care delivery

Studying your chosen disorders should enable you to investigate the **holistic** delivery of care. This is care in which the whole person is treated – the physical, intellectual, emotional and social health of the client are taken into account, for example, nutrition, exercise and mental relaxation. You should find out about the care required for your chosen disorder, from the investigation and diagnosis, through treatment and eventual outcome, whether that be recovery, long-term illness or death.

Care plans

Producing and following care plans is an important aspect of holistic care. A care plan states the client's problem(s), the objective or the expected outcome, the intervention and care that will be given, and a time scale for reaching the objectives or reviewing the service user's condition. Care plans outline what the client has a right to expect and it will be decided upon jointly by the service user and the named nurse or key worker. Care plans are reviewed at set times as the care needed may change, and the care plan should be updated to reflect any changes. Care plans are important written records which could be used in court. It is therefore important that they are

Comfort: Chest Pain
Related to:
(Check those that apply)

☐ Myocardial infarction	☐ Musculoskeletal disorders
☐ Ubstable angina	☐ Pulmonary, myocardial contusion
☐ Coronary artery disease	☐ Other: _____
☐ Chest trauma	_____
☐ Stress anxiety	_____

As evidenced by:
(Check those that apply)

Major: *(Must be present)*	☐ Person reports or demonstrates a discomfort.		
Minor: *(May be present)*	☐ Increased BP	☐ Diaphoresis	☐ Dilated pupils
	☐ Restlessness	☐ Facial mask of pain	
	☐ Crying/moaning	☐ Short of breath	☐ Anxiety

Date & signature	Plan and outcome *(Check those that apply)*	Target date	Nursing interventions *(Check those that apply)*	Date achieved
	The patient will: ☐ Verbalise relief/ control of pain ☐ Verbalise causative factors associated with chest pain ☐ Other:		☐ Assess for causative factors associated: • Activity • Stress • Eating • Bowel elimination • Previous angina attack • Other: ☐ Assess characteristing of chest pain. • Location • Intensity (scale 1–10) • Duration • Quality • Radiation	

Figure 3.25 Outline care plan for nursing a patient with chest pain

			Review history of previous pain experienced by patient and compare to current experience.	
			☐ Instruct patient to report pain immediately.	
			☐ Continuous EKG (ECG) monitoring; note and record pattern during pain.	
			☐ Provide a quiet, restful environment.	
			☐ As per physician order, administer IV analgesics in small increments until pain is relieved or maximum dose is achieved. Monitor BP during administration of pain meds. Assess pt. response to pain medication and notify physician if pain is not controlled or pt. experiences adverse reaction (decreased BP, HA, distress.	
			☐ Administer nitroglycerine as ordered by physician. Monitor as stated above.	
			☐ Titrate IV nitro to achieve pain relief as ordered by physician. Monitor hemodynamic response to medication (BP, urine output).	
			☐ Administer supplemental oxygen as ordered by physician.	
			☐ Assist with ADL's to reduce cardiac stressors.	
			☐ Assist in eliminating causative factors as identified by patient assessment.	
			☐ Other:_____	

Patient/Significant other signature

RN signature

From: http://www.rncentral.com/careplans/plans/ccp.html

Figure 3.25 Outline care plan for nursing a patient with chest pain (contd)

legible, clearly stated, and signed and dated by the care worker. Figure 3.25 shows an outline care plan for the care of a hospital patient with chest pain.

Stages in care planning

The initial assessment of needs

Any or all of the following methods may be used by a professional assessing a client:

1 **Observation** of:
  - physical condition;
  - behaviour;
  - personal circumstances.
2 **Questioning**
3 **Use of secondary sources** including:
  - medical records;
  - relatives;
  - advocates;
  - support networks.

When using any of these methods, the professional carer must bear in mind **client rights** with respect to assessment. The client has a right to:

- independence;
- choice and control;
- confidentiality.

The development of the care plan

Once the needs of the client have been assessed, and the needs which are not being met (i.e. the problems) identified, goals can then be set (i.e. the required outcome). The action required to meet these goals can then be identified and then implemented (Figure 3.25).

Implementing and monitoring

Throughout the implementation of a care plan there should be both repeated assessment of the client's needs and constant monitoring of progress so that the care plan can be adapted if necessary. A variety of sources of information can be used to enable the professional to monitor a care plan, for example:

- client interview;
- carer interview;
- client's records;
- observation of client, their care and environment.

Review and evaluation

Evaluation is a means of finding out whether the carer (or team of carers) has achieved what they set out to do when they developed the care plan. It is important that the evaluation is objective and not subjective. For this reason, where possible, professionally agreed standards and criteria are needed to guide the evaluator. In the light of the evaluation, shortcomings can be identified and, resources permitting, improvements can be made to subsequent care plans.

 Activity

> 1 Look at Figure 3.26. For each of the disorders you choose to research, copy and complete one of these for an imaginary patient suffering from the disorder.
>
> 2 If you have the opportunity to gain experience in a work placement, ask if you can see examples of care plans (remember issues of confidentiality).

Safe practice

There are health and safety risks in any job, and there are a number of particular risks which affect people who work in health-related professions.

The Health and Safety at Work Act (1974)

The Health and Safety at Work Act (1974) is based on the following principles:

- All employers and employees should be aware of health and safety matters. Personal responsibility is very important.
- There is one comprehensive framework, which includes basic legislation, regulations covering specific hazards at work and codes of practice.
- There is one unified enforcement authority (Health and Safety Executive) that carries out inspections, initiates legal proceedings and gives help and advice.

Responsibilities of carers in relation to the Health and Safety at Work Act (1974)

This is an outline of the duties of employers and employees produced by the Health and Safety Executive. As employees, carers must take personal responsibility for their own health. The highest occupational risk for many health care workers is injury from **moving and handling**. For medical and health services, 55% of all injuries that result in people being absent from work for more than three days are caused by manual-handling accidents. The sprains and strains arise from incorrect ways of lifting and moving loads. Many manual-handling injuries are cumulative, resulting from poor posture and excessive repetition of particular movements. Occasionally the injury can be attributed to a single handling incident. A full recovery is not always made, and physical impairment or even permanent disability can result.

———————————————————

→ Complete with title of disorder

☐ Actual   ☐ Potential

Related to:

→ Complete with other disorders to which the condition is related

As evidenced by:

Major:
(Must be present)

→ Complete with signs and symptoms

Minor:
(May be present)

Date & signature	Plan and outcome	Target date	Interventions	Date achieved
	The patient will:			

———————————————————
Patient/Significant other signature

———————————————————
Care worker's signature

Adapted from: http://www.rncentral.com/careplans/plans/blank.html

Figure 3.26 Blank outline of a care plan

The Manual Operations Handling Regulations (1992) were made under the Health and Safety at Work Act (1974). There is now an ergonomic approach to this aspect of work. Ergonomics is sometimes referred to as 'fitting the job to the person, rather than the person to the job'. The regulations require employers to carry out the following measures:

- avoid hazardous manual-handling operations where possible by redesigning the task, or automating or mechanising the process;
- make an assessment of any hazardous manual-handling operation that cannot be avoided;
- reduce the risk of injury from those operations by improving the task, the load and the working environment.

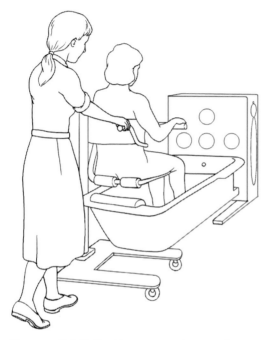

Figure 3.27 Bathing a patient using a mechanical device

Accurate records of accidents and ill-health will help identify potentially risky manual-handling operations. Mechanical assistance may be possible. Figure 3.27 shows a device used for helping patients in and out of the bath. Full training should be given to employees to ensure that they know how to safely carry out all the manual-handling operations required of them.

Health care workers are also at risk from a range of **chemical hazards**. Chemical hazards are regulated by Control of Substances Hazardous to Health 1988 (COSHH) Regulations. Substances are classed as hazardous if they cause any short- or long-term harm. They include dusts, fumes and gases, liquids, pastes, powders, oils, resins, aerosols and sprays. Liquid chemicals such as cleaning, antiseptic and sterilising fluids and solvents are often potential hazards which may affect care workers. Although **micro-organisms** are not chemicals in the sense of the rest of the substances covered by COSHH regulations, they are nonetheless included and this is of great importance in a care setting.

Employers must prevent the exposure of employees to hazardous substances. Sometimes complete prevention is not reasonably practicable, in which case it is legal to use the hazardous substance providing there are proper control measures.

Preventing exposure involves eliminating the use of the substance or substituting a less hazardous substance. **Controlling** exposure, on the other hand, includes three options:

- totally enclosing the process;
- using adequate ventilation;
- using safe systems of work and handling procedures.

The third option is the most frequently used in hospitals and other care settings, as it is not usually possible to eliminate the hazard totally. As well as making sure all employees are aware of safe working practices and handling procedures, the use of personal protective equipment and clothing is also important. Information must be given to workers about the dangers of their work, and training must take place to ensure that ways of avoiding the dangers are understood.

Precautions to be taken when making physiological measurements or taking samples

It is important that details of best practice in routine procedures are shared by health professionals. Examples of three such procedures are given below.

Testing urine

For most tests, urine should be collected first thing in the morning and strenuous exercise should be avoided by the patient before the test. Collect at least 15 cm^3 (about one tablespoon) and store in a sterile urine container. Disposable gloves should be worn by the person performing the urine test when handling urine samples. They should be informed if the patient has been taking any medications.

Obtaining venous blood samples

- Where appropriate, give a brief outline of the procedure to the patient so they know what to expect.
- Except in an emergency, apply a local anaesthetic, particularly in the case of infants and children, to minimise discomfort.
- The person taking the blood sample must wash their hands and put on sterile disposable gloves.
- Wipe the patient's skin with an antiseptic and then do not touch again with bare hands to reduce the risk of infection.

Adult patients

The correct way to obtain a blood sample:

- Apply a tourniquet to the upper arm to put pressure on the blood vessel and thus reduce the rate of blood flow. This will make the vein on the inside of the elbow joint (*antecubital fossa*) become more clearly visible. (It may sometimes be necessary to use an alternative vein, for example, on the back of the hand.)
- Use the smallest needle possible to puncture the skin over the vein and enter the vein.
- Gently withdraw the appropriate blood volume.
- Remove the tourniquet before withdrawing the needle.
- After withdrawing the needle, apply pressure with sterile cotton wool to prevent bleeding.

Infants and children

- Help will be needed. A parent must not be expected to restrain a young child or infant.
- Tourniquets are not suitable for children. Instead a firm but gentle grasp around the arm by the helper will give the necessary pressure.

- In an older child the vein on the inside of the elbow joint can be used, but in an infant it is better to use the vein in the back of the hand.
- It is important not to rush the procedure and to be gentle.

Action to be taken if problems arise

- **Bruising and haemotomas:** these may be caused by using too large a needle and by not applying pressure for long enough after the needle has been removed. Some patients who are at particular risk, for example, the elderly and patients taking anticoagulants, will need firm pressure for several minutes to prevent bleeding.
- **Puncturing an artery:** it is important to puncture a vein and not an artery. This is because the blood is under higher pressure in an artery. If it appears that an artery has been punctured, remove the needle and apply firm pressure for several minutes to prevent bleeding.
- **Needle stick injuries:** this is when a person accidently punctures their own skin, or that of another person, with a needle. It is common in emergency situations when patients and staff are under pressure. If this happens it is essential that the incident is reported and the policy of the institute is followed.

Recording blood pressure

Review the section on 'Hypertension' (high blood pressure) on pages 124–5.

Blood pressure is important in diagnosing many conditions. It is therefore important that the reading taken is as accurate as possible. Listed below are precautions that should be taken when recording blood pressure:

- Don't round off numbers.
- Don't be biased, for example, don't be influenced by the last reading to have been taken.
- Check that the patient is in the correct position. The patient should be seated with their upper arm at heart level. If the patient is lying their arm should be slightly raised. Record their position at the time of measurement.
- The patient should remain relaxed during the measurement.
- Equipment should be regularly checked and cleaned, repaired or replaced as necessary.
- Use the correct sized cuff for each patient.

Glossary

Acute An acute disease has a rapid onset, severe symptoms and is of brief duration.

Advocate Someone who speaks on behalf of, or represents the interests of, someone else, particularly those who are less able to voice their views, for example, those with learning difficulties. The advocate could be a professional, volunteer or friend.

Alveoli Air sacs in the lungs where gas exchange takes place.

Antiseptic A chemical that destroys or inhibits the growth of disease causing organisms such as bacteria.

Auto-immune disease Disorder caused by the body producing antibodies which attack its own tissues.

Blood pressure The pressure of blood in the arteries. It is expressed as two numbers; the higher number corresponds to the contraction of the heart; the lower number corresponds to the relaxation of the heart.

Body Mass Index (BMI) A simple assessment of body mass, calculated as follows:

$$\text{BMI} = \frac{\text{body mass (kg)}}{(\text{height/m})^2}.$$

Bronchioles Small tubes in the lungs that lead to the alveoli.

Bronchodilator Used to widen the air tubes in the lungs.

Care plan This states the client's problem(s), the objective or the expected outcome, the intervention and care that will be given, and a time scale for reaching the objectives or reviewing the service user's condition. It will be decided upon jointly by the service user and the named nurse or key worker.

Chronic A chronic disease often starts gradually. It lasts a long time and involves very slow changes.

Computer axial tomography (CAT scan) A series of X-rays taken at fractionally different depths which gives a detailed picture of the soft tissues of the body.

Confidentiality The preservation of secret information concerning the client that is disclosed in the professional relationship.

Disease A specific condition of ill health. Identified as actual change on the surface, or inside, some part of the body.

Endocrine gland Ductless glands that secrete hormones directly into the blood stream.

Health A person's physical, mental and social condition.

Holistic care Care in which the whole person is treated. Physical, intellectual, emotional and social health of the client are taken into account. For example, nutrition, exercise, mental relaxation and any other factors affecting health are considered.

Homeostasis The maintenance of a constant internal environment.

Illness The subjective state of feeling unwell. (i.e. how people feel).

Magnetic resonance imaging (MRI) Produces images similar to a CAT scan (see above) but without the radiation hazard.

Myocardial infarction Heart attack.

Peak flow The maximum rate at which air can be expelled. It is often used to diagnose asthma.

Progressive A condition that becomes gradually worse.

Remission The lessening or disappearance of the symptoms of the disease.

Respiratory rate Breathing rate, measured in breaths per minute.

Sickness Reported illness. Involves being treated by a professional and becoming a medical statistic.

Sign An indication of a particular disorder that is observed by the health professional but is not apparent to the patient (see **symptom**, below).

Spirometer Equipment used to measure breathing rate and lung volumes.

Sphygmomanometer Equipment used to measure blood pressure.

Stethoscope Equipment used to listen to sounds within the body.

Stool Faeces discharged from the anus.

Symptom An indication of a disease or disorder which is noticed by the patient (see **sign**, above).

Target organ An organ affected by a hormone.

Thyroid function tests Measurements of the amount of thyroid hormones in the blood that are carried out to assist with the diagnosis of disorders of the thyroid gland.

Tourniquet A device which puts pressure on a blood vessel to reduce the flow of blood.

Ultrasound An imaging technique in which sound waves are passed through the body.

Urinalysis Analysis of the blood for chemicals and cells to assist with the diagnosis of diseases.

References and resources

This unit builds on the knowledge and understanding of homeostasis and normal function as studied in Unit 3: Physical aspects of health. This is covered in Chapter 3 of 'Vocational A level Health and Social Care' Thomson et al. Published by Hodder and Stoughton (2000).

Useful websites

The Internet is a valuable source of information. A web browser such as **Altavista** or **Google** can be used to search for information on disorders. Individuals or institutions can subscribe to Internet databases such as **Medline** which provides access to the most recent biomedical literature. Useful websites include:

Department of Health
  www.doh.gov.uk
National Health Service Executive (NHSE)
  www.open.gov.uk/doh/nhs.htm
Department of Health and Social Services (DHSS) in Northern Ireland
  www.nics.gov.uk
Health and Safety Executive
  www.open.gov.uk/hsehome.htm
http://onhealth.webmd.com/conditions
This gives information on the causes, symptoms, diagnosis and treatment of various disorders and diseases. It also provides links to other useful websites.
www.rncentral.com/careplans
This gives examples of care plans and includes a blank form for writing a care plan.

Practice placements and visits

Access to clients in these situations will be exceedingly beneficial in giving the opportunity for the application of knowledge to real life situations. Visits to hospital and appropriate laboratories give the opportunity for investigations of multi-disciplinary teams and research into career opportunities.

Family and friends

You may wish to use the experiences of family and friends in your research on particular disorders. This can be a valuable resource, but you must be aware of the issues of confidentiality which will arise. Remember, sensitivity will be needed when investigating conditions and care as your fellow students may have personal or family involvement.

Answers

Chapter 3

Hypertension (p. 125)

A diet for a person with high blood pressure should be:

- high in fibre
- low in fat
- low in salt
- low in calories if the person is over weight
- low in alcohol and caffeine

Irritable bowel syndrome (p. 130)

To have a low fat diet a person may:

- use skimmed milk
- keep the use of fats such as butter and margarine to a minimum
- consume only small amounts of red meat and remove as much fat as possible

To have a high fibre diet a person may:

- eat plenty of fresh fruits and vegetables
- add bran to food

Epilepsy (p. 141)

Action to take if a person suffers a grand mal seizure:

- Call 999 if ;
  - this is the first time the person has had a seizure
  - the person has had more than one seizure in an hour
  - the seizure lasts more than two minutes
- Remember that seizures are not usually life threatening
- If a person thinks they are going to have a seizure, or begins to lose their balance they should be helped to the ground
- Put the person in the recovery position (Figure 3.28)

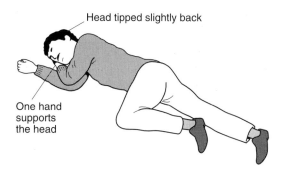

Figure 3.28 The recovery position.

- Loosen any tight clothing
- Prevent the person from injuring themselves by removing any objects they may hit, but do not restrict movements
- After the seizure the victim may be tired and confused and may fall asleep

Weight (p. 146)

Activity 1.

Palin: Overweight. Action: Increase exercise / Cut back on fats in diet

Kate: Underweight. Action: A higher energy diet is required.

Peter: OK

BMI

Activity 1.

Guy 29 BMI = (overweight)

Heather 24 BMI = (ideal weight)

Rachel 25 BMI = (ideal weight)

Activity 2.

Main advantage: Quick and easy. No calculations.

Main disadvantage: Takes no account of taller people having larger waists.

Chapter 4

Cell structure, genetics and reproduction for health care

This chapter covers:

- the organisation of the cell;
- human reproduction;
- the fundamental principles and processes underlying human inheritance;
- the issues arising from current research and practice;
- some of the most up-to-date scientific advances in genetics;
- some of the ethical and moral problems raised by the research in genetics.

The cell

The cell is the fundamental unit of living organisms. Cells can be examined with a light microscope or an electron microscope; depending on the amount of detail required.

Examining cells with a light (optical) microscope

When examining cell structure with a **light microscope** (Figure 4.1), the specimen, which is usually stained first, is mounted on a glass slide. This is placed on a stage. Light from the mirror or a built-in light source passes through the specimen. The image is magnified by a lens in an objective and a lens in the eyepiece. The total magnification is calculated by multiplying the magnification of the objective with the magnification of the eyepiece. For example, a $\times 10$ eyepiece lens and a $\times 40$ objective lens will give total magnification of $\times 400$.

The cell viewed with a light microscope

Figure 4.2 shows a typical animal cell seen with a light microscope. It is possible to see the **cell (Plasma) membrane** which encloses the **cytoplasm**. Within the cytoplasm are numerous **organelles**. These are structures in the cell which have specific functions. Most organelles are too small to be seen with typical light microscopes, but the **nucleus**, the largest organelle, is usually visible.

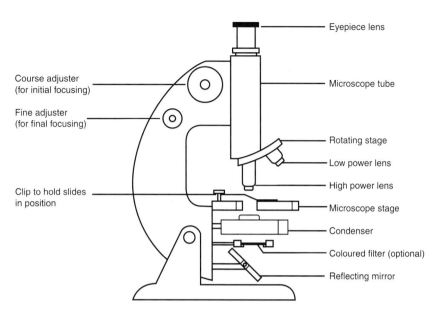

Eyepiece lens

Course adjuster
(for initial focusing)

Microscope tube

Fine adjuster
(for final focusing)

Rotating stage

Low power lens

High power lens

Clip to hold slides
in position

Microscope stage

Condenser

Coloured filter (optional)

Reflecting mirror

Figure 4.1 Light microscope

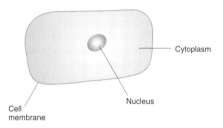

Cytoplasm

Nucleus

Cell
membrane

Figure 4.2 Typical structure of an animal cell seen with a light microscope

Activity

1   If you have access to a microscope, use Figure 4.1 to help you identify the different parts.

2   Look at a prepared slide of cheek cells. Draw a cell and label the nucleus, cytoplasm and cell membrane.

Examining cells with an electron microscope

To study the cell structure in more detail, an **electron microscope** is used (Figure 4.3). The maximum possible magnification of a light microscope is ×1500. The maximum possible magnification of an electron microscope is ×1 000 000. More important than the magnification of a microscope, is its **resolution**. If a microscope has a high resolution, it can be used to distinguish two points which are very close together. If it has a low resolution, the two points will be seen as a single point. A light microscope can be used to distinguish two points which are 200nm apart, whereas an electron microscope can be used to distinguish two points which

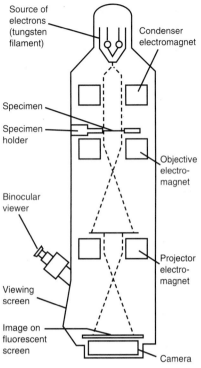

Source of electrons (tungsten filament)

Condenser electromagnet

Specimen

Specimen holder

Objective electro-magnet

Binocular viewer

Projector electro-magnet

Viewing screen

Image on fluorescent screen

Camera

Figure 4.3 Electron microscope

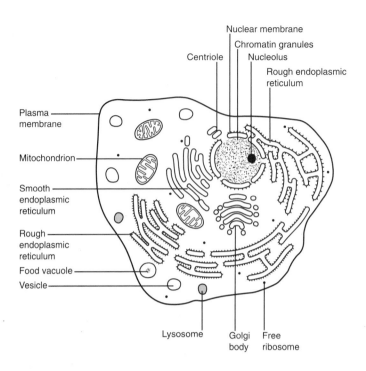

Nuclear membrane
Chromatin granules
Centriole
Nucleolus
Rough endoplasmic reticulum

Plasma membrane

Mitochondrion

Smooth endoplasmic reticulum

Rough endoplasmic reticulum

Food vacuole

Vesicle

Lysosome

Golgi body

Free ribosome

Figure 4.4 Typical structure of an animal cell seen with a transmission electron microscope

are only 0.1nm apart. This is because the electron microscope uses a beam of electrons instead of light and electrons have a much shorter wavelength than light. (**NB** There are 1 000 000 nm in 1 mm.)

The beam of electron is emitted from a source at the top of the microscope. It is focused on to the specimen with electromagnets. There is a vacuum inside the microscope to prevent molecules of air scattering the electrons. This means that all specimens viewed with this type of microscope are dead. The specimen is very thin to allow the beam of electrons to pass through. The electrons then produce an image on a fluorescent screen or photographic plate.

The electron microscope described above is a **transmission electron microscope**. It produces images such as that shown in Figure 4.4. Another type of electron microscope, a **scanning electron microscope**, scatters electrons off the surface of a specimen and can be used to produce 3-D images.

The cell viewed with an electron microscope

A number of organelles can be seen in detail when the cell is viewed with an electron microscope.

Nucleus and nuclear envelope

The nucleus is the largest organelle in the cell. It is bound by a double membrane called the nuclear envelope. There are **pores** in the nuclear envelope that allow material in and out of the nucleus. The **nucleoplasm** is denser than the cytoplasm and contains one or more **nucleoli**. These are dense structures which synthesise the ribosomes (see page 168). The nucleoplasm also contains **chromatin** which consists of DNA (see pages 169–71) and proteins. When the cell divides, this becomes organised into visible **chromosomes**. The DNA determines which proteins are made. Enzymes, which control all metabolic processes are proteins, so in this way the nucleus controls all the cell's activities.

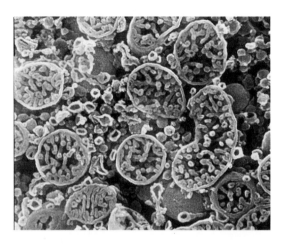

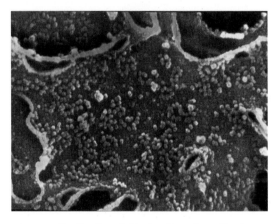

Figure 4.5 Rough (top) and smooth (bottom) Endoplasmic reticulum

Endoplasmic reticulum

The endoplasmic reticulum is a network of membranes found throughout the cell. There are two distinct forms: rough endoplasmic reticulum (RER) and smooth endoplasmic reticulum (SER). Table 4.1 gives details of their structures and functions.

Golgi apparatus

The Golgi apparatus consists of a stack of flattened sacs made of smooth endoplasmic reticulum. Materials come to one face of the Golgi apparatus in vesicles that fuse with the flattened sacs. These materials are then processed as they pass through the Golgi apparatus, before leaving in

Table 4.1 The two types of endoplasmic reticulum

Rough endoplasmic reticulum	Smooth endoplasmic reticulum
Ribosomes on membrane	No ribosomes on membrane
Flattened cavities	Tubular cavities
May be continuous with the nuclear envelope	Not continuous with the nuclear envelope
Concerned with the transport and processing of proteins	Concerned with the transport and processing of lipids and steroids

vesicles from the opposite face. For example, proteins are converted to glycoproteins, such as mucus, by the addition of carbohydrates.

Lysosomes

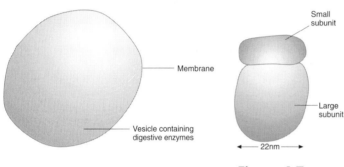

Figure 4.6 Lysosome

Figure 4.7 Lysosomes

Lysosomes are membrane-bound vesicles which contain digestive enzymes. They may digest damaged or redundant cell organelles. When the cell dies the lysosomes release their enzymes which digest the cell contents, a process known as autolysis.

Ribosomes

Ribosomes are very small organelles. They are made of protein and RNA (see page 171) and consist of two sub-units, one large and one small. They are found on the rough endoplasmic reticulum as well as free in the cytoplasm. They are the site of protein synthesis.

Centrioles

These are hollow cylinders which have a diameter of about 0.2μm. Each cell contains two centrioles at right angles to one another. When the cell is about to divide, the centrioles move to opposite sides of the cell where they are involved in the synthesis of the protein strands of the spindle (see 'Mitosis', page 175).

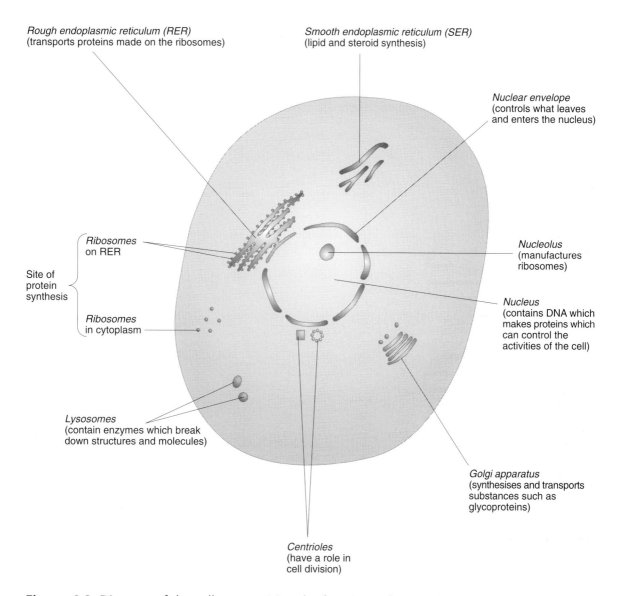

Rough endoplasmic reticulum (RER)
(transports proteins made on the ribosomes)

Smooth endoplasmic reticulum (SER)
(lipid and steroid synthesis)

Nuclear envelope
(controls what leaves
and enters the nucleus)

**Ribosomes
on RER**

Site of
protein
synthesis

**Ribosomes
in cytoplasm**

Nucleolus
(manufactures
ribosomes)

Nucleus
(contains DNA which
makes proteins which
can control the
activities of the cell)

Lysosomes
(contain enzymes which break
down structures and molecules)

Golgi apparatus
(synthesises and transports
substances such as
glycoproteins)

Centrioles
(have a role in
cell division)

Figure 4.8 Diagram of the cell summarising the functions of organelles

The structure and behaviour of DNA

DNA (deoxyribonucleic acid) carries the genetic information in the cell. As already mentioned, it codes for all the proteins made. It is found in the chromosomes which are present in each nucleus. In humans there are 46 chromosomes in each nucleus (23 pairs), except in the nuclei of gametes which only contain 23 chromosomes. The chromosomes consist of DNA and protein.

DNA structure

A DNA molecule is a double helix (Figure 4.9a). Each strand is a string of units known as nucleotides. A nucleotide (Figure 4.9b) consists of a:

- sugar;
- phosphate group;
- nitrogen-containing base.

In DNA the sugar is deoxyribose and there are four different bases:

- adenine (A);
- thymine (T);
- cytosine (C);
- guanine (G).

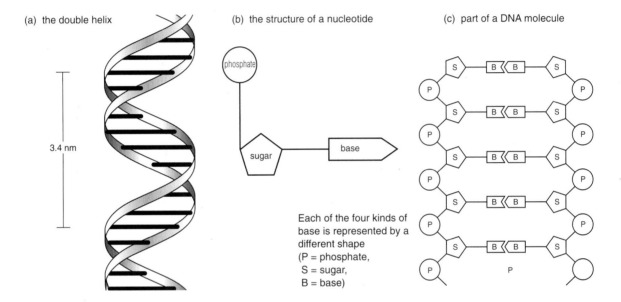

Figure 4.9 DNA structure: a) The double helix b) The structure of a nucleotide c) Part of a DNA molecule

As DNA strands are made up of many nucleotides they are known as a **polynucleotides**.

The two strands run in opposite directions and are linked together at the bases (Figure 4.9c). Adenine (A) always pairs with thymine (T); cytosine (C) always pairs with guanine (G). This is known as complementary base pairing. Two hydrogen bonds link A and T, and three hydrogen bonds link C and G.

DNA replication

When a cell divides into two, the chromosomes have to replicate, so that each of the new cells still contains the original number of 46 chromosomes. Because each chromosome is, in part, a DNA molecule, this means that the DNA molecules have to replicate. Figure 4.10 shows how this happens.

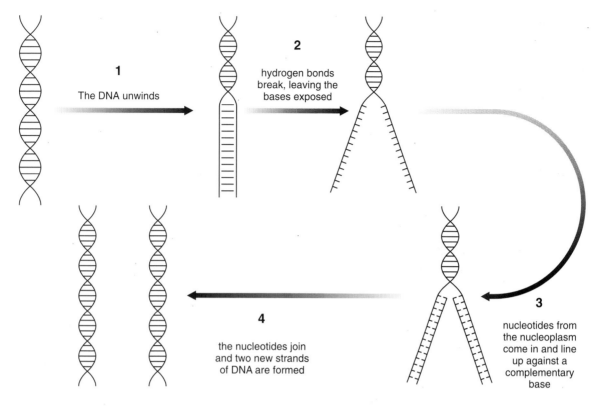

Figure 4.10 DNA replication

RNA (ribonucleic acid)

In addition to DNA, another polynucleotide is required for the synthesis of proteins. This is ribonucleic acid (RNA).

RNA structure

Although DNA and RNA are both polynucleotides (made up of nucleotides), there are a number of significant differences between the two molecules. Table 4.2 shows how the structure of RNA differs from that of DNA.

Protein synthesis

Proteins make up about 10% of our body weight. Each protein molecule only lasts for about a fortnight. To replace these proteins we have to make about 30g of protein an hour. This means we are making billions of molecules of protein every minute. Different proteins are made up of polypeptide chains which, in turn, are made up of different sequences of amino acids. The sequence of bases in the DNA molecule determines the sequence of amino acids in the proteins made in a cell. The process of protein synthesis can be divided into transcription and translation.

Table 4.2 A comparison of DNA and RNA structure

DNA	RNA
Double strand of nucleotides	Single strand of nucleotides
The sugar is deoxyribose	The sugar is ribose (Figure 4.11)
Has the base thymine	Thymine is replaced by uracil
One form	Three forms: messenger, transfer and ribosomal

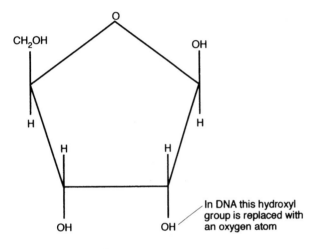

In DNA this hydroxyl group is replaced with an oxygen atom

Figure 4.11 Ribose sugar

Transcription

The DNA molecules are in the chromosomes in the nucleus of a cell. The proteins are made on the ribosomes on the rough endoplasmic reticulum or in the cytoplasm. This means that the 'message' has to be carried from the DNA out of the nucleus to the ribosomes. The message is carried in the form of **messenger RNA (mRNA)**. In the process of transcription the message is transcribed (copied) from DNA to mRNA. Figure 4.12 illustrates this process.

Translation

The mRNA leaves the nucleus through a pore in the nuclear membrane. It goes into the cytoplasm and becomes attached to a number of ribosomes. Ribosomes are made of protein and a type of RNA known as **ribosomal RNA (rRNA)**. The ribosomes 'read' the message in the mRNA. This process is known as translation (i.e. the message in the mRNA is translated into a sequence of amino acids in a polypeptide chain).

In order for translation to take place, a third type of RNA is required. This is **transfer RNA (tRNA)** (see Figure 4.13). Figure 4.14 illustrates the process of translation. The tRNA molecules join up with specific amino acids. The anticodons of the tRNA molecules join with the complementary codons (sequence of three bases) at the ribosome. In this way a particular codon codes for a particular amino acid. On the ribosome there are two mRNA codons to which tRNA molecules can attach. The first two tRNA molecules combine with the first two mRNA codons. A bond forms between the two amino acids. The first tRNA breaks away and is free to pick up another amino acid. The ribosome moves along the mRNA one codon and another tRNA attaches to the next codon. A bond forms between its amino acid and the growing chain of amino acids on the adjacent tRNA. This is repeated until the polypeptide chain is complete. It takes about 30 seconds to make a polypeptide chain about 150 amino acids long.

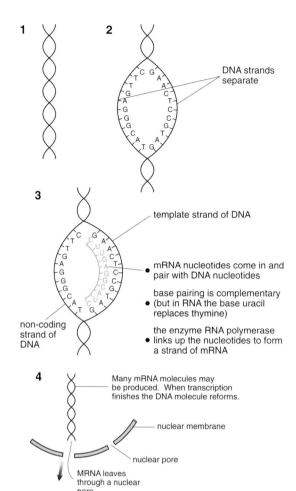

Figure 4.12 Transcription

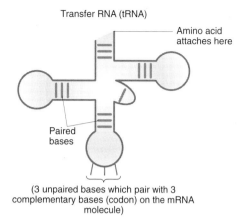

(3 unpaired bases which pair with 3 complementary bases (codon) on the mRNA molecule)

Figure 4.13 Transfer RNA (tRNA)

Reproduction

The reproductive process, which involves cell division, the production of gametes (sperm and egg), fertilisation, the development of the embryo and birth all play an important role in the continuation of life and the maintenance of the characteristics of the human race.

Cell division

Cells in the body are constantly dividing. There are two distinct forms of cell division: **mitosis** and **meiosis**.

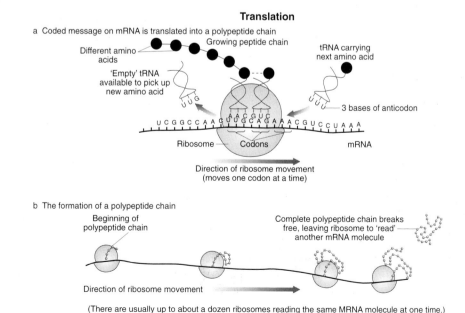

Figure 4.14 Translation

a)

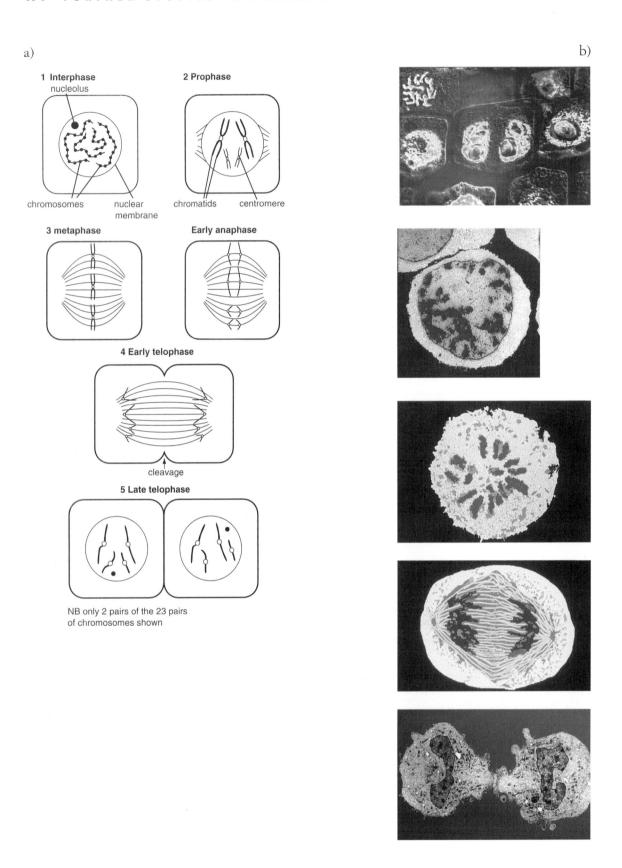

b)

Figure 4.15 Stages of mitosis, b) Seen through a electron microscope

- In **growth and repair** (**cell replacement**), it is essential that the cells produced in cell division (daughter cells):
  - have the same number of chromosomes as the parents (46 in humans)
  - are genetically identical

Cell division in growth and repair is mitosis.

- In **reproduction**, it is essential that the gametes produced (eggs and sperm) have:
  - half the number of chromosomes of the parent cells (23 in humans)
  - are genetically different

Gametes are produced by meiosis.

Mitosis

Although mitosis is a continuous process, it is easier to describe if it is divided up into a number of stages. These are shown in Figure 4.15.

1 **Interphase** Between divisions cells are in interphase. During this time the chromosomes are not visible. New cell components are being made and DNA will be replicated (see Figure 4.10).

2 **Prophase** The chromosomes gradually become visible as they shorten and thicken by twisting. Eventually they can be seen to consist of two **chromatids** joined at the **centromere**. The centrioles organise microtubules (thin protein threads) into a **spindle**. The nuclear membrane breaks down and the nucleoli disappear.

3 **Metaphase** The chromosomes become attached to the middle (equator) of the spindle.

4 **Anaphase** The chromatids separate at the centromeres and are drawn to opposite ends (poles) of the spindle.

5 **Telophase** The spindle breaks down and new nuclear membranes form around each set of chromatids to give two new nuclei. Nucleoli reform and the cytoplasm divides to form two new daughter cells.

Activity

1 Use a microscope to observe cells in the stages of mitosis (for example, use a prepared slide of an onion root tip). Try to find each of the stages shown in Figure 4.15.

2 If possible, watch a video of mitosis so that you can see the chromosomes actually moving.

Meiosis

Nearly all the cells in the human body contain 23 pairs of chromosomes. These cells are known as **diploid** cells (2n). Gametes contain only half this number and are described as **haploid** (n). When two haploid gametes fuse in fertilisation, the diploid number of chromosomes is restored. Figure 4.16 shows the role of meiosis in maintaining the correct number of chromosomes generation after generation. Figure 4.17 shows the main stages of meiosis and Table 4.3 gives a comparison of the processes of mitosis and meiosis. Whereas in mitosis there is one division of the nucleus, in meiosis there are two divisions:

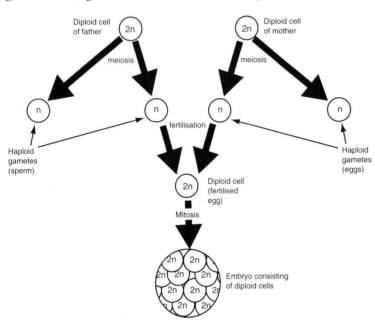

Figure 4.16 Maintenance of the diploid number of chromosomes

First meiotic division

This is sometimes known as the 'reduction division' because it is in this division that the number of chromosomes are halved.

1 **Prophase I** As in mitosis, the chromosomes gradually become visible as they shorten and thicken by twisting. However, there is a very important difference at this stage. Whereas in mitosis the pairs of chromosomes do not associate, in meiosis the matching (homologous) chromosomes pair up. The centrioles organise microtubules (thin protein threads) into a spindle. The nuclear membrane breaks down and the nucleoli disappear.

2 **Metaphase I** The pairs of chromosomes line up on the equator of the spindle as shown in Figure 4.17.

3 **Anaphase I** The homologous chromosomes separate with whole chromosomes moving towards each pole.

4 **Telophase I** The spindle breaks down and new nuclear membranes form around each set of chromosomes to give two new nuclei. Nucleoli reform and the cytoplasm divides to form two cells.

Second meiotic division

The second division is very similar to mitosis.

1 Prophase II A new spindle reforms in each cell.

2 MataphaseII The chromosomes line up on the equators as shown in Figure 4.17.

3 AnaphaseII The centromeres divide and the chromatids move towards opposite poles of the spindles.

4 Telophase II The spindles break down and new nuclear membranes form around each set of

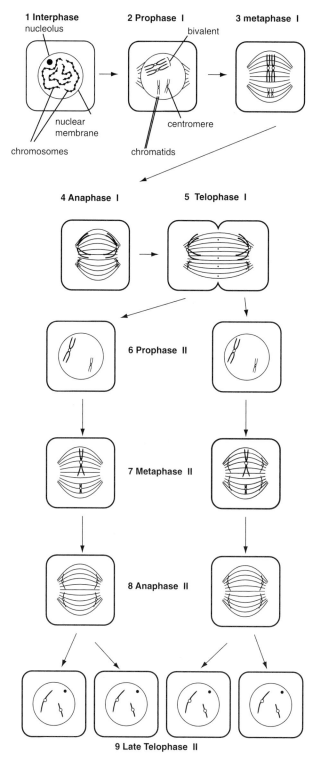

1 Interphase
nucleolus
nuclear membrane
chromosomes

2 Prophase I
bivalent
centromere
chromatids

3 metaphase I

4 Anaphase I

5 Telophase I

6 Prophase II

7 Metaphase II

8 Anaphase II

9 Late Telophase II

Figure 4.17 Stages of meiosis

chromatids. Nucleoli reform and the cytoplasm divides to give four new haploid cells.

The gametes produced by meiosis are genetically different from one another. There are two features of meiosis which bring this about:

1 **Independent assortment:** Figure 4.17 shows the separation of matching (homologous) chromosomes. One chromosome of each pair will have been inherited from the father (paternal) and one from the mother (maternal). When the homologous chromosomes draw apart in anaphase I, a mixture of the maternal and paternal chromosomes (and therefore genes) will end up in the gametes.

2 **Crossing over (or genetic recombination):** during prophase I a process known as crossing over occurs. Homologous chromosomes become joined at a number of points (**chiasmata**). There is then a breakage at these points which leads to the crossing over of genes (Figure 4.18).

Reproduction in humans

Structure and function of the female and male reproductive systems

Sexual reproduction involves the fusing of two sex cells (gametes), the male spermatazoon (sperm) and the female ovum (egg). This process is fertilisation. The reproductive system is responsible for producing the gametes and enabling internal fertilisation to occur within the body of the woman. The resulting cell is called a zygote, and this develops into an embryo and then a foetus. The female reproductive system is adapted to enable the foetus to develop to a certain stage before birth occurs.

Table 4.3 A comparison of mitosis and meiosis

	Mitosis	**Meiosis**
What products are formed?	two diploid, genetically identical daughter cells	four haploid, genetically different daughter cells
How many nuclear divisions are there?	One	Two
Do homologous chromosomes pair?	No	Yes
Is there crossing over?	No	Yes
What processes are they involved in?	Growth and cell replacement (repair)	Sexual reproduction

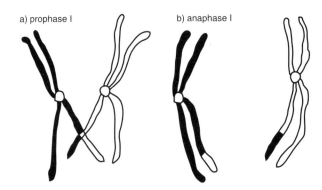

a) prophase I   b) anaphase I

Figure 4.18 Crossing over

Activity

Figure 4.19 shows the structure of the female reproductive system, and Figure 4.20 shows the structure of the male reproductive system.

Use the diagrams to trace the route taken by sperm from their production in the testes to the site of fertilisation in the oviduct or fallopian tube.

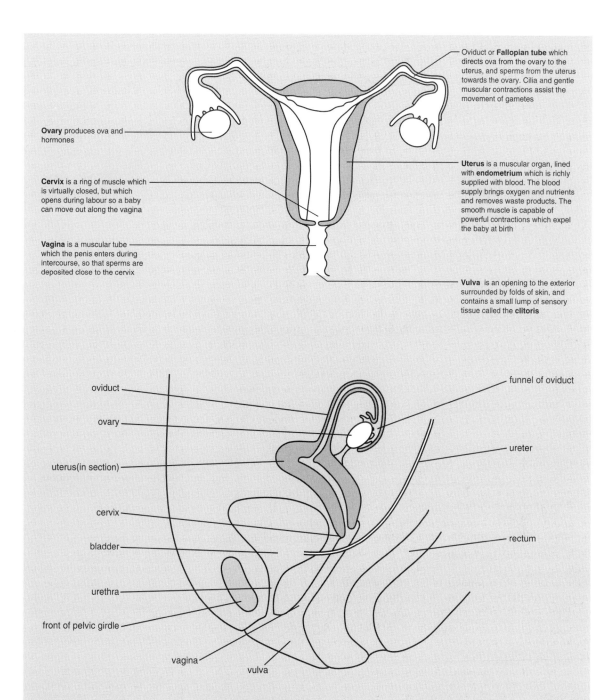

Oviduct or **Fallopian tube** which directs ova from the ovary to the uterus, and sperms from the uterus towards the ovary. Cilia and gentle muscular contractions assist the movement of gametes

Ovary produces ova and hormones

Uterus is a muscular organ, lined with **endometrium** which is richly supplied with blood. The blood supply brings oxygen and nutrients and removes waste products. The smooth muscle is capable of powerful contractions which expel the baby at birth

Cervix is a ring of muscle which is virtually closed, but which opens during labour so a baby can move out along the vagina

Vagina is a muscular tube which the penis enters during intercourse, so that sperms are deposited close to the cervix

Vulva is an opening to the exterior surrounded by folds of skin, and contains a small lump of sensory tissue called the **clitoris**

oviduct

funnel of oviduct

ovary

ureter

uterus(in section)

cervix

bladder

rectum

urethra

front of pelvic girdle

vagina

vulva

Figure 4.19 Female reproductive system

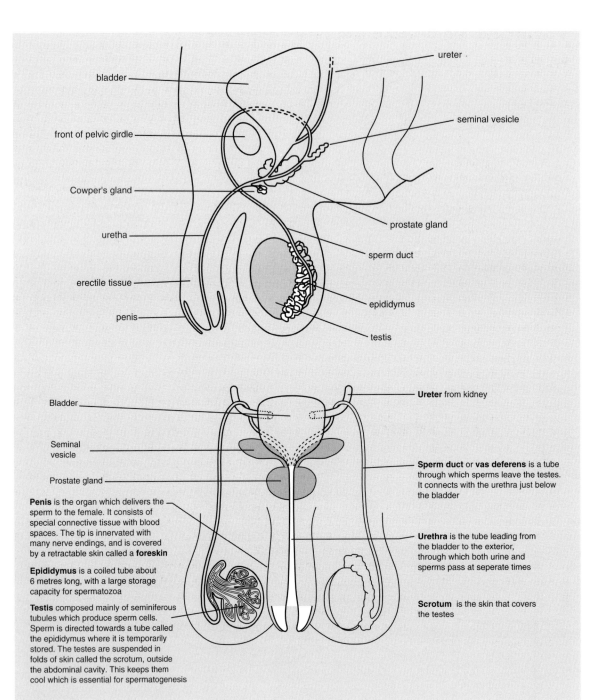

bladder

ureter

front of pelvic girdle

seminal vesicle

Cowper's gland

prostate gland

uretha

sperm duct

erectile tissue

epididymus

penis

testis

Bladder

Ureter from kidney

Seminal
vesicle

Prostate gland

Sperm duct or **vas deferens** is a tube
through which sperms leave the testes.
It connects with the urethra just below
the bladder

Penis is the organ which delivers the
sperm to the female. It consists of
special connective tissue with blood
spaces. The tip is innervated with
many nerve endings, and is covered
by a retractable skin called a **foreskin**

Urethra is the tube leading from
the bladder to the exterior,
through which both urine and
sperms pass at seperate times

Epididymus is a coiled tube about
6 metres long, with a large storage
capacity for spermatozoa

Scrotum is the skin that covers
the testes

Testis composed mainly of seminiferous
tubules which produce sperm cells.
Sperm is directed towards a tube called
the epididymus where it is temporarily
stored. The testes are suspended in
folds of skin called the scrotum, outside
the abdominal cavity. This keeps them
cool which is essential for spermatogenesis

Figure 4.20 Male reproductive system

The production of male and female gametes

Female gamete production (oogenesis)

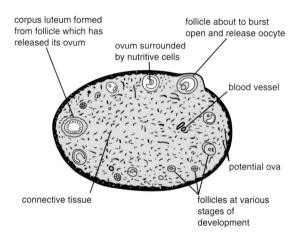

Female gametes (ova or eggs) are produced by the ovary (Figures 4.21 and 4.22 – refer to these figures while reading this section). The process of oogenesis starts when the female foetus is in her mother's uterus. Cells from the outside layer of the ovary (germinal layer) divide by mitosis to form **oogonia**. Some of these develop into **primary oocytes**. These are surrounded by a layer of cells, which is known as a primary follicle. There are many of these primary oocytes present when the baby is born, but only a small fraction will ever go on to become ova.

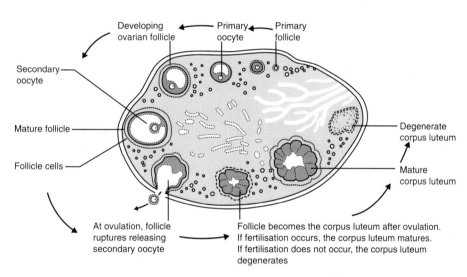

Figure 4.21 The ovary

At puberty, primary oocytes start to develop, but only one each month from alternate ovaries, will actually mature. The follicle increases in size and the oocyte undergoes the first meiotic division (see 'Meiosis', above). This is not an equal division. A large **secondary oocyte** and a smaller **polar body** are produced. The secondary oocyte starts to undergo the second meiotic division, but this process stops at metaphase II. The large follicle bursts, releasing the oocyte from the ovary. This is **ovulation**. Cilia move the oocyte along the oviduct. If the oocyte is fertilised, the second meiotic division is completed to form the haploid **ovum**. The polar body also divides, but the products degenerate.

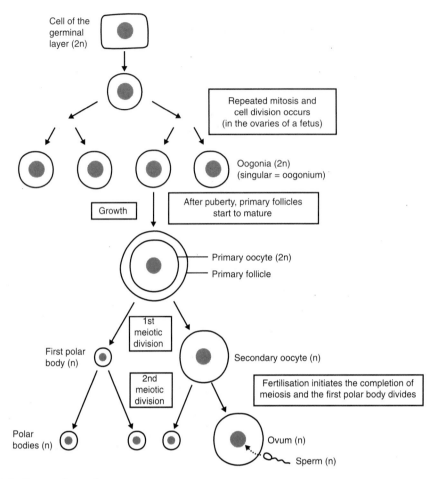

Figure 4.22 Formation of an ovum

The follicle tissue left on the surface of the ovary becomes a **corpus luteum** (yellow body). This produces the hormone, progesterone (see page 192). If fertilisation takes place, the corpus luteum remains for about three months, but if there is no fertilisation it degenerates after two weeks.

Male gamete production (spermatogenesis)

Male gametes (sperm cells) are produced by the testes (Figure 4.23 – refer to this Figure while reading this section). The process of spermatogenesis starts when a boy reaches puberty. Cells in the outside layer of the sperm tubes (germinal layer) divide by mitosis to form **spermatogonia**. These divide by mitosis and then grow to form **primary spermatocytes**. These then divide by meiosis. After the first meiotic division, haploid **secondary spermatocytes** are formed. The second meiotic division forms **spermatids**. The spermatids develop into sperm cells.

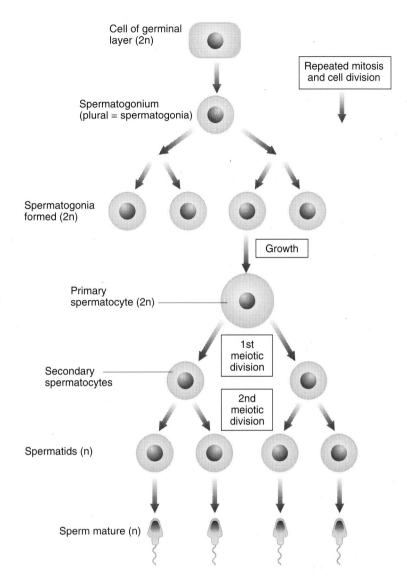

Cell of germinal layer (2n)

Repeated mitosis and cell division

Spermatogonium (plural = spermatogonia)

Spermatogonia formed (2n)

Growth

Primary spermatocyte (2n)

1st meiotic division

Secondary spermatocytes

2nd meiotic division

Spermatids (n)

Sperm mature (n)

Figure 4.23 Production of sperm cells

Activity

1 Examine microscope slides of a section of an ovary and a section of the testis. Compare these with Figures 4.21 and 4.23 and identify what you see.

2 Compare oogenesis (Figure 4.22) and spermatogenesis (Figure 4.23). What are the features of the processes that lead to:

- the production of higher numbers of sperm being produced compared with the number of eggs produced?
- the production of eggs which are much larger than sperm?

3 Why is it important that high numbers of sperm are produced?

(See page 221 for answers.)

Fertilisation

When fertilisation occurs, the sperm penetrates the ovum and their two nuclei fuse (Figure 4.24). The resulting fertilised egg is known as the zygote. This process usually takes place in the Fallopian tube (Figure 4.19) 12–24 hours after ovulation (release of the egg from the ovary).

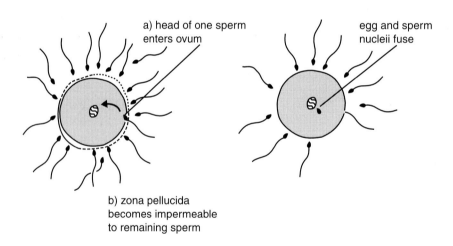

Figure 4.24 Fertilisation

Development of the zygote

Immediately after fertilisation, the zygote undergoes rapid cell division. The first division, or **cleavage**, results in the formation of two cells (see 'mitosis' on page 175) and takes about 36 hours (Figure 4.25). Within another 24 hours the second division is completed, resulting in four cells. These then divide to form eight cells which then divide to give 16 cells and so on. A few days after fertilisation, these divisions have led to the formation of a solid mass of cells known

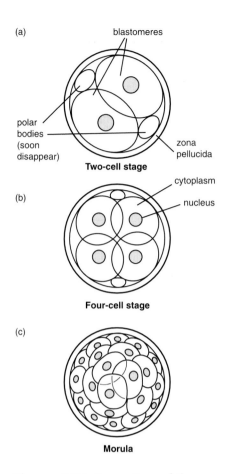

(a) blastomeres

polar bodies (soon disappear)

zona pellucida

Two-cell stage

(b) cytoplasm

nucleus

Four-cell stage

(c)

Morula

Figure 4.25 Formation of the morula

as the **morula**. Because progressively smaller cells are formed, the morula is about the same size as the original zygote. As the morula forms, waving cilia assist its movement down the Fallopian tube and into the uterus.

As cell division continues, a hollow, fluid-filled ball is formed which is known as a **blastocyst**. As the amount of fluid in the blastocyst cavity increases, the cells become separated into two parts: a flattened outer cell layer known as the **trophoblast** which eventually goes on to form the embryonic part of the placenta, and the **inner cell mass** which is the origin of the embryo (Figure 4.26). About seven to eight days after fertilisation, **implantation** takes place. This is when the blastocyst becomes attached to the **endometrium** (the lining of the uterus). During implantation, the outer cells of the blastocyst secrete enzymes that digest the cells of the endometrium. Eventually, the blastocyst becomes buried in the endometrium. The uterus lining develops a rich supply of blood vessels and becomes increasingly muscular. The outer cells of the blastocyst form finger-like projections (**chorionic villi**) through which the exchange of nutrients, oxygen and excretory materials occurs.

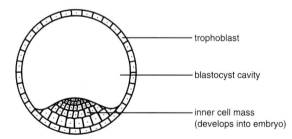

trophoblast

blastocyst cavity

inner cell mass (develops into embryo)

Figure 4.26 Simplified diagram of the human blastocyst

Activity

What is meant by an **ectopic** implantation?
(see page 221 for answer)

Development of the embryo

For the first two months of development, the developing human is called an **embryo**. During this time the beginnings of the principal organs are formed, and the embryonic membranes are developed.

Following implantation, **gastrulation** takes place. This begins at the end of the 1st week and is completed during the 3rd week. It involves the arrangement of the inner cell mass of the blastocyst into three layers:

1 the **ectoderm**, which forms the skin and nervous system;

2 the **mesoderm**, which forms the muscle, bones, blood and other connective tissues;

3 the **endoderm**, which forms the epithelial lining of the alimentary canal and respiratory tract, and a number of other organs.

(Throughout the following description of the development of the embryo and foetus, refer to Figures 4.27 and 4.28.)

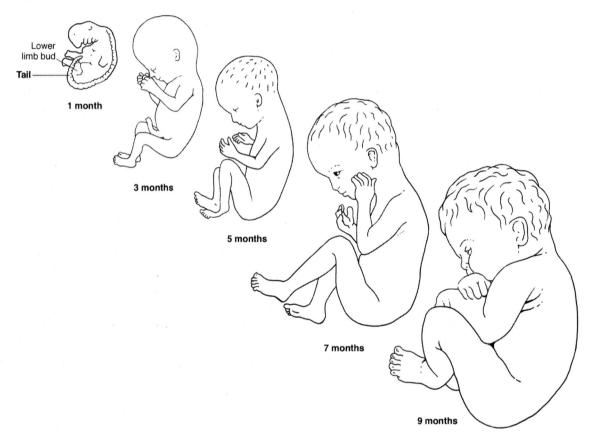

Figure 4.27 Development of the foetus and embryo in the uterus

Days: 28   31   35   48

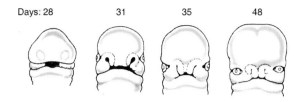

Figure 4.28 Development of the face

In the 4th week, the limb buds appear as small swellings. The embryo has a 'C-shaped' appearance, with a prominent tail.

At the end of the 5th week, the embryo is approximately 2mm long, and would therefore be visible to the naked eye. The spine is beginning to form, and the origin of the nervous system is just visible. Blood formation begins. Growth of the head is obvious due to the rapid development of the brain.

During the 6th week, the embryo grows to about 6mm long (the size of a grain of rice) and the chest and abdominal cavities start forming. The tail becomes less noticeable and the four limb buds continue to develop. By the end of the 6th week, an ultrasonic scan can detect the first heart motions. (The cardiovascular system is the first organ system to start functioning.) Blood vessels are forming within the umbilical cord and the earliest parts of the stomach and intestine are formed within the abdominal cavity. Small depressions form where the eyes and ears will be, and the mouth and jaw are also beginning to develop.

By the end of the 7th week, the limb buds are clearly distinguishable as arms and legs. Ridges can be seen where the fingers and toes will develop. Blood vessels are present throughout the head and body, and they contain blood cells. The heart beats with sufficient force to move the cells through the vessels. The liver, kidney and lungs are all developing. The brain and spinal cord and head are also all developing very quickly. The head is assuming its final shape but is bent forward over the chest and is very large compared with the body. The inner parts of the ears are forming. The eyes continue to develop, but they are still completely covered with the skin which will eventually become the eyelids. Although the nose is still not present, apertures can be seen where the nostrils will form. By now, the embryo is about 13mm long.

By the 8th week, all the major internal organs have begun to develop, but the functioning of most of these is minimal. The embryo is now about 22mm long. This is the main time of growth for the eyes and the middle and inner ears. The external ears are beginning to take on their final appearance, but they are still low set on the head. The heart is beating strongly. The lungs have grown but are still solid. The two sides of both the upper and lower jaws have fused, so that the mouth can be recognised. Shoulders, elbows, hips and knees can also be seen as the limbs continue to develop. Although the external genitalia have begun to form, sex differences are not yet obvious. The tail disappears completely.

Development of the foetus

From the beginning of the 9th week after conception until birth, the developing human is known as a foetus. This change in name is to signify that the developing human has now acquired definite human characteristics. Development during the foetal period is mainly concerned with the growth of the organs that formed during the embryonic period.

Weeks 9–12

By the 9th week, the foetus is developing muscles and so is starting to move. However, these movements are not yet detected by the mother. Bone formation (**ossification**) begins particularly in the skull and long bones.

At 9 weeks, most of the red blood cells are produced by the liver, but by 12 weeks they are being produced by the spleen. During this period, **urine** formation begins. It is excreted into the amniotic fluid, and the foetus reabsorbs some of this fluid after swallowing it.

At 9 weeks, the foetus is about 30mm long and weighs about 2g. By 12 weeks, it is about 65mm long and weighs about 18g.

Weeks 13–16

Body growth is very rapid during this period. By 16 weeks, the foetus is about 160mm long and weighs about 135g. The formation of the skeleton is taking place rapidly, and foetal movement continues to increase, although it is still not sufficiently vigorous to be detected by the mother. By 16 weeks, the ovaries will have formed in females and primitive ova can be seen. The external genital organs continue to develop, and the sex of the baby is now obvious. The head is now rounded, and the neck is developed so that it can move freely. The mouth, nose, eyes and external ears are all properly developed. Fingers, toes, fingernails and toe nails are all present. A fine downy hair (**lanugo**) covers the whole foetus, including the face, and eyebrows and eyelashes start to grow.

Weeks 17–20

The growth of the foetus slows down during this period. The limbs grow at a relatively quicker rate until they reach their final relative proportions, and muscle is rapidly increasing. The skin becomes covered with a fatty secretion (**vernix caseosa**) which protects it from the chapping that could result from continuous exposure to the amniotic fluid. **Brown fat** forms which is an important site of heat production, particularly in the newborn infant. Head hair may become visible at this time.

At the end of the 20th week, the foetus is about 255mm (25.5cm) long and weighs about 340g.

Weeks 21–25

Growth is rapid during this period, and by the end of 25 weeks the foetus is about 34cm long and weighs about 600g. By 24 weeks, the cells lining the lungs have secreted a layer of **surfactant** which facilitates the expansion of the developing **alveoli**.

Weeks 26–29

By this time, the lungs have developed sufficiently to function if the foetus is born prematurely. The central nervous system has also developed enough to bring about rhythmic breathing movements, and to control body temperature. By 28 weeks, the formation of red blood cells in the spleen ceases and begins in the bone marrow. Fat forms under the skin, which means that the foetus loses its wrinkled appearance.

Weeks 30–38

After 35 weeks, most foetuses will be plump. By 36 weeks, the circumference of the head and the abdomen are approximately equal. In a male, the testes will have descended into the **scrotum**. The lanugo will have disappeared from most of the head and body, but the foetus remains almost entirely covered with vernix except on the mouth and eyes. The colour of the iris is always blue at this stage.

The baby increases in weight by about 28g per day from the 36th week until birth. At birth, it will be about 50cm long, on average, and weigh about 3.4kg.

Activity

From the above information, make a table to show:

*   the size
*   movements
*   sensory development (i.e. the development of the brain and nerves, the eyes and the ears)

of the embryo and foetus at 1, 3, 5, 7 and 9 months after conception.

Plot a graph from the figures given to show the increase in:

*   length
*   weight

from conception to birth.

Birth

Birth, or **parturition**, usually occurs at approximately 266 days or 38 weeks after fertilisation. This is usually calculated as 280 days or 40 weeks after the last menstrual period.

In the first stage of labour, the uterus starts to contract. These contractions become more frequent and intense until the cervix is fully dilated (Figure 4.29).

In the second stage, the baby is pushed downwards, usually head first, through the vagina (**delivery**).

The third and final stage is the delivery of the placenta (**afterbirth**).

Activity

Watch a video of a baby being born, and, if possible, interview a mother informally to find out about her experience of giving birth.

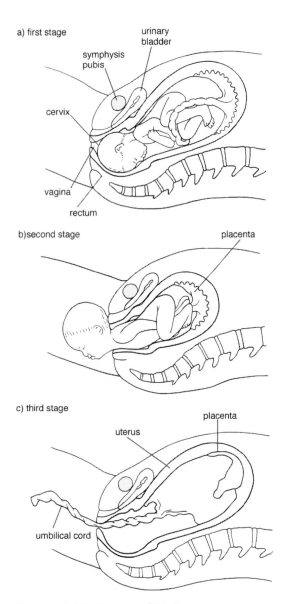

a) first stage

urinary bladder

symphysis pubis

cervix

vagina

rectum

b) second stage

placenta

c) third stage

placenta

uterus

umbilical cord

Figure 4.29 Stages of birth

The menstrual cycle

Figure 4.30 shows the events of the **menstrual** cycle. This cycle takes, on average, 28 days.

1 For the first 3–5 days of the cycle **menstruation** takes place. During her 'period' a woman loses about 60–80 cm^3 of blood that comes from the breakdown of the **endometrium** (lining of the uterus).

2 After menstruation, the endometrium becomes thicker again. The follicle develops (see 'Female gamete production' on pages 181–2) and on about the fourteenth day of the cycle ovulation occurs.

3 In the second half of the cycle the corpus luteum is formed from the empty follicle. At the end of the cycle the corpus luteum disappears.

The role of hormones in reproduction

The menstrual cycle is controlled by hormones. Hormones also have an important role to play if pregnancy occurs. The roles of the main reproductive hormones are described below, and Figure 4.31 shows the interaction of hormones in the menstrual cycle.

The role of hormones in the menstrual cycle

Follicle stimulating hormone (FSH)

FSH is produced by the pituitary gland. As its name suggests, it stimulates the development of follicles. It also stimulates the ovaries to produce oestrogen.

Oestrogen

Oestrogen stimulates the growth of the endometrium in the early stage of the menstrual cycle. It also stimulates the pituitary gland to produce luteinising hormone (LH). Oestrogen brings about a number of changes in the female at puberty.

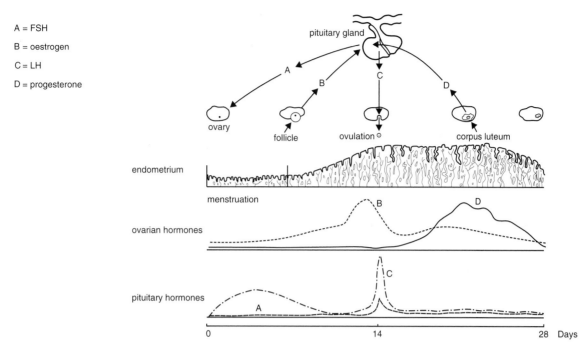

A = FSH

B = oestrogen

C = LH

D = progesterone

Figure 4.30 The menstrual cycle

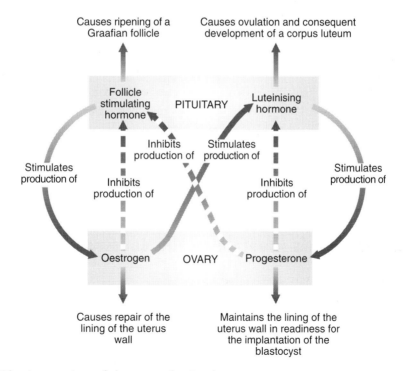

Figure 4.31 The interaction of the reproductive hormones

Luteinising hormone (LH)

LH brings about ovulation and is involved in the development and maintenance of the corpus luteum, which produces the hormone progesterone.

Progesterone

In the second half of the menstrual cycle progesterone prepares the endometrium for the possible arrival of a fertilised egg. It inhibits the production of FSH and LH. The drop in LH means the corpus luteum degenerates and the level of progesterone falls. When the level of progesterone falls, FSH production is no longer inhibited and the cycle can begin again.

The role of hormones in pregnancy

Progesterone

In the first 12 weeks of pregnancy, the corpus luteum continues to produce progesterone, which maintains the endometrium in a suitable condition for the implanted embryo. After this the placenta starts producing progesterone to maintain the uterus lining. Progesterone prepares the breasts for milk production.

Oestrogen

Together with progesterone, oestrogen helps to maintain the lining of the uterus and to prepare the breasts for milk production.

Oxytocin

Oxytocin is one of the hormones involved in birth. It is produced by the hypothalamus in response to the baby's head pressing down on the cervix. It makes the muscles of the uterus contract. (See 'Birth' on page 189). Oxytocin is also involved in the contraction of muscles in the breast to squeeze milk out when the baby is feeding.

Prolactin

This hormone is produced by the anterior pituitary gland stimulating the production of milk.

The effects of mother's lifestyle on the development of the embryo

There are a number of aspects of a mother's lifestyle that can have adverse effects on her unborn baby.

Drugs

Most drugs taken by the mother will diffuse across the placenta to the foetal circulation. Some of these may cause harm, particularly during the 12 weeks after conception. Drugs which adversely affect the development of the foetus are known as **teratogenic**. It is important, therefore, that the mother takes the correct dose of any prescribed medicines, and checks carefully whether non-prescribed drugs she may require are safe to be taken during pregnancy.

Alcohol is teratogenic if taken in excess. Babies born to mothers who drink large amounts of alcohol throughout the pregnancy may be born with **foetal alcohol syndrome**. These children have characteristic facial deformities, stunted growth and mental retardation. More moderate drinking may increase the risk of miscarriage, but many women continue to drink small amounts of alcohol throughout their pregnancy with no ill effects.

Illegal drugs, such as LSD, are teratogenic and may cause the foetus to develop more slowly. Babies born to heroin addicts are addicted themselves and likely to suffer withdrawal symptoms. They are likely to be underweight and may even die. If necessary, women should seek professional help to enable them to stop taking these drugs before conception.

Smoking

Smoking decreases the fertility of both males and females. Women who smoke during pregnancy are more likely to produce a premature or stillborn baby. Women who smoke are twice as likely to deliver a low birth weight baby as are women who do not smoke. The more a woman smokes during her pregnancy, the lower the birth weight of the baby is likely to be. There is also evidence that smoking in pregnancy causes mental and physical retardation later in the child's life. Even 'passive' smoking can harm the baby's development, so women planning a pregnancy should not only give up smoking but also encourage their partner to do likewise.

Activity

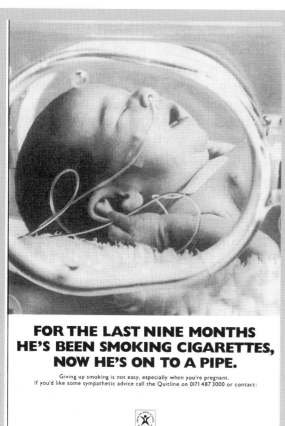

Look at Figure 4.32 and then design your own advertisement to encourage pregnant women to give up smoking. What practical advice would you give to enable them to do this?

Figure 4.32 An anti-smoking advertisement aimed at pregnant women

Promiscuous sexual behaviour

If a woman has a number of different sexual partners it will increase the likelihood that she will contract a sexually transmitted disease (STD). An example of an STD is **syphilis**, which, although a rare condition now, has such harmful effects on the foetus that a blood test is done to test for its presence. If the result is positive and treatment is given before 20 weeks, the foetus will suffer no ill effects.

The role of the placenta in the passage of potentially harmful substances

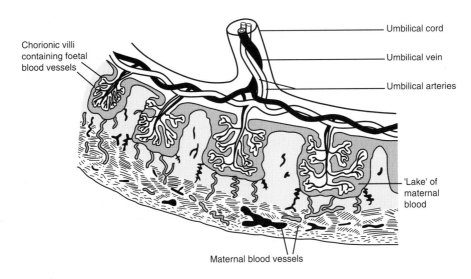

Figure 4.33 Diagram of the placenta

Figure 4.33 shows the structure of the placenta. It allows contact between maternal and foetal tissues, and is necessary for the exchange of materials between the mother and the foetus (Figure 4.34). It also produces hormones which are essential in pregnancy. As well as allowing the exchange of useful materials, the placenta also allows the passage of potentially harmful substances from mother to foetus. Examples of these harmful substances are given below.

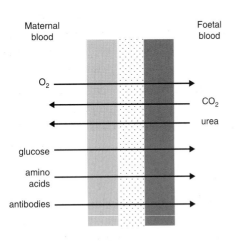

Figure 4.34 Transport across the placenta

Carbon monoxide

This is a harmful substance found in cigarette smoke. It is absorbed from the mother's lungs into her blood. It diffuses across into the foetus's blood. It combines with haemoglobin to form carboxyhaemoglobin. The carbon monoxide combines with haemoglobin 250 times more readily than oxygen, so it decreases the amount of oxygen circulating in the foetal blood. This leads to the harmful effects described in the section on 'Smoking' on page 193.

Nicotine

This is another harmful substance found in cigarette smoke which can cross the placenta from the maternal to the foetal blood. It has the effect of increasing the unborn baby's heart rate.

Viruses

Viruses are small enough to cross the placenta from mother to foetus. Some viruses can have very harmful effects on development, particularly in the first 12 weeks after conception. One such example is **rubella**. The symptoms are mild, and once the person has the disease they will not have it again. However, if a mother is infected in the first 12 weeks of her pregnancy, the virus can mean that her baby will be born deaf, blind or with heart defects. If a pregnant woman does contract the disease, she will be offered a termination because the likelihood of the baby being affected is so high (approximately 12%).

The **human immunodeficiency virus** (HIV) may be passed across the placenta from the mother to the unborn baby. However, although the virus particle is very small (less than 1.0 um in diameter) there is a low risk of this happening.

Foetal red blood corpuscles

The mother's blood will be tested to find out whether she is **Rhesus positive** or **Rhesus negative**. People who are Rhesus positive have **antigens** on the surface of their red blood cells. These cause the red blood cells from people who are Rhesus negative to produce the corresponding **Rhesus antibodies**. The antibodies bind the antigens together and so cause the clumping together of the Rhesus-positive blood cells. Sometimes, in the last few months of the pregnancy, a few fragments of the foetal red blood cells will cross the placenta into the mother's bloodstream. If the father is Rhesus positive and the baby inherits this condition, and the mother is Rhesus negative, the cells of the baby will cause the mother to produce Rhesus antibodies. Some of these antibodies will move back across the placenta to the foetal circulation. With a first baby, the antibodies do not usually form quickly enough to reach a level which could cause harm. However, because the antibodies will already be in the mother's blood, subsequent Rhesus-positive children may be affected with potentially fatal results. When the foetal red blood cells clump together, they become stuck in the **capillaries** and

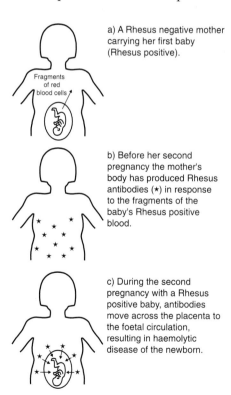

a) A Rhesus negative mother carrying her first baby (Rhesus positive).

Fragments of red blood cells

b) Before her second pregnancy the mother's body has produced Rhesus antibodies (★) in response to the fragments of the baby's Rhesus positive blood.

c) During the second pregnancy with a Rhesus positive baby, antibodies move across the placenta to the foetal circulation, resulting in haemolytic disease of the newborn.

Figure 4.35 A summary of the development of haemolytic disease of the new-born

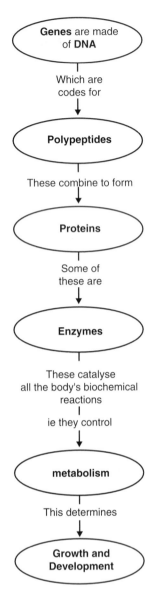

Figure 4.36 Summary of the link between genes and growth and development

eventually burst, releasing their **haemoglobin**. This is known as **haemolysis**. (See Figure 4.35 for a summary.)

If the blood tests show the mother to be Rhesus negative (about 15% of the population have this), she will have several further blood tests to check for the presence of the Rhesus antibodies during her pregnancy.

If necessary, the baby can receive a blood transfusion once it is born, or even whilst still in the uterus. Alternatively, immediately after giving birth to her first Rhesus-positive baby, the Rhesus-positive mother can be injected with a substance which will destroy any foetal blood cells in her circulation before they can trigger the immune response.

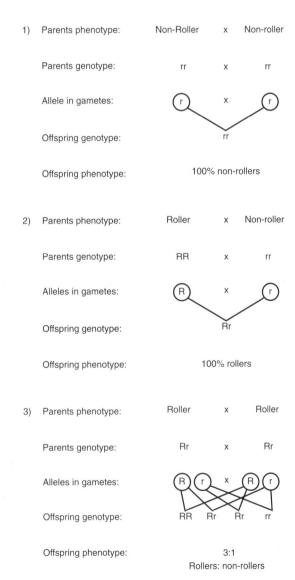

Figure 4.37 a) Examples of genetic crosses

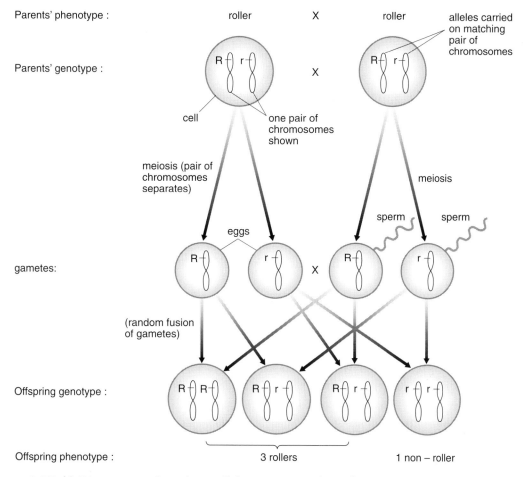

Figure 4.37 b) Diagram to show how alleles are carried on chromosomes

Basic principles of inheritance

Genetics

The genes an individual inherits from their parents will obviously affect that person's growth and development.

All the cells of the body, except for the eggs and sperm (**gametes**), contain 23 pairs of **chromosomes** (see page 169). One of each pair has come from the father, and one from the mother. The chromosomes contain DNA, which codes for all the **polypeptides** (sub-units of proteins) the body makes. The length of DNA that codes for one polypeptide is known as a gene. All biochemical reactions in the body are catalysed by **enzymes**, which are proteins. In this way, the genes control the body's metabolism and, therefore, growth and development. Figure 4.36 summarises this information.

A person's **genotype** refers to the genes they possess. The term **phenotype** describes the physical characteristics determined by the genes.

Each characteristic is determined by one or more pairs of genes; one of each pair is on the chromosome inherited from the mother, and one of each pair is on the chromosome inherited from the father. Genes exist in alternative forms known as **alleles**. For example, brown and blue are alternative forms (alleles) of the gene for eye colour. One allele is usually **dominant** over the other **recessive** allele.

For example, the ability to roll one's tongue is genetically determined. The 'rolling' allele, R, is dominant over the recessive, 'non-rolling' allele, r. (It is customary to abbreviate the dominant allele to the initial capital letter, and the recessive allele to the corresponding lower-case letter.) A person who cannot roll their tongue will have the alleles rr. A person who *can* role their tongue will have either the alleles RR or Rr. In the latter case, the dominant, 'rolling' allele masks the effect of the recessive, 'non-rolling' allele. A person with identical alleles for a characteristic (e.g. RR or rr) is known as **homozygous**, whereas a person with different alleles for a characteristic (e.g. Rr) is known as **heterozygous**. Figures 4.37a (page 196) and 4.37b (page 197) illustrate how alleles may be passed to the offspring.

The work of Gregor Mendel

Gregor Mendel (1822–84) was an Austrian monk who discovered what we now call genes. When he published his work, it was ignored for 34 years until 1900, when it was realised that his experiments on garden peas had established the basic laws of heredity. Prior to this it was thought that the heredity material was a fluid which carried characteristics from each parent to give a blend of characteristics in the offspring. Two laws have been produced from Mendel's work.

Mendel's First Law (the Law of Segregation)

'Each inherited character is determined by two alleles, only one of which can be carried by a gamete.'

This is based on the work done by Mendel using **monohybrid crosses**. These are genetic crosses in which only a single characteristic was observed, for example, the height of the pea plant which could be tall or short. Table 4.4 shows examples of other characteristics Mendel studied.

Table 4.4 Examples of characteristics of pea plants studied by Mendel

Character	Dominant trait	Recessive trait
Height	Tall	Short
Flower colour	Red	White
Pod colour	Green	Yellow
Seed shape	Round	Wrinkled
Seed colour	Yellow	Green

Parents: Tall   Short

F₁ generation: Tall (100%)

                    (F₁ plants crossed together)

F₂ generation: Tall   Short

Ratio: 3   :   1

Figure 4.38 An example of one of Mendel's monohybrid crosses

Mendel crossed tall and short parents and found that all the offspring in the first generation (known as F_1 plants) were tall. When he crossed these F_1 plants together he found a ratio of 3:1 tall plants to short plants. (This next generation was known as the F2 generation.) This is summarised in Figure 4.38.

From these monohybrid crosses, Mendel concluded that:

• one form of the characteristic was dominant to the alternative recessive form;

T = tall allele; **t** = short allele

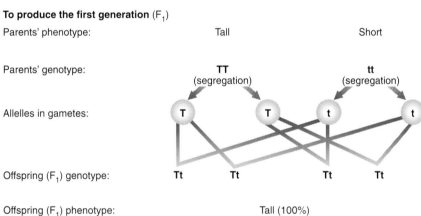

To produce the first generation (F_1)

Parents' phenotype: Tall   Short

Parents' genotype: TT   tt
                                (segregation)   (segregation)

Allelles in gametes: T   T   t   t

Offspring (F_1) genotype: Tt   Tt   Tt   Tt

Offspring (F_1) phenotype: Tall (100%)

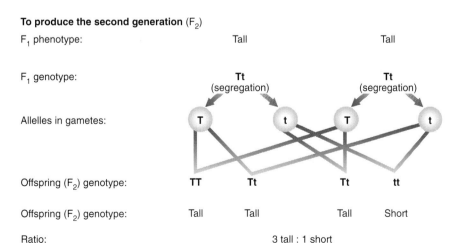

To produce the second generation (F_2)

F_1 phenotype: Tall   Tall

F_1 genotype: Tt   Tt
                                (segregation)   (segregation)

Allelles in gametes: T   t   T   t

Offspring (F_2) genotype: TT   Tt   Tt   tt

Offspring (F_2) genotype: Tall   Tall   Tall   Short

Ratio: 3 tall : 1 short

Figure 4.39 An explanation of Mendel's monohybrid crosses

- the heredity material behaved as particles, rather than a type of fluid;
- in the formation of gametes, the pair of factors (alleles) which determine a characteristic split up, or **segregate**.

Figure 4.39 explains Mendel's monohybrid crosses in terms of alleles. (**NB** Mendel did not use terms such as 'gene' and 'allele'. These were introduced later by other scientists.)

Mendel's Second Law (the Law of Independent Assortment)

'The segregation of each member of a pair of alleles is not affected by the segregation of any other pair.'

In addition to his monohybrid crosses, Mendel also carried out **dihybrid crosses** (genetic crosses in which two characteristics were observed, for example, pea plant height and seed shape.) Mendel crossed tall plants with round seeds and short plants with wrinkled seeds. He found that all the offspring in the first generation (F_1 plants) were tall with round seeds. When he crossed these F_1 plants together he found in the F_2 a ratio of :

- nine tall plants with round seeds;
- three tall plants with wrinkled seeds;
- three short plants with round seeds;
- one short plant with wrinkled seeds.

This is summarised in Figure 4.40.

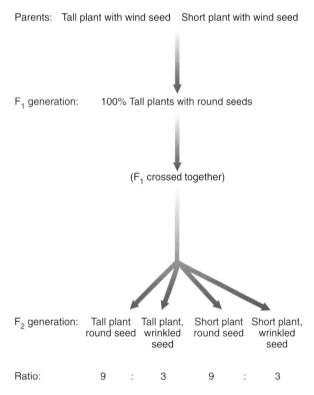

Parents: Tall plant with wind seed   Short plant with wind seed

F_1 generation: 100% Tall plants with round seeds

(F_1 crossed together)

F_2 generation: Tall plant   Tall plant,   Short plant   Short plant,
                     round seed   wrinkled   round seed   wrinkled
                                  seed   seed

Ratio: 9   :   3   9   :   3

Figure 4.40 An example of a dihybrid cross

From these dihybrid crosses, Mendel concluded that characteristics, in this case height and seed shape, are inherited independently of one another.

Figures 4.41 and 4.42 explain Mendel's dihybrid crosses in terms of alleles. When the pair factors (alleles) for each characteristic segregates (separates) in gamete formation, as described in the monohybrid cross above, it does so independently of the segregation of any other pairs. This is called **independent segregation** or **independent assortment**. For example, the pair of alleles, Tt, segregates independently of the pair of alleles Rr. This means four types of gametes (TR, Tr, tR, tr) are found in equal numbers (independent assortment of chromosomes in meiosis is described on page 177). (**NB** Mendel was studying genes that were found on different pairs of chromosomes. If genes

T = tall allele; **t** = short allele; **R** = round seed allele; **r** = wrinkled seed allele

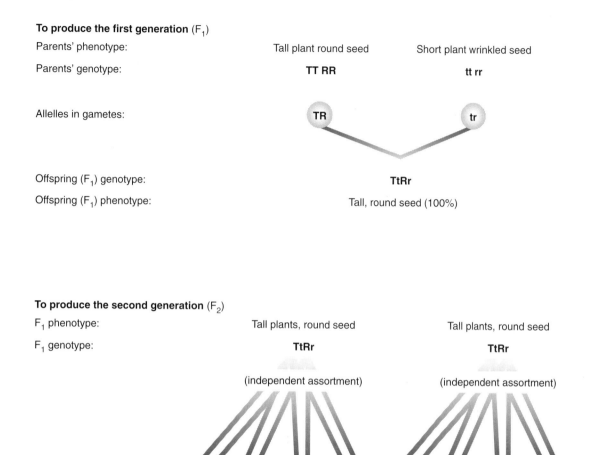

To produce the first generation (F$_1$)

Parents' phenotype: Tall plant round seed   Short plant wrinkled seed

Parents' genotype: **TT RR**   **tt rr**

Allelles in gametes: TR   tr

Offspring (F$_1$) genotype: **TtRr**

Offspring (F$_1$) phenotype: Tall, round seed (100%)

To produce the second generation (F$_2$)

F$_1$ phenotype: Tall plants, round seed   Tall plants, round seed

F$_1$ genotype: **TtRr**   **TtRr**

(independent assortment)   (independent assortment)

Allelles in gametes: TR   Tr   tR   tr   TR   Tr   tR   tr

Figure 4.41 a) An explanation of a dihybrid cross

are found on the *same* pair of chromosomes, independent segregation is less likely – see 'Autosomal linkage' on pages 208–9.)

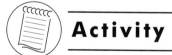

Activity

Look at Figure 4.41. What ratio of phenotypes would be found in a cross between an F$_1$ plant (TtRr) and a short plant with wrinkled seeds?

(See page 221 for the answer.)

(A punnett square is used to show how the various gametes may combine)

Offspring genotype (F$_2$)

	TR	Tr	tR	tr
TR	TTRR	TTRr	TtRR	TtRr
Tr	TTRr	TTrr	TtRr	Ttrr
tR	TtRR	TtRr	ttRR	ttRr
tr	TtRr	Ttrr	ttRr	ttrr

Offspring phenotype:	tall plant round seed	tall plant wrinkled seed	short plant round seed	short plant wrinkled seed
Ratio:	9 :	3	3 :	1

Figure 4.41 b) An explanation of a dihybrid cross

Deviations from Mendelian inheritance

There are a number of exceptions to normal Mendelian inheritance. The following conditions affect the expected Mendelian ratios.

- incomplete or co-dominance;
- multiple alleles;
- polgenic inheritance;
- sex linkage;
- autosomal linkage;
- mutations.

Incomplete or co-dominance

In all the examples of genetic crosses given so far in this chapter, in a pair of alleles, one has always been dominant and one has been recessive. However, there are exceptions to this. As we have seen, a heterozygous individual has two different alleles for a characteristic. In some cases *both* these alleles will have an effect on their phenotype. In this case, where neither allele is completely dominant or completely recessive, we say that there is **incomplete dominance** or **co-dominance**. An example of this is the inherited blood disorder, **thalassaemia**.

Thalassaemia

People who inherit this condition have abnormal haemoglobin. It is most likely to affect people of Mediterranean and South Asian descent. There are two forms of thalassaemia: **thalassaemia major** and **thalassaemia minor**.

To produce the second generation (F$_2$)

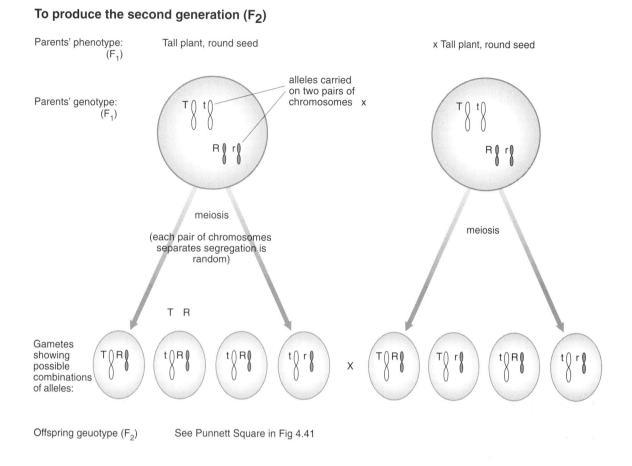

Figure 4.42 Diagram to show how alleles are carried on chromosomes in a dihybrid cross

Thalassaemia major

Sufferers of this condition cannot produce enough haemoglobin, and so they cannot produce enough red blood cells; those that they do produce are nearly empty. Babies with this condition are normal at birth, but become anaemic between the ages of three and 18 months. They become pale, do not sleep or feed well and may vomit. If they are not treated, they usually die when they are between one and eight years old. The condition can be treated with medication and regular blood transfusions (every three to four weeks), which allow those affected to lead relatively normal lives. People with this disease are homozygous (their cells contain two alleles for thalassaemia).

Thalassaemia minor

People with this condition (also known as 'trait') are usually healthy but may have slight anaemia. Usually a person is not aware that they have thalassaemia minor, but it will show up if they have a blood test as their red blood cells are not normal. People with thalassaemia minor are heterozygous (their cells contain one allele for the condition and one normal allele). Because the thalassaemia allele and the normal allele show incomplete or co-dominance, heterozygous individuals are affected slightly by the condition, but not to the extent of individuals homozygous for thalassaemia.

(For further examples of co-dominance, see the information on blood groups, below, and sickle cell anaemia, on page 214.)

Multiple alleles

In all the examples of genetic crosses given so far in this chapter, there have been two alternative forms of an allele. For example, there are rolling or non-rolling alleles for tongue rolling, tall or short alleles for pea plant height (and see other pea plant examples in Table 4.4), and thalassaemia allele or normal allele in haemoglobin production. However, there are sometimes *more* than two alternative forms of an allele and we refer to this as **multiple alleles**. (**NB** There will still only be two alleles present in a cell for a particular characteristic, because one allele is carried on each chromosome in a matching pair.) The inheritance of blood groups in humans is an example in which there are multiple alleles.

Blood groups

The ABO blood group in humans is controlled by a gene with multiple alleles. There are three alleles:

- O   (represented as i^O);
- A   (represented as I^A);
- B   (represented as I^B).

I^A and I^B are co-dominant, and both are dominant to the recessive i^O. An individual will have two of the possible three alleles. Table 4.5 shows the possible genotypes and phenotypes.

Table 4.5 Possible genotypes and phenotypes in the ABO blood group

Alleles (genotype)	Blood group (phenotype)
$I^O I^O$	O
$I^A I^A$	A
$I^A I^O$	
$I^B I^B$	B
$I^B I^O$	
$I^A I^B$	AB

Activity

Is it possible for two parents to produce children who have all four possible phenotypes i.e. O, A, B, and AB?

(See page 221 for the answer)

Polygenic inheritance (multiple factor inheritance)

In all the examples of genetic crosses described so far in this chapter, each characteristic has been controlled by a single gene (i.e. one pair of alleles). However, many characteristics are controlled by a number of genes which interact together. This is known as **polygenic inheritance**. Characteristics that are determined by polgenic inheritance include height, intelligence and skin colour. (These three characteristics are also affected by environmental factors.)

Characteristics that are controlled by only one gene show **discontinuous variation**. That is the phenotypes fit into distinct categories. For example, a person is either a tongue roller or they are not; a person has either blood group A or B or AB or O (see Figure 4.43a). Characteristics that are determined by more than one gene show **continuous variation**. That is there is a range of phenotypes in the population. If a histogram is plotted, it will show a **normal distribution** (see Figure 4.43b).

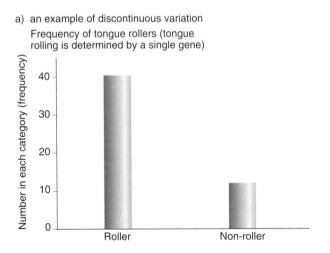

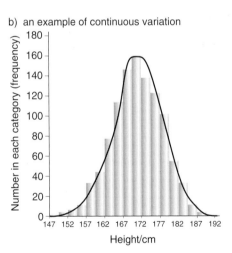

Figure 4.43 a) An example of discontinuous variation b) An example of continuous variation

The genetic determination of sex

One of the smallest of the 23 pairs of chromosomes determines a person's sex. Females have two X chromosomes whereas males have one X chromosome and one smaller Y chromosome. Figure 4.44 shows that there is an equal chance of parents producing a male or female baby.

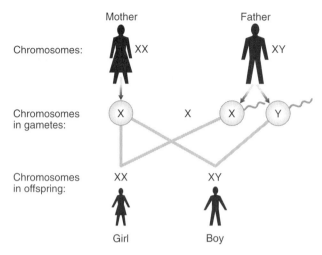

Figure 4.44 Determination of sex

Sex linkage

The genes for certain characteristics are carried on the sex chromosomes (usually the X chromosome because it is longer than the Y chromosome), and we say that these characteristics are **sex-linked**. Examples of conditions that are determined by sex-linked genes include **red-green colour blindness** and **haemophilia**.

Red-green colour blindness

This condition is caused by an allele carried on the X chromosome, which means that the cones in the retina of the eye do not function correctly. A person with the condition cannot distinguish between the two colours. About 8% of males and 0.4% of females are red-green colour blind.

Haemophilia

This is a condition in which the blood does not clot properly. If it is untreated, it leads to internal bleeding. Bleeding into the joints causes pain. It is now possible to extract the clotting factor from donated blood in order to treat the disease, but before this the condition was often fatal. It occurs in about 1 in 25,000 males and is much rarer in females.

As can be seen in the examples given above, sex-linked conditions are more common in males than in females. This is because males only have one X chromosome and, therefore, only have one allele. If they have the harmful recessive allele which causes the condition, it will not be masked by a 'normal' allele. Females who have the recessive allele which causes the condition are only likely to be **carriers** and not suffer the disease themselves. This is because on their second X chromosome they will carry the dominant 'normal' allele that will mask the effect of the harmful allele. These carriers can, of course, pass the harmful allele on to their children. Figure 4.45 shows examples of crosses involving sex-linked conditions.

1 (N = 'normal' allele;   n = colour blind allele)

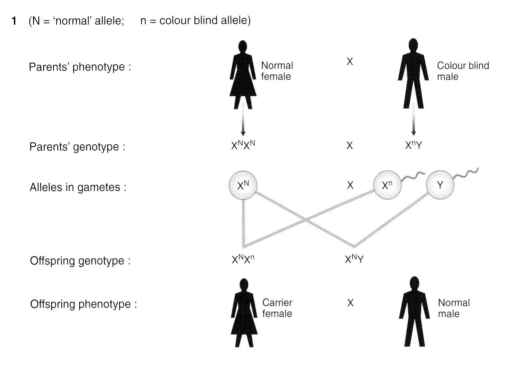

NB Affected males pass the harmful allele to their daughters.

2 (N = 'normal' allele;   n = 'haemophilia' allele)

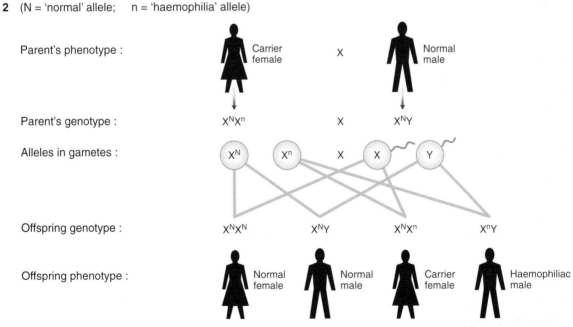

NB A carrier female has a 50% chance that any sons she produces will be affected.

Figure 4.45 Crosses involving sex linked conditions

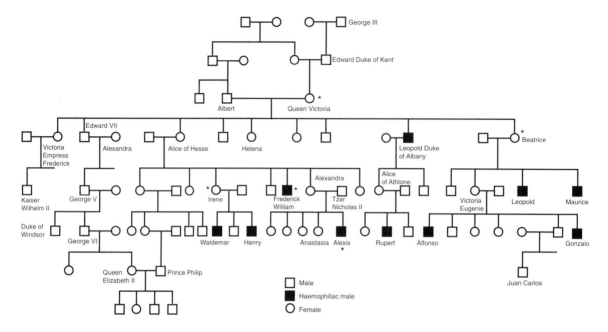

Figure 4.46 Family tree showing inheritance of haemophillia in the Royal Family

Activity

1 Look at the crosses shown in Figure 4.45. A female with red-green colour blindness would have the genotype X^nX^n. Write out a genetic cross to show the phenotype and genotype of her parents.

2 Look at Figure 4.46 which shows the inheritance of haemophilia in the Royal Family.

Work out the genotypes of the marked (*) individuals. (Remember, because the allele is carried on the X chromosome, males only carry one allele, and haemophilia is a recessive condition.)

(See page 222 for the answers.)

Autosomal linkage

In the description of dihybrid inheritance above (pages 200–2), it was explained that Mendel's Law of Independent Assortment only applies if the alleles for the two characteristics are found on separate pairs of chromosomes as shown in Figure 4.42. If, however, the alleles are found on the *same* pair of chromosomes, a different pattern of inheritance will be seen. Alleles on the same chromosome are more likely to be inherited together and will not show independent assortment. Figure 4.47 shows an example of this.

In fruit flies the genes for wing shape (Normal, N, or 'dumpy', n) and eye colour (Red, R, or brown, r) are found on the same pair of chromosomes

Crossing individuals to obtain F$_1$ generation

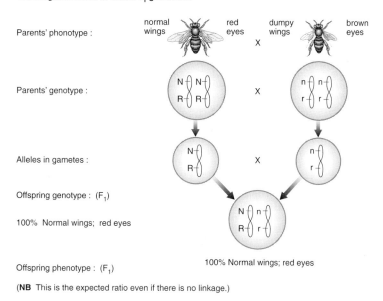

Parents' phonotype :

Parents' genotype :

Alleles in gametes :

Offspring genotype : (F$_1$)

100% Normal wings; red eyes

Offspring phenotype : (F$_1$)

100% Normal wings; red eyes

(**NB** This is the expected ratio even if there is no linkage.)

Crossing an F$_1$ individual with a homozygous

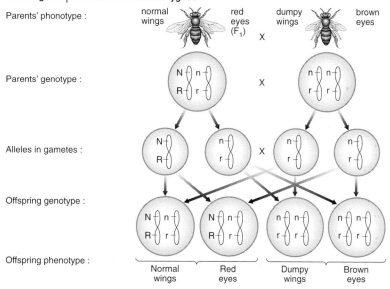

Parents' phonotype :

Parents' genotype :

Alleles in gametes :

Offspring genotype :

Offspring phenotype :

Normal wings | Red eyes | Dumpy wings | Brown eyes

(**NB** If there is no linkage a ratio of normal wings, red eyes; normal wings, brown eyes; 1 dumpy wings, red eyes; dumpy wings, brown eyes would be obtained.)

Figure 4.47 Examples of autosomal linkage

Alleles which are found on the same chromosome will not *always* be inherited together. The process of **crossing over** in meiosis was described on pages 176–7. This allows alleles on the same chromosome to be separated in gamete formation. The further apart on a chromosome the two alleles are, the more likely crossing over will occur between them, and so the more likely they are to be separated.

Mutations

Occasionally there are 'mistakes' in cell division which change the genetic material. This change in genetic material is known as a **mutation** and may be:

- an alteration in the number of chromosomes;
- an alteration in the structure of one or more chromosomes;
- an alteration in the sequence of bases (see 'DNA structure' on pages 169–70).

If the mutation occurs in the process of meiosis, it will be present in the gametes produced. All the cells of an individual produced from such a gamete will carry the same mutation and will be unable to code for the correct proteins. The mutation may be passed on to their children and subsequent generations.

The causes and effects of mutations

Mutations are changes which arise spontaneously, although there are a number of factors which are known to increase the rate at which they occur. Examples of these **mutagens** are listed below:

- types of **radiation**, for example, x-rays and ultraviolet radiation;
- some **chemicals**, for example, nitrous acid, formaldehyde and mustard gas;
- some **viruses**.

Most mutations are harmful. There are about 5000 diseases which are caused by mutations. Examples of these include cystic fibrosis, haemophilia, sickle cell anaemia and Down's syndrome.

Chromosomal disorders

Chromosomal disorders are caused by either changes in the *structure* of chromosomes or changes in the *number* of chromosomes. These are **chromosome mutations**.

1 **Changes in chromosome structure.** Figure 4.48 shows the changes which can occur in chromosome structure. In each of these changes a number of genes are affected.

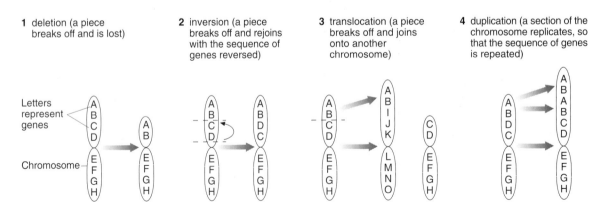

1 deletion (a piece breaks off and is lost)

2 inversion (a piece breaks off and rejoins with the sequence of genes reversed)

3 translocation (a piece breaks off and joins onto another chromosome)

4 duplication (a section of the chromosome replicates, so that the sequence of genes is repeated)

Figure 4.48 Changes in chromosome structure

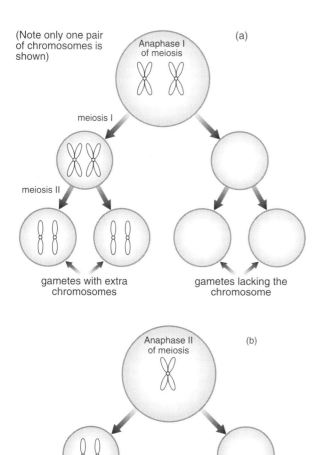

(Note only one pair of chromosomes is shown)

Anaphase I of meiosis (a)

meiosis I

meiosis II

gametes with extra chromosomes

gametes lacking the chromosome

Anaphase II of meiosis (b)

gamete with extra chromosomes

gamete lacking chromosome

Figure 4.49 Non-disjunction

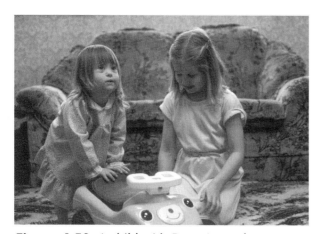

Figure 4.50 A child with Down's syndrome

2 Changes in chromosome number.
Changes in chromosome number result from an unequal separation of chromosomes in cell division. In anaphase I of meiosis the homologous chromosomes may fail to separate, or in anaphase II (see 'Meiosis' on pages 176–7) both chromatids may move towards one pole. These both result in one gamete having one too many chromosomes, and one gamete having one too few. This failure of the chromosomes or chromatids to separate is known as **non-disjunction** (Figure 4.49). When a gamete with an extra chromosome joins with another gamete in fertilisation, this results in a zygote with three of that chromosome instead of a pair. This condition is known as **trisomy**. All the cells in the individual developing from this zygote will be affected. Many affected foetuses will be miscarried but it can give rise to various genetic diseases depending on which chromosome is affected. Three examples are described below.

Down's syndrome

About 1 in 650 babies are born with Down's syndrome (Figure 4.50). The condition is caused by trisomy of chromosome number 21 (Figure 4.51). There are characteristic features of a person with Down's syndrome:

- the face tends to be flat;
- eyes tend to slant;
- growth may be retarded;
- there may be congenital heart disease;
- there is an increased incidence of respiratory disease;
- learning difficulties range from mild to severe;
- children are usually very affectionate and happy.

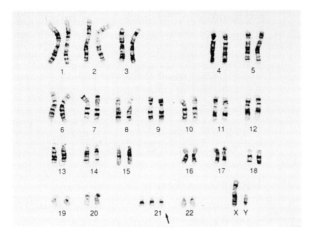

Figure 4.51 Karyotype of a female with Down's syndrome showing trisomy of chromosome number 21

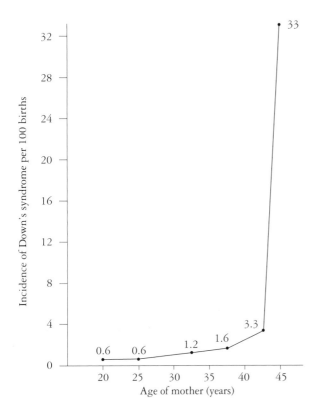

Figure 4.52 The relationship between Down's syndrome and maternal age

The risk of having a baby with Down's syndrome increases significantly for older mothers (Figure 4.52). Pre-natal testing is available (see pages 215–7).

Klinefelter's syndrome

Klinefelter's syndrome occurs in about 1 in 500 to 1 in 1000 male births. People with this condition have XXY sex chromosomes instead of the usual XX or XY. The extra X chromosome could have come from either the egg or the sperm (Figure 4.53). People with XXY chromosomes are male, but tend to have the following characteristics:

- small testes;
- no sperm production;
- little development of facial hair;
- to a certain extent body shape may be female;
- normal IQ (although there may be some language difficulties).

Turner's syndrome

Turner's syndrome occurs in about 1 in 2000 female births. People with this condition have just one X sex chromosome instead of the usual XX or XY (Figure 4.54). People with this syndrome are female, but tend to have the following characteristics:

- undeveloped sex organs;
- small stature;
- 'webbed' neck.

Other problems may include learning difficulties, skeletal abnormalities, hearing loss, liver dysfunction, and heart and kidney abnormalities.

Genetic disorders

Genetic disorders are caused by changes in the sequence of base pairs in part of a DNA molecule which codes for a protein. These changes are **gene mutations**. As explained in the section 'Protein synthesis' on pages 171–3, each triplet of bases (codon) codes for an amino acid (triplet code). A change in the sequence of bases changes the genetic code, so that the wrong sequence

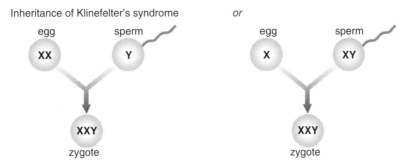

Figure 4.53 The inheritance of Klinefelter's syndrome

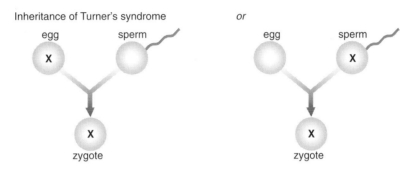

Figure 4.54 Inheritance of Turner's syndrome

of amino acids may be formed. Figure 4.55 shows examples of types of gene mutation. Gene mutations may:

- have no effect at all – most amino acids are coded for by a number of triplets, so a change in a single base may still code for the same amino acid. For example, if the DNA triplet TGA changes to TGC it still codes for the amino acid threonine.
- Give rise to a disorder, for example, sickle cell anaemia (described below) .
- Be fatal.

Frameshift mutations are particularly harmful. This is what happens when one base is added or lost (insertion or deletion), which changes all the subsequent triplets. In substitution, only a limited number of triplets are affected. The following example illustrates how a message can be changed by a small alteration.

Correct message:

THE FAT CAT AND DOG SAT AND ATE THE BIG RAT

If one letter is substituted for another there is a small change:

THE FAT CAT AND DOG SAT AND ATE THE BIG BAT

If, however, one letter is added or taken away (the equivalent of a frameshift mutation) the whole message changes:

THE ATC ATA NDT HED OGS ATA NDA TET HEB IGR AT

Changes in base pairs (gene mutations)

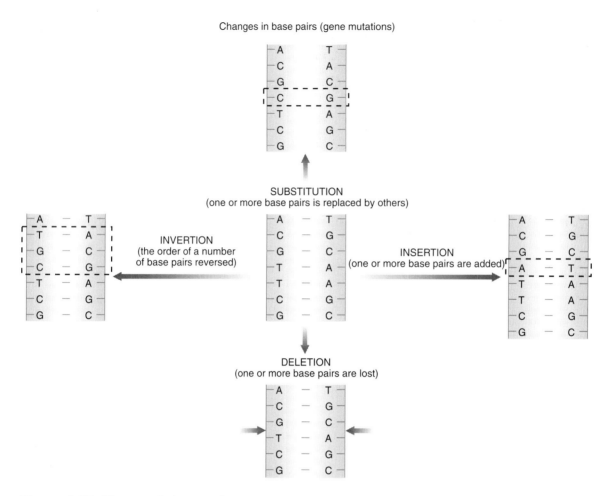

Figure 4.55 Changes in base pairs

Examples of diseases caused by gene mutations are haemophilia (described in the section on 'Sex linkage' on pages 206–8), and sickle cell anaemia.

Sickle cell anaemia

This disease is caused by a substitution. Normally , when haemoglobin is formed, the sixth amino acid in the B chain is coded for by the DNA triplets CTT or CTC. These code for the amino acid glutamic acid. However, if the code CTT becomes CAT, or CTC becomes CAG, the amino acid valine is coded for instead.

This small change has drastic effects. The red blood cells can become sickle shaped (Figure 4.56). In this condition the cells become inefficient at carrying oxygen and can block the capillaries. The lack of oxygen reaching parts of the body can cause severe pain, and this is know as a crisis. Heart and kidney failure are common and many sufferers die young.

Sickle cell anaemia is an example of co-dominance (see pages 202–4). People with the disease are homozygous for the condition (that is, they have two sickle cell alleles). People who are heterozygous for the condition (that is, have one sickle cell and one 'normal' allele) have sickle

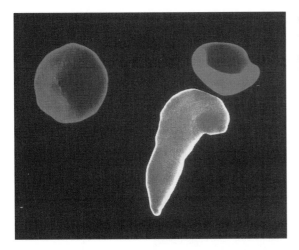

cell trait. This means that more than half of their red blood cells are normal (not sickle shaped). They may suffer from slight anaemia, but they have the advantage of being resistant to the most dangerous form of malaria.

Figure 4.56 Red blood cells from a person with sickle cell

The detection and prevention of genetic disorders

Prenatal screening

Several techniques and screening methods are used between conception and birth to detect and prevent a number of genetic disorders. A **screening technique** is used to identify if the foetus is at increased risk of having a disorder. When a screening test is positive, or abnormal, then a **diagnostic test** is used to determine if the disorder is present. For example, a blood test (see 'Specialised blood tests', below) would be used to screen for babies at increased risk of Down's syndrome, and then amniocentesis or chorionic villus sampling (see page 217) would then be used in these 'at risk' cases to diagnose whether the condition was actually present.

Specialised blood tests

At about 15–16 weeks into pregnancy, women in the UK are offered a blood test to determine whether or not there is an increased risk of having a baby with Down's syndrome or other chromosomal abnormalities. (The test also screens for other non-genetic conditions.) The test measures the amount of two substances in the mother's blood: **alphafetoprotein (AFP)**, a protein produced by the foetal liver, and **human chorionic gonadatrophin (hCG)**, a hormone. The test carries no risk to either the mother or the baby and the results are usually ready within a few days.

In pregnancies with Down's syndrome, the AFP level tends to be lower than average and the hCG level tends to be higher than average. These measurements are used, together with the mother's age, to calculate the risk of her baby having Down's syndrome. If this indicates a significant risk (greater than 1 in 250), the result is called 'screen positive' and she will be offered amniocentesis (see below).

Ultrasound

Tissues of the body can be examined by the use of **ultrasound** (high frequency sound waves). The ultrasound is transmitted into the body, where it is reflected at the boundaries between different types of tissue. The time lapse and intensity loss of the reflected ultrasound (returning signal) allows the nature and position of the tissues to be deduced. The sound waves are generated by a hand-held device which is placed over the area to be scanned (Figure 4.57). The echo of the returning waves is recorded and analysed by a computer which forms a screen image.

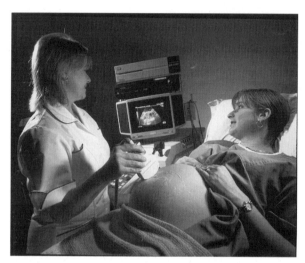

Figure 4.57 A pregnant woman undergoing a ultrasound scan

Ultrasound scans are completely painless and cause no damage to the tissues. For these reasons they are routinely given to pregnant women to monitor the foetal development. The scans reveal the size and stage of development and therefore the age of the foetus; the position of the foetus; multiple births; and foetal or placental defects. Ultrasound cannot be used to diagnose Down's syndrome. However, it can show up abnormalities such as a thick pad of skin behind the neck, and heart or gut defects which are common in individuals with Down's syndrome, which will suggest that the condition may be present. Further diagnostic testing such as amniocentesis can then be carried out. Ultrasound is used to guide the needle into the uterus during amniocentesis.

Amniocentesis

If blood tests (see above) indicate that a woman has an increased risk of having a baby with Down's syndrome, she will be offered amniocentesis. An ultrasound scan is used to check the position of the baby in the uterus. A fine needle is then inserted through the abdominal wall into the uterus to take a sample of amniotic fluid. This sample contains cells shed by the baby. These cells can be grown for about 7–14 days and then their chromosomes are examined under a microscope. The chromosomes are counted, matched up in pairs, and examined for missing or extra pieces. There will normally be 22 pairs, plus the two sex chromosomes, giving a total of 46 chromosomes, but a Down's syndrome baby will have a total of 47 chromosomes (Figure 4.51). Amniocentesis can also detect other problems caused by changes in chromosome number such as Klinefelter's syndrome or Turner's syndrome. The test will also show whether the baby is male or female.

Amniocentesis is generally carried out in the 16th to 18th week of pregnancy and takes 3–4 weeks to give a result. Amniocentesis carries the risk of causing miscarriage and it is estimated that up to 1 in 100 women who have the test will miscarry as a result. For this reason, amniocentesis is not offered routinely, but only when factors such as the mother's age or specialised blood tests (see above) suggest that there is an increased risk of chromosomal abnormality.

Chorionic villus sampling

This test involves taking a sample of the developing placenta (**chorionic villi**). It is usually done at about 10–11 weeks into the pregnancy. Using ultrasound to guide it, a fine needle is inserted, either through the vagina or through the wall of the abdomen and about 10–15mg of tissue is withdrawn. The foetal tissue is separated from the maternal tissue and the foetal cells are grown. The chromosomes are then examined as in amniocentesis. The results are usually available after about 1–3 weeks. The advantage of this test over amniocentesis is that results can be obtained much earlier in the pregnancy. However, there is a slightly higher risk of miscarriage.

Chromosomal analysis of foetal fluid

Blood can be taken directly from the foetus and analysed for chromosomal defects. The technique is known as Percutaneous Umbilical Blood Sampling (PUBS). A needle is inserted through the mother's abdomen and a blood sample is withdrawn from the umbilical vein which runs through the umbilical cord. Ultrasound is used to check the position of the needle. The results from this test can be obtained more quickly than from amniocentesis.

Genetic counselling

Genetic counsellors give advice to couples planning to have a child on the probability of their producing a child with a genetic disease. They may use any of the following sources of information:

- If the parents already have an affected child, it is easier for them to predict the likelihood of the next child being affected. For example, if an unaffected couple have a child with cystic fibrosis, there is a one in four chance that their next child will be affected.
- **Pedigree analysis** involves the examination of a family tree showing affected members of the family (see Figure 4.46).
- The frequency of the gene in the population as a whole indicates the likely genotype of the partner.
- If the prospective parents are related to each other, they are more likely to have inherited the same gene.
- For some genetic diseases, a sample of blood or cheek cells can be tested with a **DNA probe** to test for the presence of the harmful allele. In this way, carriers of the disease can be identified.

Genetic counsellors will also give advice to parents prior to screening of the foetus (see 'Prenatal Screening' above).

Once any risks have been identified, the genetic counsellor will discuss the options available to a couple, to enable them to make an informed decision. These options will be influenced by the moral and religious beliefs of the couple and their cultural background. They may include:

- not having children;
- using in vitro fertilisation (**test-tube baby**) so that the cells of the embryo can be screened for genetic abnormalities before implantation. With sex-linked diseases (see pages 206–8), a female embryo may be selected for implantation;
- using egg, sperm or embryo donation;
- terminating the pregnancy if foetal screening shows abnormalities.

Ethical issues associated with genetic screening

The genetic screening techniques described in 'Prenatal screening' on pages 215–7, may reduce the frequency of genetic and chromosomal disorders. However, genetic screening also creates ethical and moral dilemmas. Personal, social and cultural issues will determine what is considered acceptable or non-acceptable.

Activity

Below are a number of discussion points which highlight some of the ethical issues associated with genetic screening. These may be used as the basis for group discussions, debates or role plays.

Discussion points

- Who should be screened for genetic disorders, for example: all individuals, foetuses and new born babies for all diseases possible; anyone who requests it or only those considered at risk of a particular disorder?

- If screening and diagnostic techniques show that a foetus has a genetic disorder, do parents have the right to terminate the pregnancy (i.e. have an abortion)?

- For some parents termination is not considered an option. Would screening the foetus for genetic disorders have any advantages for these parents?

(See page 222 for suggestions.)

- Increasingly it is being shown that many diseases have some genetic basis, for example, people may have genes which make it more likely that they will develop breast cancer or heart disease. This may affect their ability to obtain life insurance or a mortgage. Who do you think should have information from screening – only the individual concerned, family members who may also be genetically affected, financial institutions?

- Individuals with the condition Huntingdon's chorea usually do not show symptoms until middle age. Then gradually they will lose co-ordination until they can no longer walk or talk. They will die within a few years. It is a dominant condition which means that the children of sufferers have a 50% chance of being affected. Sufferers usually have children before they know that they themselves are affected. If you had a parent who was diagnosed with this condition, would you wish to be tested?

- The law has recently changed so that all new-born babies will be screened for cystic fibrosis. Can you think of advantages and disadvantages associated with this?

Glossary

Amniocentesis   A process in which a sample of amniotic fluid is withdrawn in order to check the cells of the foetus for chromosomal abnormalities.

Cell   The fundamental unit of living organisms.

Centrioles   Tiny cylindrical granules in the cell which appear to have a role in spindle formation in cell division.

Chromosome   Thread-like structures in the nucleus made of protein and DNA on which the genes are found.

Congenital   A non-inherited abnormality present at birth.

Deoxyribonucleic acid (DNA)   The chemical of which our genes are made.

Diploid   Term used to describe cells which have pairs of chromosomes. There are 46 chromosomes in a diploid human cell.

Electron microscope   A microscope that shows more detail than the light microscope (see below). A beam of electrons is focused on the specimen by electromagnets.

Embryo   The term used for the developing human in the first two months after conception.

Endoplasmic reticulum   The network of membranes found throughout a cell. There are two types: rough endoplasmic reticulum (RER) and smooth endoplasmic reticulum (SER).

Fertilisation   The fusion of the sperm nucleus and egg nucleus.

Foetus   The term used for the developing human from the beginning of the ninth week after conception until birth.

Gametes   Sperm and ova (eggs).

Gene   The length of DNA that codes for the sequence of amino acids in a polypeptide chain.

Genetic counselling   A service which explains genetic disorders and the probability of their transmission.

Genotype   The alleles present in an individual.

Golgi apparatus   A stack of membrane bound flattened sacs in the cell which transports and modifies proteins.

Haemoglobin   The protein found in red blood cells which carries oxygen.

Haploid   The term used to describe cells which have half the number of chromosomes of a diploid cell. Gametes are haploid.

Incomplete or co-dominance   The type of inheritance where one allele is not completely dominant over another allele.

Karyotype   The sum total of an organism's chromosomal characteristics, usually shown as a photo of all the pairs of chromosomes in a cell (**karyogram**).

Light (optical) microscope   A microscope in which light passes through the specimen and the image is magnified by a glass lens in the objective and a glass lens in the eyepiece.

Lysosomes   Membrane bound vesicles in the cell which contain digestive enzymes.

Meiosis   Cell division which results in the daughter cells having only half the number of chromosomes found in the parent cell. Produces the gametes.

Micrometer (μm)   There are 1000 micrometers in a millimetre.

Mitosis   Cell division which results in all daughter cells having the same number of chromosomes as the parent cell.

Multiple alleles   Type of inheritance in which there are more than two alternative forms of a gene.

Mutation   An unpredictable change in the genetic material.

Nanometer (nm)   There are 1000 nanometers in a micrometer (see above).

Nuclear envelope   The double membrane that surrounds the nucleus.

Nucleus   The largest organelle in the cell. It contains the chromosomes.

Organelle   A structure found within a cell that has a particular function.

Ovum (plural ova)   Egg.

Oogenesis   Production of the ova (eggs).

Phenotype   The appearance of an organism.

Polygenic inheritance   The type of inheritance in which more than one gene determines a particular characteristic.

Polypeptide chain   Made up of amino acids; one or more polypeptide chains are folded together to form a protein.

Ribonucleic acid (RNA)   A chemical that is found in three different forms: messenger RNA; ribosomal RNA; and transfer RNA. All are essential for protein synthesis.

Ribososmes   Small organelles that are the site of protein synthesis.

Sex linkage   Describes genes carried on the X chromosome, for example, colour blindness and haemophilia. These conditions are more common in males than females.

Spermatogenesis   The production of sperm cells.

Ultrasound   A process used for, among other things, the monitoring of the age and development of the unborn baby, and to check for multiple births.

Zygote   The fertilised egg.

Resources

There is some commonality in the content of this unit with GCE Advanced level Human Biology, so A/AS level Biology or Human Biology textbooks will be useful. Science parks and museums often have excellent genetics exhibitions, so it's worth investigating what is available locally. If possible, a GP, genetic counsellor or visiting midwife could be invited to discuss some of the medical conditions, prenatal screening and some of the ethical issues faced by individuals as the knowledge provided by medical science grows and evolves. Ethical issues could be considered in group discussions.

Useful websites

www.jeansforgenes.com
This website gives details of the annual appeal which raises funds for genetic research. It also provides personal stories of people who suffer from genetic diseases and activities to help students develop an understanding of genetics and inheritance.

www.progress.org.uk
The Progress Educational Trust provides information on biological ethical issues such as genetic screening.

Answers

Chapter 4

The production of gametes

Activity 2 (Comparing male and female gamete production)

- More sperm than eggs are produced because there are more mitotic cell divisions in sperm production and four sperm are formed from each primary spermatocyte. In egg production only one ovum is formed from each primary oocyte.

- Eggs are larger than sperm because there is more growth and unequal meiotic cell divisions produce large ova.

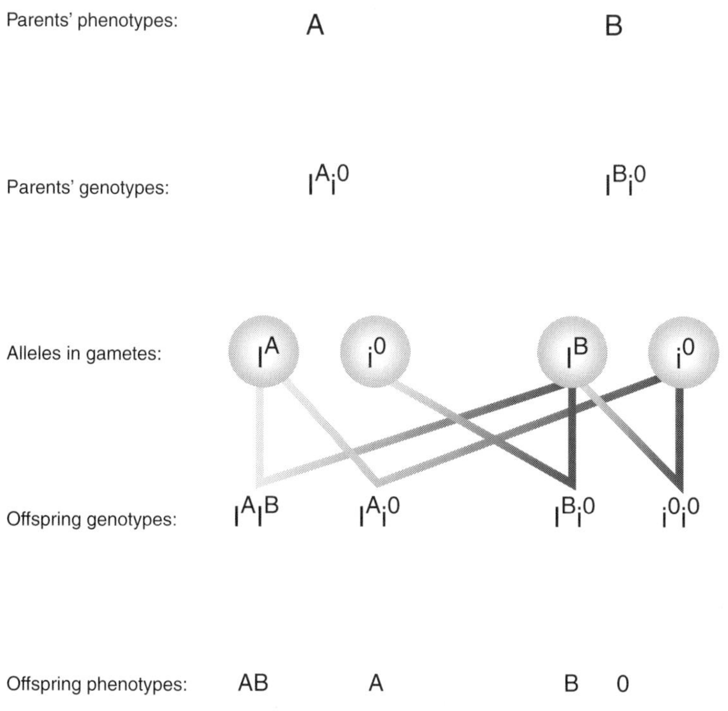

Parents' phenotypes: A   B

Parents' genotypes: $I^A i^0$ $I^B i^0$

Alleles in gametes: I^A i^0 I^B i^0

Offspring genotypes: $I^A I^B$ $I^A i^0$ $I^B i^0$ $i^0 i^0$

Offspring phenotypes: AB   A   B   0

Figure 4.59

Activity 3 (Comparing numbers of male and female gametes)

- High numbers of sperm are produced because very few will survive the journey to the ovum.

Fertilisation

Ectopic implantation: this is when the blastocyst becomes attached to the fallopian tube instead of the uterus lining.

Dihybrid cross

1 Tall plants, round seeds:

1 Tall plants, wrinkled seeds:

1 Short plants, round seeds:

1 Short plant, wrinkled seeds

Multiple alleles

Yes, it is possible for two parents to produce children with all four possible ABO blood group phenotypes. See figure 4.59 (above).

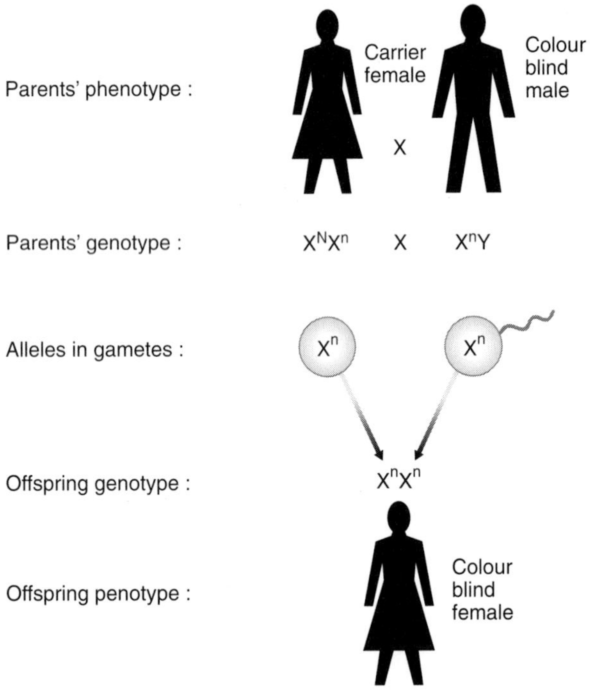

Parents' phenotype : Carrier female X Colour blind male

Parents' genotype : $X^N X^n$ X $X^n Y$

Alleles in gametes : X^n X^n

Offspring genotype : $X^n X^n$

Offspring penotype : Colour blind female

Figure 4.60 How a female inherits red-green colour blindness

Sex linkage

2) Look at Figure 4.58.

- Queen Victoria $X^N X^n$ (she must have been a carrier because she produced an affected son).
- Beatrice $X^N X^n$ (she must have been a carrier because she produced affected sons).
- Irene $X^N X^n$ (she must have been a carrier because she produced affected sons).
- Fredrick William $X^n Y$ (he was haemophiliac).
- Alexis $X^n Y$ (he was haemophiliac).

Ethical issues associated with genetic screening

Parents who would not consider termination may still benefit from genetic screening of their foetus because:

- it would allow necessary medical treatment to be available to the baby from birth;
- it would give the parents time to start coming to terms with the condition of the baby before the birth.

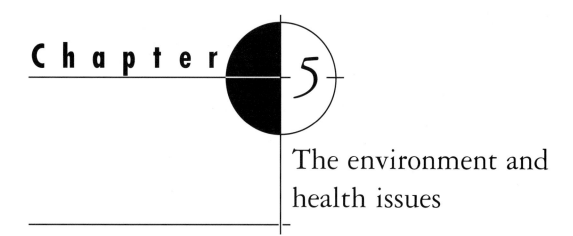

Chapter 5

The environment and health issues

This chapter covers:

- how some human activities cause harm to the environment and to people's health;
- strategies that have been developed to improve the environment;
- policies and legislation that have reduced the harmful effects of urbanisation;
- health and social care workers who are involved in environmental health issues.

Harmful effects of human activity on the environment and health

As populations increase, particularly in large towns and cities, pressures on the environment and citizens increase. There are issues surrounding basic needs such as shelter, food, warmth, security and accumulation of waste. Rural environments are also affected as the drive to produce more food to supply an ever-growing population becomes more intense. There are issues surrounding the use of fertilisers and pesticides, soil erosion and compaction, the destruction of wildlife habitats and pollution of the waterways.

Urbanisation and population density leading to overcrowding, poverty and waste accumulation

Urbanisation is the term used to describe the process where the proportion of people living in towns and cities increases. This may happen because:

- there is more migration from rural to urban areas than from urban to rural areas (Table 5.1 gives reasons for migration from rural to urban areas);
- life expectancy is greater in urban areas than rural areas;
- there is a higher birth rate in urban areas than rural areas.

Rapid urbanisation took place in the UK in the nineteenth century, but over the last century, the number of people living in cities in Economically More Developed Countries (EMDCs) has decreased. The numbers living in cities in Economically Less Developed Countries (ELDCs) is

Table 5.1 The push-pull model of migration

Push factors (factors driving people away from the countryside)		Pull factors (factors attracting people to the city)
Poor health care	→	Better health care
Poor education	→	Better education
Poor transport	→	Better transport
Low employment	→	Higher employment
Low wages	→	Higher wages
Irregular wages	→	More regular wages

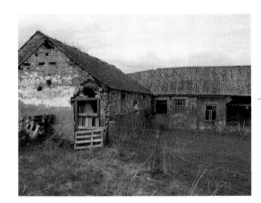 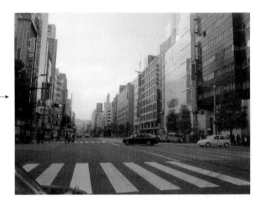

Table 5.2 The population of the world's ten largest cities in 1950, 1980 and 2000 (ELDC cities are given in italics) (Figures for 2000 are estimates) (From 'The Human Environment' Series Editor Bob Digby 1996 publ. Heinemann Fig. 3.1, page 59)

City	1950 (million)	City	1980 (million)	City	2000 (million)
New York	12.3	Tokyo	16.9	*Mexico City*	25.6
London	8.7	New York	15.6	*São Paulo*	22.1
Tokyo	6.7	*Mexico City*	14.5	Tokyo	19.0
Paris	5.4	*São Paulo*	21.1	*Shanghai*	17.0
Shanghai	5.3	*Shanghai*	11.7	New York	16.8
Buenos Aires	5.0	*Buenos Aires*	9.9	*Calcutta*	15.7
Chicago	4.9	Los Angeles	9.5	*Bombay*	15.4
Moscow	4.8	*Calcutta*	9.0	*Beijing*	14.0
Calcutta	4.4	*Beijing*	9.0	Los Angeles	13.9
Los Angeles	4.0	*Rio de Janeiro*	8.8	*Jakarta*	13.7

rapidly increasing. Table 5.2 shows the changes in populations in the world's ten largest cities in the past 50 years.

Activity

Look at Table 5.2. How many of the world's 10 largest cities were in ELDCs in:

a   1950

b   2000?

Globally, more people will be living in towns and cities than in the countryside by the year 2010. This increase in the urban population can lead to a number of problems which are described below.

Overcrowding

If there is a high level of migration into an urban area, there will not be adequate housing. People will have to resort to renting single rooms for a whole family, sleeping on the street or building their own shelters illegally on land they do not own. This latter option leads to the growth of **shanty towns** or **squatter settlements**. Every major city in ELDCs has these and in some urban regions up to 50% of the population live in these areas. When there is overcrowding sewage disposal is often inadequate, which leads to disease. Crime is a problem and there is likely to be insufficient education, health care or power supplies. The pressure on transport systems means that the roads become very congested.

However, a high population density does not necessarily lead to a lower standard of living. There are more people per unit area living in Chelsea, London, than there are in slums in Delhi, India.

Poverty

If there is a high level of migration into cities, it is likely that there will not be enough jobs available. This leads to poverty. It is difficult to define exactly what should be classed as poverty, but the following are sometimes used to identify the poor:

- insufficient food supply;
- low income worked out on a *per capita* (per person) basis;
- insufficient access to clean drinking water and sewage disposal;
- lack of access to primary health care facilities;
- low adult literacy rates.

Economic conditions deteriorated in ELDCs in the last decade because of the debt owed by these countries to other countries and recession. Generally this has had a greater effect on urban areas than rural areas. The price of food, water, energy and housing has increased, but inflation and unemployment have meant that real wages have fallen.

Waste accumulation

The amount of waste produced globally has increased. This is partly because of the increase in population and partly because of an increase in the buying of consumer products. The large amounts of packaging and the short life-span of many of these products has led to the expression, 'throwaway society'. The more wealthy a country is, the higher the waste production per person. In an urban environment waste accumulation becomes a particular problem because of the concentration of a large number of people in a comparatively small area.

Domestic waste

Domestic rubbish contains mostly plastics, organic material and paper. Disposal is vital as rubbish can be toxic and emit bad odours, and can become infested with flies and vermin. Bacteria will grow and some of these could cause disease.

Methods of waste disposal

- In many ELDCs a high proportion of the waste is disposed of in **rubbish dumps**.
- In EMDCs waste is put into **landfill** sites. The waste is spread in a layer and then covered with top soil. Table 5.3 shows the advantages and disadvantages of this method of waste disposal.
- Some countries **incinerate** their waste. In some cases the heat produced is used for energy production. However, poisonous substances may be released in the smoke. For example, if plastics are burnt at less than 900°C they release dioxins which are some of the most toxic substances known. There is often considerable local opposition to incinerators.
- One of the cheapest options of waste disposal is **dumping at sea**. However, there has been considerable opposition to this by environmental groups such as Greenpeace.

 # Activity

Walk around a supermarket.

- List the uses of packaging.
- Note down examples of products which could be classed as 'over-packaged' (i.e. there is an unnecessary amount of packaging)

Industrial waste

A vast quantity of industrial solid waste is produced every year in the UK. Most of this is dumped in pits or heaps. **Spoil heaps** consist of waste material from activities such as gravel extraction. These are unsightly but they do not present a direct threat to health. **Slag heaps** are the result of ore-digging and metal-refining activities, particularly from the mining of coal. These can contain toxic materials, such as metals, which may be leached into water supplies. Copper, zinc and cadmium are examples of toxic waste from mining operations. Vegetation is difficult to grow, and slag heaps can become unstable. The Aberafan disaster in Wales in 1966

Table 5.3 The advantages and disadvantages of disposing of waste in a landfill site

Advantages	Disadvantages
Cheap	Uses valuable land
Waste is hidden from view	Sites attract rats
Eventually the site can be landscaped and used for other purposes	Increase in traffic (delivery lorries)
Methane gas released in decomposition can be burnt to provide energy	Water draining through the site may become polluted and local water courses may become contaminated
	Methane gas may build up creating a fire risk
	The site may smell while rubbish is decomposing
	Subsidence may lead to problems in subsequent land use

occurred when a slag heap became destabilised by heavy rain and engulfed a school and houses, killing 116 children and 28 adults.

There are many toxic materials produced as waste by industrial processes. These pose difficult problems for safe disposal. There are special regulated disposal sites and treatment plants around the country, but accidents and problems with transport are not uncommon.

The following are some toxic wastes:

- cyanides;
- asbestos;
- organic solvents;
- acids;
- alkalines;
- metals;
- oils;
- tar;
- paint sludge;
- phenols.

The polluting effects on the environment can be great. Plants and animals are affected both on land and in water as the toxic material may reach rivers and then the sea.

The poisonous effects on humans are various. Examples include:

- Mercury which accumulates particularly in the kidney, liver and brain. Eventually paralysis and death occur.
- Asbestos fibres, which can be breathed in and can cause the destruction of lung tissues and cancer.

Toxic waste materials may also be flammable or explosive. Specialist treatment plants which render the toxic waste safe and incineration are both methods used to reduce contamination. However, some toxic waste is dumped without treatment. Sites for dumping include old mine shafts and marshy land. The contamination of underground water is a possible problem.

The impact of intensification of agriculture on environment and health

Intensive agriculture can be described as food production in which there are high inputs of capital and/or labour per unit area of land. Its aim is to produce high yields per unit area. Examples of intensive agriculture (Figure 5.1) include:

- the production of rice in the paddy fields of South East Asia;
- dairy farming;
- battery hen units (hens in small cages);
- market gardening.

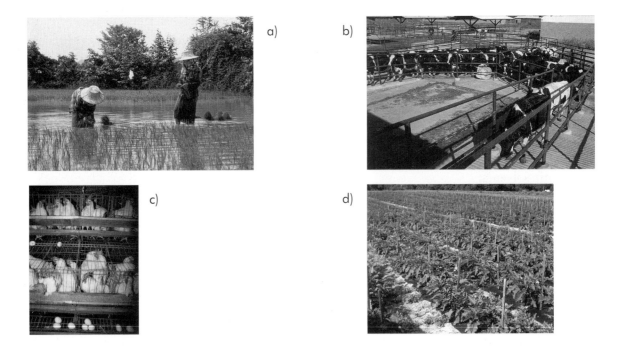

Figure 5.1 Examples of intensive agriculture: a) rice production in paddy fields in South East Asia b) dairy farming c) battery hen units d) market gardening

There are several reasons why there may be pressure on farmers to farm intensively, for example:

* land shortage;
* a high population density;
* a need to supply an urban population with highly perishable foods.

The advantage of intensive agriculture is that it should provide a plentiful supply of food, but there are a number of problems associated with it that can have a harmful effect on the rural environment and health. Some of these are described below.

The increased use of fertilisers

Fertilisers can be used to increase the supply of nutrients, such as nitrogen, to plants. This can increase their rate of growth and yield. As crops grow, they take up nutrients from the soil. When these crops are harvested, these nutrients are lost from the system and fertilisers can be used to replace them. Farmyard manure can be used as a fertiliser. This adds nitrogen and improves the structure of the soil. Inorganic chemicals, usually compounds containing nitrogen, potassium and phosphorous can also be used as fertiliser.

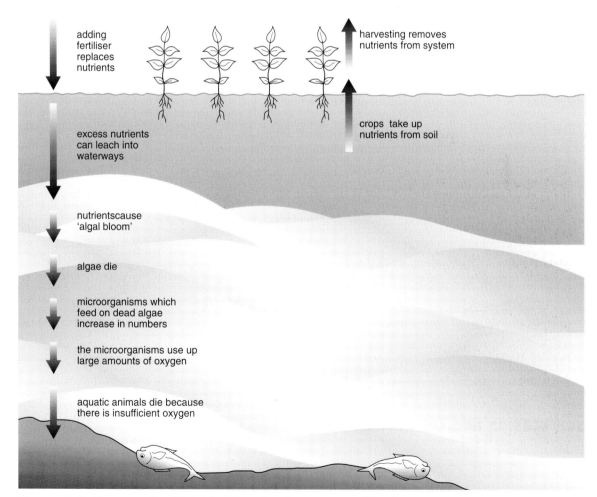

Figure 5.2 The use of artificial fertiliser leading to eutrophication

However, the application of excess fertiliser, either as manure or in an inorganic form, can lead to **eutrophication** (Figure 5.2). Nitrogen is leached out of the soil and then carried to lakes in water run off from the land. Once in the lake, the nitrogen causes an increase in algal growth that becomes so dense on the surface waters that light is unable to penetrate to the layers beneath. As a result, algae lower down in the water cannot photosynthesise and eventually die. Bacteria that decompose these dead algae multiply and use large amounts of oxygen in their activities, thus causing an increase in the **biological oxygen demand** (BOD). The oxygen level in the water is then severely depleted, and fish and other animals die. Anaerobic bacteria, which can thrive in the absence of oxygen, feed on the decaying material and produce ammonia, methane and hydrogen sulphide. This process is eutrification. The water is made unfit for most forms of life and is certainly not fit for human consumption. It is usually still bodies of water that undergo eutrophication, but this can also happen in short stretches of river and even in seas.

If there are very high levels of nitrogen in drinking water, this can cause 'blue-baby' syndrome. A baby who has this syndrome has blue lips and body and suffers from respiratory failure. There is also some evidence that high nitrate levels may cause stomach cancer.

The increased use of pesticides

A wide range of toxic chemicals are used to control or eradicate pests and weeds. Whilst helping to increase yield, these pesticides may have harmful effects. Pesticides decrease the number of species in an area (**biodiversity**). They may do this by actually killing a species or by affecting the food source of a species. For example, the number of grey partridges has dropped by approximately 80% over the past three decades partly because pesticides have killed off much of their food source in the fields and hedgerows where they breed.

There is a risk that a pesticide could be passed through food chains to humans. Some examples of pesticides include:

- Mercuric chloride: a fungicide used for dusting seeds. Mercury is toxic.
- Copper compounds: fungicides that are in general use. Copper is toxic.
- Sodium chlorate: a herbicide used to clear paths of weeds. Not very toxic.
- Organo-phosphorous compounds, e.g. Parathion: insecticides that are very toxic but not persistent. Can kill useful insects such as bees.
- Organo-chlorine compounds, e.g. DDT, dieldrin: these are insecticides. DDT is persistent and accumulates in food chains. It makes egg shells thin which led to a decline in the numbers of birds of prey. However, the phasing out of DDT has now led to a recovery in numbers.
- 2.4 D (dichlorophenoxyacetic acid and 2.4.5 T (trichlorophenoxyacetic acid). They attack broadleaved plants, leaving cereals to grow.

Soil erosion and compaction

Humans began to change the environment when they adopted agriculture as a way of life. Forest, woodland and scrub were cleared to provide the land required to grow enough food for the growing population.

Deforestation still goes on today. For example, vast tracts of tropical forest in the Amazon basin have been cleared in recent decades (Figure 5.3), and poor Brazilian families have been given financial inducements to settle as farmers in the cleared areas. The removal of vegetation exposes the soil to erosion by wind or water; in many of these areas tropical storms have washed away most of the bare soil that had previously been held in place by tree roots.

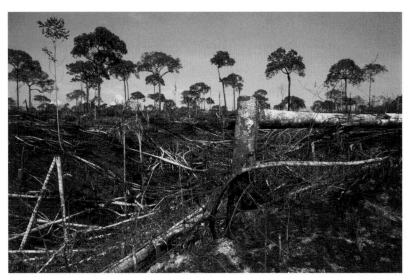

Figure 5.3 Deforestation in Brazil

Soil erosion is now world-wide. The Yellow River in China is so called because its colour comes from soil washed away from the surrounding land. In dry areas the wind has eroded soil from farmland, creating dust storms – this occurred in the USA in the 1930s. Wind and rain have also caused erosion in North Africa, where goats and cattle have over-grazed the vegetation for centuries.

Destruction of wildlife habitats

We have seen that in many parts of the world **forests** have been removed to provide land for agriculture. Wetlands have been drained for the same reason and, as a result, fens and bogs have disappeared. In the UK East Anglia is an example of this.

Intensive methods of farming require large machines such as combine harvesters to work efficiently and so **hedgerows** have been removed to allow extra space. The large fields created are used to raise **monocultures**, that is, crops of a single species such as wheat.

This destruction of habitats and production of monocultures has led to a decrease in the number of species of wild plants and animals.

- In the last 30 years there have been alarming declines in populations of a number of **birds**. Common birds such as the skylark, song thrush, grey partridge and tree sparrow have declined by over half in a very short period of time, and have completely disappeared from some areas.
- **Mammal species**, such as the brown hare and pipistrelle bat, have also undergone serious declines.

- There have been declines in the numbers of over 700 **invertebrate species** such as insects and spiders.
- A number of **plant species** have declined, and in some cases, disappeared altogether.

Pollution of waterways

Over half the prosecutions in the UK for the serious pollution of rivers are now against farmers. Certain products of modern farming are particularly to blame:

- **Slurry** is the heavy liquid excrement from poultry, cattle or pigs kept indoors. This is kept in storage tanks for safe disposal but leakage may contaminate rivers.
- **Silage** is grass cut while still green and left to ferment, often in silos. It is used as animal feed. It creates a highly acid liquid effluent which can be very toxic if it pollutes water ways.
- **Fertilisers** can cause eutrophication (see page 230).

Pollution

The effect of human activities on the environment is proportional to the size of the human population, which is increasing at the rate of about 100,000,000 each year. The waste products that result from these activities are often added to the environment at a rate faster than it can accommodate. Sometimes these products are substances that are already naturally present in the environment, but we call then **pollutants** if they reach critical levels and if they are potentially harmful to life. Waste products that are potential pollutants can be in solid, liquid or gaseous form. But waste does not always consist of **materials**: forms of energy such as sound, heat and radioactive particles can be pollutants as well.

It is convenient to divide the environment into air, water and land to investigate pollution, but all parts of the environment are linked, and a substance produced as a waste product from a process on land may pollute both air and water.

Air pollution

The **atmosphere** is a layer around the earth of approximately 2000km. Most of this layer comprises the **stratosphere**. The **trophosphere** extends 8km above the earth, and the proportions of gases in it are as follows:

Nitrogen	78.08%
Oxygen	20.96%
Argon	0.93%
Carbon dioxide	0.03%

There are also variable amounts of carbon monoxide, ammonia, methane, helium, krypton, sulphur dioxide, hydrogen sulphide and nitric and nitrous oxides. These are present as part of natural recycling processes.

Table 5.4 The health effects of vehicle pollution

Pollutant	Source	Health effect
Nitrogen dioxide (NO_2)	One of the nitrogen oxides emitted in vehicle exhaust	May exacerbate asthma and possibly increase susceptibility to infections
Sulphur dioxide (SO_2)	Mostly produced by burning coal. Some SO_2 is emitted by diesel vehicles	May provoke wheezing and exacerbate asthma. It is also associated with chronic bronchitis
Particulates PM10, total suspended particulates, black smoke	Includes a wide range of solid and liquid particles in air. Those less than 10 µm in diameter (PM10) penetrate the lung fairly efficiently and are most hazardous to health. Diesel vehicles produce proportionally more particulates than petrol vehicles	Associated with a wide range of respiratory symptoms. Long-term exposure is associated with an increased risk of death from heart and lung disease. Particulates can carry carcinogenic materials into the lungs
Acid aerosols	Airborne acid formed from common pollutants including sulphur and nitrogen oxides	May exacerbate asthma and increase susceptibility to respiratory infection. May reduce lung function in those with asthma
Carbon monoxide (CO)	Comes mainly from petrol car exhaust	Lethal at high doses. At low doses, can impair concentration and neuro-behavioural function. Increases the likelihood of exercise-related heart pain in people with coronary heart disease. May present a risk to the foetus
Ozone (O_1)	Secondary pollutant produced from nitrogen oxides and volatile organic compounds in the air	Irritates the eyes and air passages. Increases the sensitivity of the airways to allergic triggers in people with asthma. May increase susceptibility to infection
Lead	Compound present in leaded petrol to help the engine run smoothly	Impairs the normal intellectual development and learning ability of children
Volatile organic compounds (VOCs)	A group of chemicals emitted from the evaporation of solvents and distribution of petrol fuel. Also present in vehicle exhaust	Benzene has given most cause for concern in this group of chemicals. It is a cancer-causing agent which can cause leukaemia at higher doses than are present in the normal environment
Polycyclic aromatic hydrocarbons (PAHs)	Produced by the incomplete combustion of fuel. PAHs become attached to particulates	Includes a complex range of chemicals, some of which are carcinogens. It is likely that exposure to PAHs in traffic exhaust poses a low cancer risk to the general population
Asbestos	May be present in brake pads and clutch linings, especially in heavy-duty vehicles. Asbestos fibres and dust are released into the atmosphere when vehicles brake	Asbestos can cause lung cancer and mesothelioma, cancer of the lung lining. The consequences of the low levels of exposure from braking vehicles are not known

Source 'How vehicle pollution affects our health', Dr C. Read (ed.) London Symposium of 20 May 1994, supported by the Ashden Trust

Burning fossil fuel in the home, in industry and in internal-combustion engines (Table 5.4) has altered the proportions of atmospheric natural gases. New technology has added new gases to the atmosphere that are destroying the ozone layer (in the stratosphere). The ozone layer is important because it absorbs ultraviolet and infra-red radiation and thus prevents damage to living organisms from this radiation. Ultraviolet rays can cause mutations and infra-red rays can cause an increase in body temperature.

Children are particularly susceptible to air pollution, partly because of their large lung surface area: body volume ratio, which is a factor of their small size.

Asthma is a condition resulting largely from air pollution, particularly traffic emissions.

Some asthma facts:

- Asthma affects 1 in 7 children.
- It is the most important cause of emergency hospital admissions.
- Respiratory diseases account for a third of children's GP visits.
- Asthma accounts for 1 in 20 childhood deaths.
- Hospital admissions for childhood asthma have increased 13-fold since the early 1960s.

Smoke and other particles

Smoke comprises very small particles of carbon. Larger particles include soot and ash. These are produced by burning coal and oil, and are released into the air. Smoke can affect the alveoli of the lungs by damaging their epithelial linings. It causes respiratory problems and aggravates bronchitis. It can reduce light intensity at ground level and lower the rate of photosynthesis in plants, which may be even further decreased if there are deposits of soot coating leaves and blocking stomata, thereby preventing gaseous exchange.

Tiny particles of pollutants that measure less than 250 micrometers in diameter (**microparticles**) and come mainly from the engines of diesel vehicles, may be responsible for perhaps tens of thousands of premature deaths a year in the UK. They are now regarded as the most life-threatening form of air pollution. It is thought that the particles are small enough to slip through the normal defence mechanisms in the lungs.

Sulphur dioxide

Sulphur dioxide is released into the air both when fossil fuels are burnt and during the smelting of ores. It is normally present in concentrations of 0.3–1.0 µg m^{-3}, and is produced both by volcanoes and from other natural processes. In industrial areas it can reach a concentration of 3,000 µg m^{-3}. Sulphur dioxide is oxidised to sulphate ions in the air. When it returns to the earth in rain, it can enrich deficient soils, and plants can take up the sulphates through their roots. However, sulphur dioxide in air is mostly damaging to plants as it combines with water to form **sulphurous** and **sulphuric acid**. This is then precipitated as 'acid rain', so called because it is rain with a low pH. This damages trees and kills life in lakes. The most damage has occurred in Scandinavia since the prevailing winds carry the sulphur dioxide from the UK and the rest of Europe to that area. (Figure 5.5 shows conifers with acid-rain damage.)

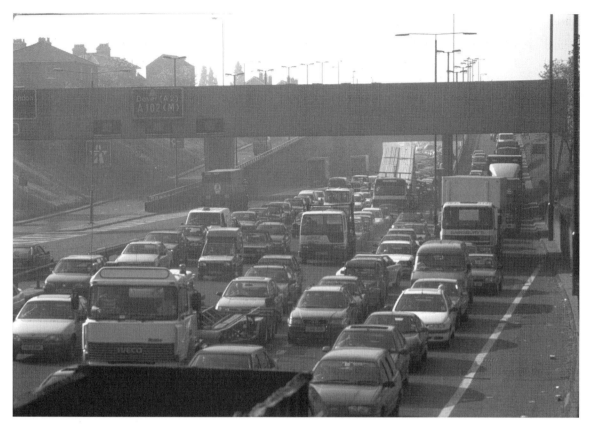

Figure 5.4 A health threat: the increase in traffic emissions

The human respiratory system also is affected by sulphur dioxide: extra mucus is produced by the goblet cells in the linings of the bronchi and bronchioles. Also, the cilia stop beating and are now no longer able to remove the mucus with the particles and bacteria it contains (normally, this is constantly removed from the lungs). This mucus then prevents gaseous exchange occurring in the alveoli where the epithelial linings can also be damaged.

Bronchial conditions can result from an exposure to sulphur dioxide. Figure 5.6 shows the effects of sulphur dioxide on the respiratory system.

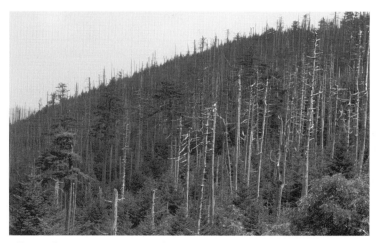

Figure 5.5 The effect of acid rain on conifer trees in North Carolina

Smog

Smog occurs in special environmental conditions that cause fog to remain static and hang over an area. In a large urban area where fossil fuels are being burnt, smoke and sulphur dioxide are produced. These pollutants then become trapped in the fog, causing damp and dirty smog. These were common in London in the 1950s. In 1952 there was an especially bad one, during which there were many deaths (see Table 5.5). This was the trigger for the modern air-pollution-control legislation.

Table 5.5 The health effects of sulphur dioxide and smoke in December 1952 during the London smog

Date in December	Deaths per day	Smoke µg/m^{-3} air	Sulphur dioxide µg/m^{-3}
1	250	200	350
2	260	300	400
3	300	400	620
4	260	350	520
5	325	1,100	1,000
6	600	1,600	1,520
7	875	1,700	1,850
8	900	1,580	2,000
9	850	1,000	1,500
10	600	300	350
11	550	200	360
12	500	200	350
13	520	300	350
14	450	300	375
15	400	250	350

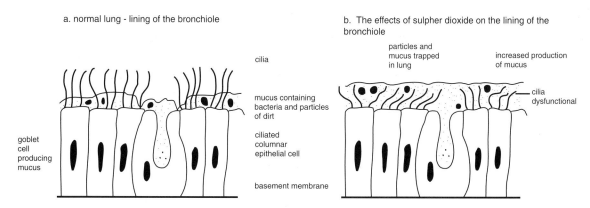

a. normal lung - lining of the bronchiole

cilia

mucus containing
bacteria and particles
of dirt

ciliated
columnar
epithelial cell

goblet
cell
producing
mucus

basement membrane

b. The effects of sulpher dioxide on the lining of the
bronchiole

particles and
mucus trapped
in lung

increased production
of mucus

cilia
dysfunctional

Figure 5.6 The effects of sulphur dioxide on the respiratory system

Activity

Look at the data in Table 5.5. Illustrate this in graphical form, and then answer the following question:

What conclusions can be drawn from the data?

(See page 287 for answer)

Carbon dioxide

The burning of fossil fuels such as coal, oil and natural gas releases carbon dioxide. Data collected from different sites around the world shows that the level of this gas has been steadily increasing.

Carbon dioxide is known as a 'greenhouse gas' as it enables the atmosphere to absorb the earth's heat and re-radiate it back to earth. If it were not for this 'greenhouse effect', the earth would be too cold to sustain life. However, if the level of carbon dioxide increases too much, then too much global warming could result (Figure 5.7).

Other greenhouse gases and ozone depletion

Other greenhouse gases include:
- chlorofluorocarbons (CFCs) from aerosol sprays, refrigerators and bubbles in plastic foams;
- methane from bacterial activities and the use of natural gas;
- nitrous oxide from fertilisers;
- ozone from car-exhaust fumes.

CFCs are also responsible for destroying ozone in the stratosphere. There are now holes in the ozone layer over the Arctic and Antarctic. As a result, damaging ultraviolet and infrared light can come

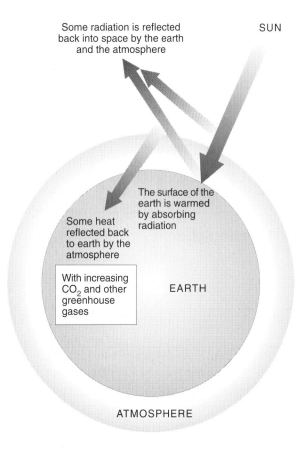

Figure 5.7 The greenhouse effect

through. This causes skin cancer in humans, and damages plant and marine life. There are now signs, however, that the reduction in the use of CFCs since 1987 means that the hole in the ozone layer is starting to shrink.

Carbon monoxide

Carbon monoxide occurs in car-exhaust fumes and cigarette smoke. It has an affinity for haemoglobin which is 250 times greater than that of oxygen. It forms a stable compound with haemoglobin and prevents oxygen combining with it.

Nitrogen oxides

Nitrogen oxides, such as nitrogen dioxide and nitric oxide, are produced by the burning of fuel in car engines, and are emitted in car exhausts. They can combine with other chemicals in sunlight and form **peroxyacyl nitrates** (PANS) that result in photochemical smogs. These nitrogen-containing gases are all very poisonous, and cause breathing difficulties.

Lead

This is the most serious heavy-metal pollutant in the atmosphere. The lead in car-exhaust fumes accounts for 80% of this. It is added to petrol as **tetraethyl lead** (TEL), which serves as an anti-knock compound, and it comes out as **lead chlorobromide**. There is an increasing worry about lead affecting the brains of children. Lead is also taken into the body in food, and it is possible that the lead that contaminated the food originally came from car exhausts.

Activity

TEST THE AIR

1 The card test

You can check levels of air pollution in your area with a 'white-card test'. Obtain four pieces of white card (each 15cm²) with at least one shiny side. Number the cards 1 to 4 and smear the shiny side of each with a thin layer of Vaseline.

- Leave Card 1 indoors.
- Leave Card 2 near a busy road.
- Leave Card 3 in a garden or your school grounds.
- Leave Card 4 underneath a tree.

Stand each card upright with the Vaseline side facing outwards. Secure the cards with string or sticky tape and make a note of the time, date and place you left them. After three or four days, fetch the cards and compare each with Card 1 to decide which is the dirtiest. Most air pollution is caused by cars and factories. This may help to explain your results.

Using the white-card test, it is easy to make a pollution map of your area. Simply draw a local map, or take a copy of a printed one, and mark the places where you left cards using different colours to represent the level of pollution.

A quicker way to test for pollution in public areas is gently to wipe some dirt from a surface – a park bench, for example – with a clean, damp piece of cotton wool. Wipe the surface only once and place the cotton wool in a clear polythene bag. Remember to use a new piece of cotton wool for each test and to keep a record of your tests in order to compare the dirtiness of the samples. You could use colours on your pollution map to show different levels of pollution.

2   Leaf-washing

Leaves in badly polluted areas often appear covered in soot and grime. This can be a problem because plants need sunlight in order to make food. The sunlight falling on the leaves may be blocked out if they are covered with too much dirt.

When the weather is dry, you can investigate this problem further with a 'leaf washing test'. Collect a filter paper and funnel, jamjar, pencil, clean paintbrush and notepad, and half-fill the jam jar with water. Identify some leaves to wash: the best ones to choose are those on plants, trees, bushes or hedges that do not lose their leaves in winter.

a)   Choose a leaf which is neither too high nor too near the ground. Dip it into the water and gently wash both sides using the paintbrush. Try not to remove the leaf from the plant.

b)   Now repeat the process with 14 more leaves.

c)   Pour the dirty water through the filter paper. When the water has drained away, remove the filter paper and allow it to dry.

The dirt that you have washed from the leaves will be left on the paper. You could repeat the leaf-washing test to compare plants growing in different places, such as near a busy road or in your school grounds. Be careful when you are collecting leaves on or near roads. Add your results to your pollution map. (Note: It is only a fair test if you use plants with leaves of similar size.)

Adapted from *The Guardian*, 14 May 1991

Water pollution

Pure water rarely exists naturally: rainwater absorbs chemicals as it passes through the air; water that runs into rivers carries with it materials that have been leached from the soil; and as rivers flow towards the sea, organic matter and silt are picked up. The sea itself contains salt, other minerals and organic materials. Many additives are therefore natural products. Often, though, materials in quite high concentrations are released directly or indirectly into water as the result of human activity, and these additives are considered as pollutants. (The problems of acid rain were discussed on page 235.) Domestic, industrial and agricultural effluents are released into rivers and seas. These include sewage, toxic chemicals and farm wastes.

Activity

1   Design a poster to show the natural water cycle, including rain, rivers and the seas. Show the role both of vegetation and of the human removal and return of water. When you have read this section on water pollution, you can add the sources of human pollution to your poster.

2   List at least eight uses of water by humans. Remember that each individual in the UK uses about 150 litres of water a day for domestic use alone.

Why we need clean water

Humans need water for a wide variety of uses. It must be clean, and not be contaminated with pollutants, in order to prevent infectious disease and poisoning. Water-borne disease-causing organisms include various parasitic worms and also **protozoa** such as *Entamoeba histolytica*, which causes **amoebic dysentery**. **Pathogenic bacteria** carried in water may cause intestinal infections, and more serious diseases such as cholera and typhoid. Many pathogenic viruses are carried in water, e.g., the **poliomyelitis** virus. In the Third World, over 4 million children die a year from drinking unclean water, mainly because it is contaminated with pathogens.

Toxic chemicals in industrial waste are common pollutants of water. These are poisonous to humans as well as to aquatic flora and fauna. They may enter humans directly, in water, or they may be in our food. Chemicals such as heavy metals accumulate in food chains and become concentrated in organisms that we eat, such as fish.

Animals and plants that live in water are in balance, and rely on each other to remain alive. Plants capture the energy from the sun via photosynthesis to make nutrients, some of which will feed animals. There is a balance of oxygen and carbon dioxide brought about through the processes of respiration and photosynthesis. Both organic and inorganic pollutants upset this balance, and ecosystems will be damaged. In some cases of pollution, the relative levels of plants, animals and decomposers change, and the death of most of the plants and animals involved will eventually occur. This is not only a serious environmental consequence: in addition, the water will be rendered unacceptable for use by humans.

Purification is carried out before water is used, but although the treatment can remove organic waste and some bacterial contamination, it cannot cope with heavy chemical pollution.

Industrial pollutants

Water pollution by industrial waste can reach water either directly or indirectly, leached from landfill waste deposits. Examples include:

1 Mercury can be changed to **dimethyl mercury**, a neurotoxin. This accumulates in marine food chains and becomes concentrated in fish. When this is then eaten by humans, it concentrates in the kidneys, liver and brain. It can cause paralysis, numbness, convulsions and blindness, and even death. In Japan in the 1950s, there was a mercury poisoning incident in which over 160 people died.

2 Lead is taken into humans via air, food and water. It concentrates in the liver, kidneys and bones. There is evidence that it can cause mental retardation.

3 Aluminium poisoning causes many symptoms. It is thought that Alzheimer's disease may be linked to aluminium in water, taken in over a long period.

In 1988 there was an incident in Camelford, Cornwall, when 20 tonnes of aluminium sulphate was accidentally poured into the town's water supplies instead of into a special tank for the storage of toxic chemicals. In 2001, because of the number of complaints from local residents, an inquiry into the long-term health effects was announced.

Sewage

Sewage-treatment works exist throughout the country to deal with sewage before it is released into water courses. However, leakage, overflow and general inefficiency causes sewage to enter rivers. In some parts of the country untreated sewage is still released directly into the sea. Sewage does eventually break down, but if too much enters the water at one time, bacteria present in the sewage reduces oxygen to a low level, causing aquatic wildlife to suffer. Eutrophication can occur in stretches of a river below the outfall where the sewage comes in.

Even where sewage is treated successfully, large quantities of sludge are still left behind. This can be dumped on land and is sometimes used as fertiliser, though this is not always possible because it can contain high levels of toxic heavy metals such as lead, if industrial waste is processed along with domestic waste at the sewage works. Some sludge is taken to the sea and dumped under government licence. Sludge can be digested to release methane, which can be used to make electricity, but this process is not very common.

For water pollution from farming, see page 232.

Marine pollution

Sea water moves continuously, and pollutants can be carried away and dispersed provided they are not too concentrated. Polluting effects are more likely in shallow, enclosed seas where eutrophication can occur as a result of sewage or fertiliser pollution.

Organochloride insecticides are thought to be responsible for the decline in marine predatory birds such as the herring gull, osprey and brown pelican. DDT (dichlorodiphenyl-trichloroethane) is such an insecticide, and it can be concentrated by as much as 70,000 times in oysters – as little as 0.001ppm can reduce their growth. DDT concentrates in the tissues in predatory birds at the top of the food chain and reduces their reproductive capacity.

Oil pollution is also a hazard: up to 10 million tonnes of crude oil are released annually into the sea. Sometimes there are large spillages. Examples include the *Torrey Canyon*, which went aground off Land's End in 1967; the *Amoco Cadiz*, which foundered off the coast of France in 1978; the big disaster of the *Braer*, which released 85,000 tonnes of oil off the Shetlands; and the *Sea Empress* disaster, in which over 70,000 tonnes of crude oil seeped into the Pembrokeshire sea. The worst casualties are the fish-eating birds: the birds settle off the slick of oil and their feathers become clogged. Seaweeds, molluscs and crustaceans are also killed by oil.

Heat

The thermal pollution of rivers and lakes occurs when hot water is released from the cooling processes of electricity generation in power stations. Water is discharged at a temperature 10–15°C higher than when it was removed from the river or lake. Since most aquatic organisms live within a fairly narrow range of temperatures, this can have the effect of favouring warm-water species at the expense of cold-water ones. Coarse fish such as roach and perch may replace salmon and trout. Plant growth is also affected by warm water. The number of algae may increase leading to eutrophication (see page 230).

Detergents

Back in the 1950s, detergents with synthetic ingredients (derived from petroleum) caused banks of foam to float down rivers and streams. The problem largely went away when the detergent manufacturers changed to biodegradable products. However, detergents still contain phosphates as a water-softening agent, and such detergents enter rivers in domestic sewage and industrial waste. Eutrophication is a result.

Activity

Measuring pollution

1   Is your river polluted? Experiments to test the purity of river water.

One way to measure the purity of a water sample is to find out how much dissolved oxygen is present: the more pollution, the less oxygen. Organic matter can enter water in sewage or farm waste pollution. We have seen that bacteria use up the oxygen in water as they decompose organic matter. Because organic matter provides food for bacteria, its presence will stimulate their growth. Therefore, the levels of oxygen present are related to the amounts of polluting organic matter present. Low levels of oxygen indicate high levels of polluting organic matter and bacteria.

Collect samples of water to be tested in 500cm³ bottles. For example, you could collect samples from a river at points above and below a sewage outfall or near a farm. Collect two bottles full of water at each collection site.

(N B Ensure that all the possible safety hazards are considered before you start work.)

a The measurement of biological oxygen demand (BOD)

The BOD is defined as the amount of dissolved oxygen, in grammes per cubic metre, taken out of solution by a sample over five days at 20°C. It can be measured using a dissolved oxygen electrode or oxygen meter. Take measurements as soon as you bring your samples back into the laboratory. Then, store the samples in the dark at 20°C for five days. Repeat the measurements. Calculate the differences in oxygen levels in your two measurements, and work out the BOD of the samples. Is there any difference in the samples you have collected? Can you explain any differences? (Sewage effluent should not exhibit a BOD of more than $20g/m^{3}$ over five days. The BOD of the river water below the sewage effluent outfall should not be more than $4g/m^{-3}$.)

b The methylene blue test to indicate oxygen levels

This is a simpler test, and can be carried out if you have not got access to an oxygen meter. Methylene blue is added to a water sample. The solution remains blue if there is a high level of oxygen but will go colourless with low levels of oxygen.

Pipette $50cm^3$ quantities from each of your samples into suitable-sized flasks or bottles which can be corked. Add $5cm^3$ methylene blue and incubate the bottles at 20°C for five days. Observe the colour changes over these five days. In clean water with a high-dissolved oxygen content, little polluting organic matter and few bacteria, the methylene blue will retain its blue colour over the five days. This water can be said to have passed the stability test. Where water has a high organic content, on the other hand, bacteria will thrive and use up the oxygen, and the blue colour will disappear more rapidly.

2 How clean is your stream?

You will need:

- hand net;
- white tray;
- hand lens;
- wide-mouthed pipette;
- petri dishes and specimen tubes;
- record sheet;

- key to freshwater animals.

Method

Divide into pairs and take different parts of the stream to study. Look carefully to see if there is any effluent running into it. Record exactly where your samples will be taken. Using the hand net, take 10 samples from the water. Sweep close to the bottom of the stream. You will probably collect mud and debris as well as samples of small freshwater animals. Tip all the samples into the tray. You can take the animals out and put them into petri dishes with the pipettes for identification.

Results

Look carefully at your samples and count the numbers of each species. Compare the results with the following tables of species able to live in very poor, poor, moderate or only very clean water.

Animals found only in very clean water:

- mayfly larvae;
- freshwater shrimps;
- flatworms;
- frogs;
- stonefly larvae;
- caddis larvae;
- newts;
- toads.

Animals tolerating water of moderate quality:

- spire-shell nail;
- orb shell;
- damselfly larvae;
- beetles;
- fish;
- ramshorn snail;
- pea shell;
- greater waterboatman;
- beetle larvae.

Animals tolerating poor-quality water (recovering from pollution):

- other pond snails;
- alderfly larvae;
- water flea;
- pond skater;
- waterlouse;
- lesser waterboatman;
- leech;
- pond measurer.

Animals found in water of very poor quality (polluted):

- sludge worm;
- cranefly larvae;
- midge larvae.

Collect all the class results together and decide what conclusions you can come to. Prepare an exhibition of your findings.

Land pollution

See pages 226–8 on 'Industrial waste' and pages 314–6 in Chapter 6 on 'Nuclear waste'.

What are sound and noise?

Sound and noise are really the same phenomenon. Noise can be defined as an unwanted sound. We detect sound using our ears. We are sensitive to changes in sounds in our environment, and we are able to react in an appropriate way. We can communicate with each other through sound and also recognise and react to dangerous sounds. These are only two examples of the importance of sound in our lives.

Sound levels

Sound is caused by a change in air pressure that is detected by the ear and registered in the brain. Normal atmospheric pressure is at about 100,000 newtons per metre.[2] The ear is a very sensitive detector, and registers a pressure change of only 0.00001 N/m^2 as a very quiet sound. Pressure changes as great as 1,000 N/m^2, on the other hand, are recognised as a loud sound, and very loud sounds can damage ears. A special way of indicating sound levels has had to be devised because the ear can detect such a very great range of pressure changes. Sound levels are given in decibels (dB) – see Figure 5.8 for some examples.

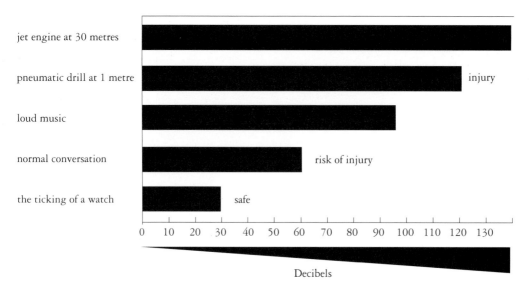

Figure 5.8 Comparative noise levels

Since the decibel scale is based on logarithms, a sound of 60 dB is not twice as loud as a sound of 30 dB: it is very much louder. Very roughly, a sound increase of 10 dB is heard by the ear as a sound about twice as loud. If there is one sound of 30 dB and another of 60 dB, then the 60 dB sound is very approximately $2 \times 2 \times 2 = 8$ times louder than the 30 dB sound.

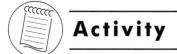

Activity

1 Discuss reasons (other than the two examples given above) why it is important for humans to be able to respond to sounds.

Noise pollution

Sound is required for human life. However, unwanted sounds or noise can be a health hazard. It is for this reason that noise can be considered as a form of pollution.

Look at Table 5.6. This shows which sounds will not cause damage to hearing (0–80 dB) and which sounds are in the danger range (90–110 dB). These louder sounds can cause permanent damage and deafness if exposure is over a long period. The effect on hearing is greater, the longer the exposure to the loud noise. 140 dB is at the threshold of pain. Really loud sounds can cause physical damage: 190 dB will cause rupture of the eardrums and damage the ossicles. On the other hand, low-intensity sounds that are not likely to cause damage to hearing may nonetheless be psychologically damaging and cause stress. Then there can be tiredness, loss of concentration and even sickness. At work, a lack of concentration could cause accidents.

Table 5.6 The sound intensity level (dB) for selected sources

db	Source	
140	Jet engine (at 25 m)	
130	Rivet gun	Injurious range
120	Propeller aircraft (at 50 m)	
110	Road drill	
100	Metal-working shop/foundry	Danger range
80–90	Heavy lorry	
80	Busy street	
60–70	Private car	
60	Ordinary conversation (at 1 m)	
50	Low conversation (at 1 m)	Safe range
40	Soft music	
30	Whisper (at 1 m)	
20	Quiet town dwelling	
10	Rustling leaf	

Some of the main noise 'polluters' are aircraft, motor vehicles, greatly amplified music and many types of machinery, including factory and domestic appliances. There is evidence that noise in the workplace can cause damage to hearing.

Noise maps produced by the Council for the Protection of Rural England show that there are very few tranquil areas remaining in England. With forecasts of huge traffic increases in the next 20 years, the noise levels are set to increase further.

Activity

Read the extract below from an article from The *Financial Times*, 9 July 1998.

- What health problems associated with excess noise are mentioned?
- What suggestions are given for preventing these harmful effects?

Noise Pollution

Source *The Financial Times*, 9 July, 1998

Noise, the combined cacophony of industry and transport, not to mention people and their toys, is one of the most serious environmental problems after air and water pollution. As well as upping blood pressure, increasing heart problems, causing headaches and ruining concentration, noise causes up to one-fifth of all hearing impairment in industrialised nations.

The World Health Organisation calculates that job-related hearing loss is the largest single compensatable illness in the world. In the UK, where it costs an estimated £35 per worker per year to meet EU standards, there are around 1,200 new cases of permanent occupational deafness each year and nearly 200,000 people suffer from work-related conditions such as tinnitus and temporary hearing loss.

Education, ear protectors and strictly policed environmental noise standards can have a considerable impact on incidence of hearing loss arising from long-term exposure to sounds of between 85 decibels (city traffic) and 120 dB (chain saw).

Homelessness

Homeless people may be housed in hotel or bed and breakfast accommodation by their local authority. However, in practice, many people either do not approach their local authority or are turned away by them. These individuals or families, who do not appear in official statistics, may be helped by voluntary organisations such as Shelter or may end up living rough.

Families living in hotels are often overcrowded, with poor access to cooking facilities. If they have to move from one bed and breakfast establishment to another, children will be disadvantaged as their education will be disrupted as they move from school to school. Homeless people are not able to register with a GP unless they have a postal address. The homeless are up to 25 times more likely to die than the average citizen, and are more likely to suffer from both physical and mental illnesses.

Every year, as many as 40,000 children run away from home or care. Research by National Children's Home Action for Children found that between 5% and 10% of these are likely to be harmed by being involved in activities such as drugs and sexual abuse and prostitution.

Strategies to improve the environment

There are a number of national and local strategies to prevent further decline in the environment. A number of these are described below.

- specialist treatments to reduce harm to the environment;
- the control of water pollution;
- the organisations responsible.

The **Department of the Environment, Food and Rural Affairs (DEFRA)** is the government department responsible for all aspects of water policy, including water supply and resources, and the regulatory systems for the water environment and the water industry. These cover:

- drinking water quality
- the quality of water in rivers lakes and estuaries
- coastal and marine waters
- sewage treatment
- reservoir safety

DEFRA works closely with the **Environment Agency**. This was set up under the **Environment Act 1995** to bring together the functions of the National Rivers Authority, Her Majesty's Inspectorate of Pollution and the waste regulation functions of local authorities. This public body employs more than 10,000 staff and is the most important environmental regulator in England and Wales. Its pollution work covers:

- land quality;
- pollution prevention and control;
- responding to pollution incidents;
- radioactive substances regulation;

- waste management;
- water quality.

The ten water and sewerage companies and the 15 water only companies in England and Wales (often known as the 'Water Industry') are responsible for the supply of drinking water and the collection, treatment and disposal of sewage. **The Office of Water Services (OFWAT)** is the regulator responsible for making sure that they provide an efficient, reliable service, for which customers pay a fair price.

The **European Union (EU)** consists of 15 member states who are responsible for deciding on legislation drafted by the **European Commission (EC)**. The **European Parliament** also has powers to influence European legislation.

Legislation

The **Environmental Protection Act 1990** controls many aspects of environment protection. In addition, the **Water Resources Act 1991** consolidated previous water legislation in respect of both the quality and quantity of water resources. There are various regulations linked to this Act that relate to specific water-pollution problems. One example is a regulation which allows areas to be designated as nitrate sensitive and the entry of nitrates into the water in these areas can then be controlled by law. Industrialists, farmers and others who cause pollution are given advice from water inspectors from The Environment Agency. If they do not respond, they may be prosecuted under the Water Resources Act 1991.

The **Water Industry Act 1991** consolidated legislation relating to the supply of water and the provision of sewerage services. As well as establishing the Environment Agency, the **Environment Act 1995** introduced measures to enhance the protection of the environment, including further powers for the prevention and remediation of water pollution.

Many quality standards are set at a European level. For example, the EC Nitrate Directive requires member states to reduce the nitrate pollution in water that arises from agricultural inputs, and the EC Dangerous Substances Directive requires control of inputs of dangerous substances into water.

Water treatments

In order to maintain clean rivers and to prevent the spread of disease, it is necessary to have:

- a source of clean water for domestic, industrial and agricultural purposes;
- an effective sewage disposal system.

A clean water supply

Companies who supply water are called 'water undertakers', and they have to conform to the rules in the Water Industries Act 1991 to make sure that the water is clean and pure. This Act states that it is the duty of a water undertaker to develop and maintain an efficient and economical system of water supply in its area. Water must be taken to premises requiring it, and mains and service pipes must be provided. Furthermore, water must be laid on constantly, in sufficient quantity and with enough pressure to reach every site. There are powers to prohibit the use of water for watering gardens or washing cars if a deficiency of water is threatened.

The water provided must be of good quality, wholesome and without contamination. There are regulations about the permitted levels of substances in the water. The fluoridation of water is permitted when a health authority has requested this as a measure to promote dental health. Water taken from a river, reservoir or underground aquifer undergoes treatment before it is pumped to users through mains and service pipes.

Regulations exist relating to payment and the powers to disconnect (Water Industry Act 1999).

The stages in water treatment

The various stages of water treatment involve the following elements of equipment:

1 **Primary grid.** This prevents large objects from the river entering the system.
2 **Settlement tank.** Water is pumped here to allow large particles and debris to drop out.
3 **Filter beds.** These vary in type. Some are *slow* sand filters that rely on a gelatinous film, which develops on the sand. It is produced by millions of protozoa and other micro-organisms which live on the sand. This filter will trap bacteria which provide food for the protozoa. *Rapid* sand filters are similar in principle, but the jelly is artificial and made from aluminium oxide.
4 **Contact tank.** This is where chlorination takes place. Any remaining bacteria are killed. The amount of chlorine added depends on the number of bacteria present, and may vary. The chlorine itself is destroyed as it kills the bacteria, and water companies must be careful not to add too much chlorine so that there is a surplus.
5 **Storage tanks.** The water is stored until required and then pumped to users through the mains supply.

Activity

Arrange a visit to a local water-treatment works. Write a report on your visit. In the report, include a flow diagram of the processes involved in the treatment of water in your area. Do the processes differ from the one outlined above?

Sewage treatment

The Water Industry Act 1991 is also concerned with the provision of sewerage systems. In this Act, sewerage undertakers are required to maintain a system of public sewers and sewage-disposal works. There are regulations about the quality of sewage effluents which can be discharged into rivers. Provision is also made for the treatment of trade effluents from industry.

There are different types of sewage-treatment works. In all cases, however, the process starts with **screening**, which traps large objects, and a process which separates road grid from the sewage.

The next stage is **sedimentation**, when solid matter settles out while the sewage stands in large tanks. The sedimented matter is called **sludge**, whilst the clearer liquid above it is called **settled sewage**.

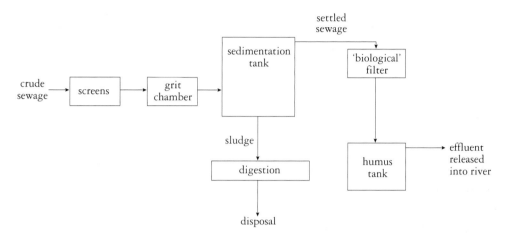

Figure 5.9 The biological filter method of sewage treatment

Further treatment follows one of two courses. The simpler, older method uses 'biological filters' (see Figure 5.9) where the settled sewage is sprinkled over **clinker**. Layers of bacteria and protozoa live on the clinker, and these feed on the organic matter suspended and dissolved in the settled sewage. The liquid is now safe to discharge into the river, after the humus has settled out. Most of the bacteria will have died during the latter processes as the organic material on which they feed is removed. However, there are still many bacteria present in sewage effluent.

Sludge from the sedimentation tank is transferred to a large tank for digestion. It is then disposed, in either dried or liquid form. Some is spread in land, or it may be deposited at sea.

More modern sewage works, on the other hand, use a method of sewage treatment known as the 'activated sludge' method. In this method, the liquid, following sedimentation, is pumped into long channels together with a small quantity of sludge containing a variety of bacteria and protozoa. Along the bottom of each channel is a perforated pipe, a diffuser, and air is bubbled into the sewage under pressure. This air has two functions. It agitates and mixes the sewage and it also maintains a high level of oxygen so that the aerobic micro-organisms present can thrive. These digest the organic material in the sewage very quickly, so this method of treatment allows a much faster processing of sewage than the biological filter process.

The principles of this process are very similar to those in the biological filter method. In more modern sewage works, the problem of sludge disposal is partially solved by digesting it and using the methane produced to make electricity.

Activity

Plan a visit to your local sewage treatment works. Which type of process is employed here, biological filter or activated sludge? Write a report on your visit. Especially note any precautions that are taken to test the quality of the effluent before it is released into the river. Does this sewage works deal with any trade or industrial waste?

The control of air pollution

The legislation

The **Environment Act 1995**, the **Environmental Protection Act 1990** and the **Clean Air Act 1993** all contain important laws on the control of air pollution. Regulations establishing the **National Air Quality Strategy** were made at the end of 1997. This requires local authorities to monitor the air quality in their area and assess whether the objectives will be met by 2005. In areas in which objectives are not likely to be met, the local authority is required to designate an **Air Quality Management Area (AQMA)** and to produce an action plan to show how they will work towards meeting the targets. The Environment Agency (see page 249) has an important role in this process as it provides information and regulates the emissions to the atmosphere of major industrial processes.

The **Health and Safety at Work Act 1974** is also relevant as it grants powers to impose restrictions on emissions from industrial premises. European law has also had a major impact on the control of air pollution in Europe.

National air quality standards have been set for eight priority pollutants:

- carbon monoxide;
- lead;
- nitrogen dioxide;
- ozone;
- fine particles;
- sulphur dioxide;
- benzene;
- 1,3-butadiene.

The standards are set on the basis of scientific evidence on the health effects of each pollution. Regulations require local authorities to assess air quality in their area. If standards are not being met, the local authority must put an action plan in place to reduce the level of the pollutant. You can find out about air pollution levels in your area from your local authority health department. Air quality is also monitored nationally in; 'Resources' on page 283 there are details of where you can find this information.

Air treatments

Tall chimneys

Chimneys which emit pollutants from industrial processes, by law, have to have certain minimum heights. Tall chimneys, which can stop noxious gases from building up locally, disperse pollution. However, they encourage the transport of sulphur dioxide and other pollutants over long distances, causing regional hazes and acid rain.

It is an offence for these chimneys to emit dark smoke except when it is unavoidable, for example, when lighting up. The amount of dust and grit emitted from chimneys is also limited by law. Power stations now have equipment fitted to remove sulphur dioxide from their waste gases (Figure 5.10).

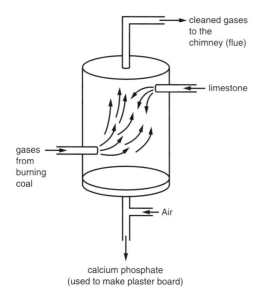

Figure 5.10 Flue-gas desulphurisation

Cutting down pollution from motor vehicles

Since 1970 the European Union has agreed a number of Directives which have progressively lowered vehicle emission limits. There are regulations which set standards for the exhaust emissions of new cars and since 1991 vehicle exhaust testing has been included in the annual MOT. Roadside emission testing is also being considered. In some areas, local authority officers can carry out testing and issue a fixed penalty to motorists whose vehicles exceed the standards.

The smaller and lighter a car is, the less fuel it uses and, therefore, the lower the emissions of carbon dioxide. A lower road tax has been introduced for smaller cars to encourage people to choose them in preference to larger cars. All petrol vehicles now run on lead free fuel. The selling of leaded fuel was banned from the beginning of 2000.

There are a number of technologies which can help reduce pollutant emissions from cars:

Catalytic converters

These have been fitted to all petrol engine cars since 1993. They convert unburned hydrocarbons and carbon monoxide to carbon dioxide and water, and nitrogen oxides to nitrogen. This allows them to reduce nitrogen oxides by 95%, hydrocarbons by 90% and carbon monoxide by 80%. There are, however, a number of disadvantages:

- The engine must be regularly serviced to allow the converter to remain working efficiently.

- They may result in cars using more fuel and, therefore, producing more CO_2.
- Catalysts contain expensive rare metals.
- Fitting catalysts to existing cars is not always possible and involves major work.

Oxidation catalyst

These can be fitted to either diesel or petrol cars. They are effective in reducing the emissions of hydrocarbons, aldehydes, carbon monoxide and particulates. They do not reduce nitrogen oxides.

Carbon canisters

These can be fitted to cars to reduce hydrocarbon emissions from the evaporation of petrol from the fuel system.

Lean burn

These engines burn cleaner than existing engines fitted with catalysts.

Alternative fuels

Table 5.7 shows some of the disadvantages of the use of petrol and diesel. Research is going on to develop engines that use less polluting fuels. Examples include methanol, ethanol, methane, liquid gas, hydrogen and electricity.

Improved aerodynamics and lighter materials

These are factors that will increase fuel efficiency.

Table 5.7 The disadvantages of petrol and diesel fuels

Petrol	Diesel
Petrol contains less energy per litre than diesel	Diesel engines have much higher emissions of particulates
Combustion in petrol engines is less efficient than in diesel engines	Diesel engines have higher emissions of nitrogen oxides
A petrol engine is less likely to stay in tune which further reduces its efficiency compared with diesel	Diesel fuel contains more carbon, so produces more CO_2 when burnt
A petrol engine warms up slower than a diesel engine which makes it worse for short journeys	

Activity

The best way to cut down on the air pollution from cars is to reduce their use.

- Can you think of ways in which you or your family could reduce your number of car journeys?

- Can you think of ways of encouraging other people to reduce their dependence on cars?

Environmental health

The legislation on Environmental Health is the responsibility of central government, but the enforcement of laws is devolved to local government. **Environmental Health Officers** (EHOs) employed by local authorities have the responsibility of protecting the people living and working in their area. Their work covers four linked areas:

- food control;
- Health and Safety at work;
- housing;
- pollution and environmental protection.

Food control

The need for legislation

Legislation on food safety has three major functions:

- the protection of the consumer;
- the protection of the honest trader;
- the promotion of freedom of choice and fair competition.

The protection of the consumer by preventing illness and the spread of disease is a very important aspect of this legislation. Food-poisoning bacteria and viruses, as well as micro-organisms causing more serious illnesses such as typhoid, may be carried by food. Contamination by metals such as lead and mercury can also cause poisoning and serious damage.

Other measures designed to ensure food safety involve regulations relating to the composition of food, including controls of ingredients – especially food additives. Procedures for processing and preserving food are also strictly controlled. There are restrictions on the amounts and types of chemicals that may be added to food. Storage methods are also covered by the laws.

As well as protecting the public from disease and damage to health, the legislation also ensures that the food is of the expected quality. It should not be damaged or spoiled. Advertising, the labelling on packets and other descriptions of food should properly describe the food and not be misleading in any way. The quantities of the ingredients should also be recorded accurately. The public is entitled to accurate nutritional information.

These laws will also protect the honest food trader as it will obviously cost more to produce and store good-quality food. Illegal actions, for example adding large amounts of preservative, will cut costs, as will substituting inexpensive ingredients.

The Department for the Environment, Food and Rural Affairs is responsible for food laws, but their enforcement is devolved to local government. Local authorities employ Environmental Health Officers (EHOs) to carry out this work.

The **Food Safety Act 1990** contains most of the legislation relating to the safety and quality of the food we buy. The Act is based on the fact that the producers and distributors of food are held responsible for the safety and quality of food on sale to the public.

The **Food Standards Act 1999** established the **Food Standards Agency**. The main objective of this body is to protect public health from risks caused by food. The Agency is responsible for developing policies relating to food safety or other interests of consumers in relation to food. It also provides advice, information and assistance to public authorities and members of the public. The article from *The Sunday Times* describes an example of police and the Food Standards Agency working together when food standard rules have been broken.

Source *The Sunday Times*, April 29th 2001

Thousands of tons of poultry meat fit only for pet food have been sold for human consumption after being "laundered" by unscrupulous traders.

Last week enviromental health inspectors raided a warehouse in Liverpool as part of investigations into a growing food scandal. They seized 40 tons of unfit meat and are continuing to trace further batches of suspect produce.

Across the country evidence is emerging that meat certified unfit for humans has been sold to supermarkets, restaurants and takeaways and also served upin schools, hospitals and old people's homes.

The meat has been used in chicken burgers and meat pastes. It has also been packaged as leg and breast portions distributed across Britain.

At least six major investigations are being conducted by police and environmental health inspectors into frauds involving "waste" chicken and turkey from slaughterhouses being repackaged for the human food chain. Some of the unfit meat is bruised or poor quality. Other meat is contaminated with infections or abcessess and is not even legally fit for pet food.

Contaminated poultry, if not properly cooked, can cause food poisoning such as salmonella and campylobacter, which in extreme cases can kill. The very young and old are especially vulnerable.

The trade has been fuelled by the growing demand for chicken, sales of which have soared because of fears over BSE and foot and mouth.

The Liverpool raid is understood to have resulted from an investigation being led by Derbyshire police and the government's Food Standards Agency

EHOs are concerned with ensuring the safety of food at all stages from production until it reaches the consumer. They inspect food premises and advise managers on hygiene and safety. If the conditions in a premises are considered a risk to health, the EHO may take legal action by serving an improvement notice. In extreme cases, the premises may be closed until the problems are put right. In 2000 nearly half of the restaurants and other catering outlets inspected were found not to be meeting food hygiene and safety standards. Many EHOs run courses to educate food handlers and also produce materials to prevent food poisoning in the home (Figure 5.11).

Health and safety at work

EHOs are responsible for enforcing the Health and Safety at Work Act 1974 (see pages 275–6) in more than one million commercial and recreational premises, employing about nine million people. The EHOs inspect premises and offer advice on how to protect employees and members of the public who use the premises. In cases of negligence, they may bring about a prosecution.

Housing

EHOs monitor housing standards. They can take action to ensure that repairs to properties are carried out where necessary to make a house suitable for habitation. In rented shared accommodation EHOs are responsible for making sure that the residents are protected from fire and public health hazards. EHOs may also be involved in housing issues such as urban renewal and generation, residential and non-residential caravan and camping, and travellers and gypsies.

Pollution and environmental protection

EHOs have an important role in monitoring and controlling pollution levels. They measure levels of air, water, soil, and noise pollution and communicate the results to the public. They are responsible for monitoring the levels of airborne emissions from small- and medium-sized industrial processes and taking action if pollution exceeds certain minimum standards. EHOs also educate the public to raise environmental awareness.

Local authority action

Although central government is responsible for the legislation produced, the responsibility for implementing the standards set falls to the local authorities.

At the Rio Earth Summit in Brazil in 1992, world leaders agreed on a plan of action to move towards a more sustainable future for the planet, balancing environmental, economic and social needs. In order to find local solutions to global environmental problems, they called upon local governments throughout the world to work with the community to produce a strategy for sustainable development. This local focus for the twenty-first century is known as **Local Agenda 21**.

There are a number of actions local authorities take in order to improve the local environment. Examples of these are given below.

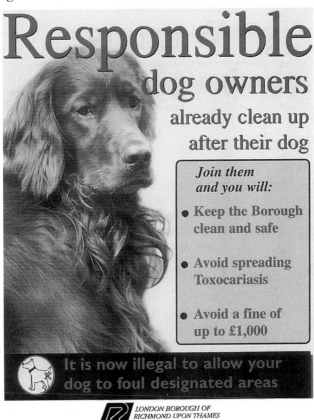

Figure 5.11 Leaflet to discourage dog fouling produced by London Borough of Richmond upon Thames leisure services

Dog fouling penalties

The Dogs (Fouling of Land) Act 1996 made it illegal for an owner to allow their dog to foul designated areas. The Act means that the owner can be fined £25, or be prosecuted for £1000 plus costs, if they do not clear up after their dog, even if there are no warning signs or waste bins present. Parks and open spaces are examples of areas which may be designated areas. Local authorities may ban dogs from some areas such as playgrounds, sports pitches and allotments (Figure 5.11).

One of the reasons dog fouling is taken so seriously is because dog faeces may contain the microscopic eggs of *toxocara*, a parasitic worm. These can be passed to humans by contact with contaminated soil. They can cause stomach disorders and blindness. Children and sports players are particularly likely to come into contact with contaminated soil.

Activity

In your locality find out in which areas your local authority has banned dogs and what steps they have taken to prevent dog fouling in other areas. Do dog owners generally respect restrictions and requests to clean up after their dogs?

Waste collection and disposal

Each year in the UK we produce over 100 million tonnes from households, commerce and industry. Waste management, recycling, waste licensing and related technical and legal subjects are covered by DEFRA's (Department for Environment, Food and Rural Affairs) Waste Policy and Waste Strategy Divisions.

The Environmental Protection Act 1990 outlines the duty of the local authority to make arrangements for the safe collection and disposal of waste by creating a Local Authority Waste Disposal Company (LAWDC) or by using the private sector. The aim of taking the responsibility away from the local authority and giving it to a separate company was to introduce competition for waste disposal contracts and to identify fully the costs for waste disposal.

In the past, waste collection and waste disposal have been organised separately, but recently the Government has started to encourage waste collection and disposal companies to work together.

At the time of The Environmental Protection Act 1990, local authorities were responsible for regulating waste disposal sites, but in 1996 these responsibilities were transferred to the Environment Agency.

Waste from households and certain industrial and commercial premises is called 'controlled waste', and it must be collected. No charge should be made for the disposal of household waste provided it does not exceed 25kg in weight, or include garden waste, clinical waste – such as syringes or dirty dressings – or dead pets. Charges can, however be made for the disposal of other household rubbish.

Although most domestic and commercial waste is not very toxic, it can only be disposed of at licensed sites: it is an offence for anyone to dump waste at unlicensed sites. Most waste is **landfilled**. There are many regulations related to the type of sites that can be used, so that common hazards such as the leaching of contaminants into water supplies and methane production are reduced. The Government taxes landfill to encourage **recycling**. It is the duty of every waste collection authority to recycle waste in their area. (See below, 'Recycling of useful materials').

Household waste can also be **incinerated** (see page 226 for 'Methods of Waste Disposal'). Figure 5.12 shows the relative proportions of the different types of waste disposal.

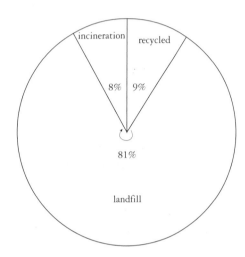

Figure 5.12 The relative proportions of the different types of waste disposal in the UK

There are very stringent regulations relating to the treatment, carriage and disposal of toxic and dangerous waste from industry. Special licensed sites exist for the disposal of such waste, including old mine shafts and land-infill sites. The main problem is that this waste may enter water supplies. In some cases, however, it is possible to make the waste safe before disposal.

Each year the Department for Environment, Food and Rural Affairs publishes statistics based on a waste management survey. For example, the 1999/2000 survey showed:

- 26.3 million tonnes of household waste was produced. This includes regular pick-ups from households (refuse collection), waste collected for recycling and composting, and waste from special collections.
- This represents 1.21 tonnes of waste per household per annum.
- 2.7 million tonnes of household waste was collected for recycling.

Recycling of useful materials

Many materials can be recycled and used again. This cuts down the amount of waste which has to be taken to landfill sites. At present only 11% of household waste is recycled. However, in their Waste Strategy 2000 for England and Wales the Government has set the following targets to increase the recycling of waste:

- to recycle or compost at least 25% of household waste by 2005;
- to recycle or compost at least 30% of household waste by 2010;
- to recycle or compost at least 33% of household waste by 2015.

Some local authorities have set an even more challenging target of sending no waste to landfill sites by the year 2015. This is known as a 'Zero Waste' policy. It is considered to be achievable by following the three Rs – reduce, reuse, recycle.

There are different ways in which local authorities can encourage recycling:

- Consumers can undertake recycling themselves by separating their recyclable waste materials and taking them to recycling centres provided by the local authority.
- Local authorities may provide bags or boxes for house-to-house collections of particular materials such as newspaper.

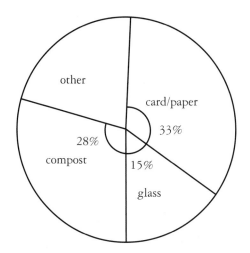

Figure 5.13 The relative proportions of the materials which were recycled from household rubbish 1999/2000

- Local authorities may provide bins in which residents dispose of materials which can be recycled such as newspaper, cardboard, plastic, cloth and cans. These are taken away for the materials to be sorted at a recycling centre (In 1999/2000, 43% of households had their recycled waste collected from their kerbsides).
- Local authorities may provide free or subsidised compost bins for recycling garden and kitchen waste.
- Local authorities may run or subsidise schemes in which residents donate unwanted items such as furniture, paint, wood and other building materials. These can then be offered to people on low incomes.

Figure 5.13 shows the relative proportions of the materials that were recycled from household rubbish 1999/2000.

Activity

Find out what encouragement your local authority gives residents to recycle their waste.

Control of Green Belt and Brownfield Site land

Green Belts

In 1935 the Greater London regional Planning Committee proposed 'to provide a reserve supply of public open spaces and of recreational areas and to establish a Green Belt or girdle of open space'. The 1947 Town and Country Planning Act allowed local authorities to incorporate Green Belt proposals in their development plans and in 1955 local planning authorities were invited to consider the establishment of Green Belts. Now Green Belts cover approximately 1,556,000 hectares, about 12% of England (Figure 5.14). There are 14 separate Green Belts, varying in size from 486,000 around London to just 700 hectares around Burton-on-Trent.

The aim of Green Belt policy is to prevent urban sprawl by keeping land permanently open.

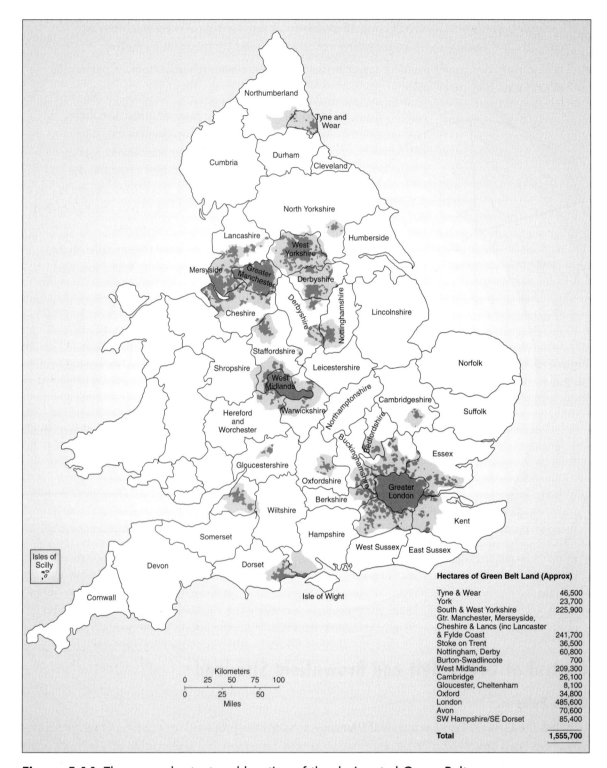

Hectares of Green Belt Land (Approx)	
Tyne & Wear	46,500
York	23,700
South & West Yorkshire	225,900
Gtr. Manchester, Merseyside, Cheshire & Lancs (inc Lancaster & Fylde Coast	241,700
Stoke on Trent	36,500
Nottingham, Derby	60,800
Burton-Swadlincote	700
West Midlands	209,300
Cambridge	26,100
Gloucester, Cheltenham	8,100
Oxford	34,800
London	485,600
Avon	70,600
SW Hampshire/SE Dorset	85,400
Total	**1,555,700**

Figure 5.14 The general extent and location of the designated Green Belt areas

There are five purposes of including land in Green Belts:

- to check the unrestricted sprawl of large built up areas;
- to prevent neighbouring towns from merging into one another;
- to assist in safeguarding the countryside from encroachment;
- to preserve the setting and special character of historic towns;
- to assist in urban regeneration of derelict and other urban land.

Once Green Belts have been defined, the land is used:

- to provide opportunities for access to the open countryside for the urban population;
- to provide opportunities for outdoor sport and recreation near urban areas;
- to retain attractive landscapes near to where people live;
- to improve damaged and derelict land around towns;
- for nature conservation;
- to retain land for agriculture and forestry.

An established Green Belt should only be changed in exceptional circumstances. If an alteration is proposed, the Secretary of State must be satisfied that the local authority has considered opportunities for development either beyond the Green Belt, or within the urban areas inside the Green Belt.

The construction of new buildings in a Green Belt is considered inappropriate unless it is for one of the following purposes:

- agriculture or forestry;
- facilities for outdoor sport or recreation;
- limited extension, alteration or a replacement of an existing dwelling;
- limited 'infilling' (building between existing houses) in villages;
- limited affordable housing for local community needs.

The Department for Transport, Local Government and the Regions issues Planning Policy Guidance notes (PPGs) which set out the Government's policies on different aspects of planning. Local planning authorities must take their contents into consideration when preparing their development plans. In July 2001 PPG notes confirmed that the Government attaches great importance to Green Belts and that they must be protected as far as can be seen ahead.

Brownfield Sites

A Brownfield Site is an area of land which has been previously developed. It is defined as 'an area of land which is or was occupied by a permanent structure (excluding agriculture or forestry buildings), and associated fixed surface infrastructure'. This type of land may be situated in either built-up or rural settings, although most of it is found in an urban setting. It includes land that has been used for mineral extraction or waste disposal. In England there are about 58,000 hectares of Brownfield land, either vacant, derelict, or available for redevelopment.

Building on Brownfield Sites is a way of recycling land. Local authorities are encouraged by the

Department of the Environment, Transport and Regions and the European Commission to build on Brownfield Sites to reduce the need for green field (undeveloped) land use.

Activity

1   Draw a map to show the extent of your nearest Green Belt.

2   Read the purposes and uses of Green Belts listed above. To what extent is your local Green Belt fulfilling these objectives?

Park and ride facilities

Local authorities are encouraged by the Government Department for Transport, Local Government and the Regions to include in their local transport plans to provide car parks on the outskirts of cities or large towns from which people can take a bus or train into the centre. These are known as Park and Ride schemes and give advantages for both the environment and the users of the schemes:

Advantages for the environment

- less air pollution;
- less congested town centres;
- more attractive town centres.

Advantages for users

- no parking charges or problems;
- better pedestrian access in town centre;
- less time wasted sitting in traffic jams.

Schemes can vary considerably in size and purpose. The Government has given the following advice to local authorities on the implementation of Park and Ride schemes:

- They should be designed to avoid encouraging additional travel, especially commuting, by car.
- The total parking available in a town should not be increased by the scheme.
- They should be designed for use by disabled people.
- They should be designed for walking, cycling, and motorcycle journeys to and from the site.
- The countryside immediately around urban areas will often be the preferred area for Park and Ride schemes, but in many cases this will be designated Green Belt land (see above). The Government encourages local planning authorities to consider non-Green Belt land first, but allow that in some circumstances a Green Belt location may be the most suitable option.

Activity

Providing Park and Ride facilities is one way in which local authorities may try to reduce traffic in towns and cities. What other steps is your local authority taking to encourage people out of their cars? How effective are their efforts in reducing traffic and air pollution?

Educational pressure groups

There are many educational pressure groups: **Friends of the Earth** and **Greenpeace** are two of the most well-known ones. Publicising environmental issues and running campaigns to develop public understanding are their main functions. As well as aiming to influence governments, these groups encourage individuals to take their *own* green action.

Friends of the Earth

This is the largest international network of environmental groups in the world, representing 68 countries. In England, Wales and Northern Ireland there are 250 local Friends of the Earth groups. Ninety per cent of their income comes from individual donations; the rest comes from special fund-raising events, grants and trading. It is a charity that provides extensive information and educational materials, and also commissions environmental research. Friends of the Earth run campaigns aimed at:

- protecting wildlife habitats and the countryside;
- encouraging sustainable agriculture;
- stopping the destruction of tropical rain forests;
- preventing air pollution and acid rain;
- promoting waste reduction and reducing over-consumption;
- forcing the clean-up of rivers and drinking water;
- stopping hazardous waste dumping;
- controlling dangerous chemicals, including pesticides;
- reducing traffic levels and improving public transport;
- stopping climate change;
- protecting the ozone layer;
- phasing out nuclear power, and promoting energy efficiency and renewable energy.

Greenpeace

This international organisation promotes environmental awareness and addresses environmental abuse through direct, non-violent confrontations with governments and companies. It was founded in 1971 to oppose US nuclear testing in Alaska. It fights to protect endangered species; to stop the dumping of hazardous waste; and to strengthen national and international laws that regulate environmental affairs.

Activity

Find out about your local Friends of the Earth group. What campaigns are they involved in?

The World Health Organisation

The World Health Organisation can also be considered to have a role as an educational pressure group. It was set up in 1948 and is defined as 'the directing and co-ordinating authority on international health work'. It promotes health beyond national or local boundaries and its aim is 'the attainment by all peoples of the highest possible level of health'. It allows governments to work together, not only to protect their own people from imported diseases, but to work in favour of protection and promotion of positive health.

Its Constitution lists a number of responsibilities. These include:

* working towards wiping out epidemic, endemic and other diseases;
* promoting improved nutrition, housing, sanitation, working conditions and other aspects of environmental hygiene;
* encouraging co-operation among scientific and professional groups to contribute to the advancement of health;
* proposing international conventions and agreements in health matters;
* promoting and conducting health research;
* developing international standards for food, biological and pharmaceutical products;
* helping in developing an informed public opinion among all people on matters of health.

The WHO is part of the United Nations and has its headquarters in Geneva in Switzerland. The member states each make a regular contribution, with additional voluntary contributions coming from governmental and non-governmental sources. There are about 4500 WHO staff. About 30% are based in Geneva, with the remaining 70% in countries all over the world.

Organic farming

Since farming began, animal manure, compost from rotting vegetation and ashes from burnt vegetation have been used by farmers to keep soils healthy. In the eighteenth century, the idea of **crop rotation** was developed by Charles 'Turnip' Townshend. Different crops take different sorts and amounts of nutrients from the soil. If the same crops are grown in the same field year after year, the soil becomes exhausted. If crops are rotated, however, the soil has a chance to recover. Peas, beans and clover put nitrogen back into the soil. A typical four-crop rotation cycle would involve turnips, wheat, barley and clover.

In the last 50 years, farmers have turned to intensive farming methods, with the same crops grown in the same fields every year. Chemicals have been used as fertilisers and pesticides. The environmental effects of these were discussed earlier in this chapter). Recently, there has been a growing concern about the use of chemicals, not only because of the environmental damage but also because it is claimed by some that pesticides remain in the crop plants. Since we then eat these plants, our own health is at risk.

Now, there is a renewed interest in organic farming methods. This approach relies on less support from chemical fertilisers, pesticides and energy. Natural fertilisers such as animal manure are used. Pests are controlled biologically, for example, by encouraging ladybirds which eat greenfly, or mechanically, for example, by protecting crops with netting. However, organic fertilisers work more slowly than chemical ones, and yields are less spectacular. The biological and mechanical control of pests is less effective than chemical control.

The scale of production is smaller, and organically produced crops can be more expensive to produce for the farmer, which means that the consumer pays more.

The article from *The Independent* shows that some unsubstantiated claims have been made for organic food.

Source *The Independent*, 24 July, 2001

THE ADVERTISING watchdog has issued a tough set of guidelines to companies producing and selling organic food after a string of false claims.

The authority hopes to counter the behaviour of companies accused of misleading the public about the health and environmental benefits of organic produce and who have consistently failed to substantiate claims made in their advertising.

As the appeal of organic food has increased over the past two years and become more widely available, the Advertising Standards Authority (ASA) in conjunction with the Committee of Advertising Practice, felt consumers had a right to make informed choices based on accurate information.

From now on, advertisers will not be able to claim that organic food production is free from chemicals, fertilisers, herbicides or pesticides.

They have also been instructed they can claim products are organic only if they come from farmers, processors or importers who follow the minimum standards in European Union regulation.

The use of words and phrases such as "environmentally friendly" or "sustainable" have been vetoed after it was decided that all food production systems cause at least some damage to the environment.

Activity

Debate whether organic farming is a better method of food production than non-organic farming. You may wish to role play this as, for example, an organic farmer, a non-organic farmer, consumers on high incomes and consumers on low incomes.

Policies and legislation for reducing the harmful effects of urbanisation

See 'Legislation' in the 'Resources' section on pages 286–7.

European and United Kingdom parliaments have developed policies and devised laws in an effort to reduce the decline in the environment caused by urbanisation.

Housing policies

Aspects of health related to housing are considered earlier in this chapter. Policies are developed by each local authority to ensure that housing in the area is adequate. Legislation exists to provide a framework within which policies can be implemented. The housing and building legislation lays down standards to try to ensure good housing conditions. The structure of new buildings is controlled by very strict regulations, and there are measures to rectify defects in older properties.

The conditions that form the basis for good housing, as outlined in the legislation, are as follows:

- The dwelling should be in a good state of repair and substantially free from damp.
- Each room should be properly lit and ventilated.
- There should be an adequate supply of wholesome water laid on inside the dwelling.
- An adequate supply of hot water should be provided.
- There should be an internal water-closet.
- There should be a fixed bath or shower, preferably in a separate room.
- A sink should be provided with suitable arrangements for the disposal of waste water.
- There should be a proper drainage system.
- Each room should have adequate points for electricity for lighting.
- There should be adequate facilities for heating.
- There should be satisfactory facilities for the storage, preparation and cooking of food.
- There should be proper provision for the storage of fuel where appropriate.

Housing legislation

There have been several important Housing Acts; the most important one is the Housing Act 1985. There was also a separate Housing Associations Act, introduced in the same year; and the Local Government and Housing Act of 1989 introduced a new system of grants for improved housing.

The Acts are very wide ranging and give many powers to the local authority, which carries them out through the housing department.

The Housing Act 1985 (council housing)

Under the 1985 Act, housing accommodation may be provided by the local authority and land may be purchased, compulsorily if necessary, to build dwellings. People who are homeless or who occupy insanitary, overcrowded homes or who have large families in unsatisfactory accommodation should be given preference in the allocation of council homes. Reasonable rents may be charged. The 1985 Act allowed local authorities to continue to sell council houses; and now the national stock of homes to rent from local authorities is severely depleted, since this provision first entered legislation in 1980. The sold homes have not been replaced by new buildings.

Homelessness

Local authorities have a responsibility to house homeless people. This first entered the statute book in a previous Housing Act of 1977, but is now covered by the 1985 Act. Certain categories have priority. These include a pregnant woman, or a person with whom a pregnant woman resides; a person with whom dependent children reside; and a person who is vulnerable on account of old age, mental illness, disability or other special reason. People who are made homeless through an emergency, like food or fire, should also be housed.

Dealing with substandard housing

Under the Housing Act of 1985, local authorities are empowered to issue repair notices to owners of dwelling houses that are defective or unfit for human habitation. The owner is required to carry out repairs so that the dwelling is of a reasonable standard, and dates are set for the completion of work. This Act also enables local authorities to improve whole areas of housing by declaring housing action areas, general improvement areas and renewal areas. Central government funds can be made available. Slum clearance is also possible: local authorities can demolish buildings that are deemed to be unfit for human habitation or dangerous or injurious to health. Compulsory purchase orders are made, and the courts have considerable powers of enforcement in this respect. Entry to premises for the purpose of valuation must be allowed, and any obstruction to the procedures leading to demolition is an offence.

Slum clearance has been a feature of housing policy for many years. Whilst slum clearances in cities such as Manchester certainly removed enormous numbers of unfit houses from our housing stock, and reduced pollution from burning coal, the high-rise flats that were often built to replace the slum houses were not without their own problems. The quality of building in the 1960s was not good, and the social effects of breaking up communities and putting people into blocks of flats had been underestimated.

Overcrowding

Overcrowding is prohibited under the 1985 Housing Act. Standards are laid down that define overcrowding.

1 When two children, over the age of 10 years and of opposite sexes, must sleep in the same room.
2 When the room:person ratio exceeds one room:two people, two rooms:three people, three rooms:five people, four rooms:seven and a half people, or five rooms or more:10 people, with two then added for every room over five.
3 When the floor-area:person ratio exceeds $10.2m^2$:two people.

(Children under one year are ignored for the purposes of assessing overcrowding). These limits are recognised as being unrealistic.

An occupier or landlord who permits overcrowding commits an offence. The local authority can require the occupier of a dwelling to provide information as to the numbers and sexes of people sleeping in the dwelling, and housing officers may enter a premises to investigate and measure rooms. If overcrowding is found, then a notice of abatement may be issued: this means that the overcrowding must cease within 14 days. Application may be made to a county court if the notice is not carried out, and eventually the occupier can be turned out if they do not comply.

The same Act also deals with houses in multiple occupation. There are regulations which ensure that premises are suitable for the number of people living there, and powers exist to take offenders to court.

The Housing Associations Act 1985

This allowed housing associations to be set up and registered. A housing association may be broadly defined as a society, body of trustees or company that is established for the purpose of providing, constructing, improving or managing housing accommodation. It does not exist to make a profit. One of the advantages of being a registered housing association is that such an association then becomes eligible for grants. Local authority assistance is sometimes available to help housing associations. The aim is to help people obtain housing through a scheme that is designed to replace simple renting from a local authority.

The Local Government and Housing Act 1989

There was a comprehensive system for grants for improving dwellings in place of many of the earlier Housing Acts. Nonetheless, the Local Government and Housing Act 1989 created an entirely new system for grants to be paid to private owners by the local authority. Resources are now only available for essential repair work and improvements where the need is greatest. There are also grants to enable disasabled people to adapt their homes.

The Housing Act 1996

The Housing Act 1996 included legislation concerning:

- the social rented sector;
- houses in multiple occupation;
- landlord and tenant matters;
- the administration of housing benefit;
- the conduct of tenants;
- the allocation of housing accommodation by local housing authorities;
- homelessness.

Housing Green Paper 2000

A Green Paper is published in order to invite comments on proposed Government strategy. Some of the key proposals the Government made were:

- a stronger role for local authorities in public and private housing;
- to raise the standards of private rented housing;
- a target to bring all social housing up to a decent standard by 2010;

- to establish a fairer system of rents for tenants of local authorities;
- to simplify the administration of housing benefit.

The response to these proposals will affect subsequent Government policies.

Transport policies

The Department for Transport, Local Government and the Regions (DTLR) is responsible for transport. The local authorities play a co-ordinating role in balancing transportation, planning and environmental issues within their areas. Policies are adopted that seek to reduce congestion and pollution whilst improving the economy and quality of life for those who live, work and shop there. Some places rely on tourism, and have to keep the area an attractive place to visit.

National policies

The Transport Act 1985 reduced the ability of local authorities to co-ordinate the provision of public transport services. This led to a number of private bus operators, which critics said provided increasingly patchy and unco-ordinated local bus services.

The Road Traffic Reduction Act 1997 and **The Road Traffic Reduction (National Targets) Act 1998** aimed to reduce the adverse environmental, social and economic impacts of road traffic. These adverse impacts included:

- the emission of gases contributing to climate change;
- effects on air quality;
- effects on health;
- traffic congestion;
- effects on land and biodiversity;
- danger to other road users; and
- social impacts.

The Transport Act 2000 included legislation to deliver the Government's transport priorities, which were to:

- reduce congestion
- improve integration
- give a wider choice of quicker, safer, more reliable travel on road, rail and other public transport

Measures were introduced to improve local bus services, including the introduction of mandatory half-fares for pensioners and disabled people.

In an effort to reduce the number of cars on the road, local authorities were provided with powers to introduce schemes in which people could be charged for using certain roads or for parking in the workplace, where this would help reduce road congestion and pollution. The money raised by these schemes can be used to help fund other transport improvements.

The **Strategic Rail Authority** was created to reduce the problems of fragmented rail services and to promote the use of railways. By 2010 the Government want rail use to increase by 50%, measured by passenger kilometres, and rail freight to increase by 80%.

Local policies

The Transport Act 2000 required local authorities to produce **Local Transport Plans,** which set out their strategies for transport and their long term targets for improving air quality, road safety and public transport and for reducing road traffic. Local authorities have to consider:

- widening travel choices;
- traffic management and demand restraint;
- integrating transport;
- planning and managing the highway network;
- rural transport; and
- integration with wider policies.

Energy policies

The Department for the Environment, Food and Rural Affairs (DEFRA) provides information on energy efficiency, but other government departments also have a role in the implementation of energy policies. For example, transport and housing policies produced by the Department for Transport, Local Government and the Regions (DTLR) may include aspects relating to energy conservation.

The **Home Energy Conservation Act 1995** and the **Energy Conservation Act 1996** required all UK local authorities with housing responsibilities to identify energy conservation measures to improve the energy efficiency of all residential accommodation in their area.

As a result of the **Kyoto Protocol**, an international agreement on global warming, developed countries have agreed that they will cut their overall emissions of greenhouse gases (see pages 237–8) by 5.2% below 1990 levels by 2008–12. These targets are legally binding and countries have different targets depending on their circumstances. The UK's target is to cut its emissions by 12.5% below 1990 levels by 2008–12. However, the Government has set goals to go further than this and to cut carbon dioxide emissions by 20% below 1990 levels by 2010. The **UK Climate Change Programme** has been produced, which sets out policies and measures across all sectors of the economy in order to reach this target.

Gas and electricity use in the home is responsible for 25% of the UK's carbon dioxide emissions. To reduce the amount of domestic energy used, a number of measures have been introduced. For example:

- **The Home Energy Efficiency Scheme (HEES)** provides grants of up to £2000 to improve the insulation and heating efficiency of low income households.
- **The Energy Efficiency Commitment for 2002–5 (EEC)** requires gas and electricity suppliers to achieve targets for the promotion of improvements in domestic energy efficiency. The EEC builds on the Energy Efficiency Standards of Performance (EESOPs), which have operated successfully since 1994.

To reduce the amount of non-domestic energy used, in 2001 the Government introduced a **Climate Change Levy**, which applies to energy used by businesses and the public sector.

Activity

1   What steps have your gas and electricity suppliers taken to encourage you to improve energy efficiency in your home?

2   The Government is proposing that 5% of UK electricity needs to be met from renewable energy sources by the end of 2003 and 10% by 2010 as long as the cost to consumers is acceptable. What are the renewable sources of energy and are any of these being used to generate electricity in your area?.

Policies and procedures to meet the requirements of health and safety in care settings

The government department responsible for Health and Safety is The Department for Transport, Local Government and the Regions (DTLR). The Health and Safety at Work Act 1974 (see below) set up the Health and Safety Commission (HSC) and the Health and Safety Executive (HSE).

Health and Safety Commission

The HSC is responsible for advising the Government on health and safety matters, and for putting the principles of health and safety law into practice. Its functions are:

- to secure the health, safety and welfare of persons at work;
- to protect the public generally against risks to health or safety arising out of work activities, and to control the keeping and use of explosives, highly flammable and other dangerous substances;
- to conduct and sponsor research;
- to promote training;
- to provide an information and advisory service;
- to review the adequacy of health and safety legislation, and to submit proposals for new or revised regulations to the Government.

Health and Safety Executive

The HSE is the enforcement body appointed by the HSC to help with carrying out these duties. The HSE and local authorities work together to make sure that health and safety law is put into practice. Their activities include:

- inspecting work places;
- investigating accidents and cases of ill health;
- enforcing good standards, usually by advising people how to comply with the law but sometimes ordering them to make improvements and, if necessary, by prosecuting them;
- carrying out and funding research;
- publishing guidance and advice.

In general, the local authorities are responsible for service industry workplaces such as shops, offices and catering facilities, and the HSE is responsible for industrial processes and manufacturing workplaces. The HSE collects and publishes health and safety statistics.

There are a number of pieces of legislation that affect professionals working in care settings and cover aspects such as fire drills, cross-infection control, manual handling and lifting regulations. Details of the most important pieces of legislation are given below.

The Fire Precautions Act 1971

This is an Act that was passed to protect people from fire risks in almost every environment to which the public has access, except their own homes. The fire authority, almost always the local authority, is able to grant fire certificates where premises reach specific safety standards relating to fire risks. All the following places are covered by this legislation:

- institutions providing treatment or care;
- places of work;
- premises used for entertainment, recreation or instruction, or for clubs and societies;
- hotels, hostels and anywhere providing sleeping accommodation;
- schools and premises used for training or research.;
- any building to which members of the public have access, including shops.

Applications for fire certificates have to contain full details of the premises and the intended purpose, and the protection provided for people against fire risks must be fully described.

The most important fire safety points mentioned in the Act are as follows:

- the means of escape in cases of fire;
- the means of fighting fires, and how this equipment will be maintained in efficient working order;
- how fire warnings will be given to people in the building;
- the training that people employed in the building must receive in what to do in the case of fire.

The fire-authority inspector will visit the premises to make an assessment of fire safety, and will either grant the fire certificate or, if they are not satisfied that the safety standards have been reached, refuse it. If the application is turned down, then advice will be provided about what steps have to be taken in order to gain a certificate. If, on the other hand, the fire certificate is granted, it will specify the precise functions of the premises covered and give details of all the fire precautions expected to be found there.

Inspection and the enforcement of fire safety legislation

Inspections of places of work for fire safety purposes are often arranged in conjunction with the Health and Safety Commission. Such inspections can also be carried out by officers of the fire brigade if so authorised by the fire authority.

Inspectors have powers to enter premises and require the production of a fire certificate. They can carry out fire safety checks to make sure that all the requirements of the certificate are in place. It is an offence to obstruct a fire inspector who is trying to carry out an inspection. The occupier of premises which should have a fire certificate commits an offence if such a certificate has not been obtained. It is also an offence to contravene any of the conditions and requirements laid down in the fire certificate. Fines or imprisonment may be imposed.

In addition to prosecuting offenders, the Act also enables codes of practice to be produced to help occupiers make their premises safe against fire hazards. Furthermore, improvement notices may be issued if fire precautions need upgrading or are slightly deficient. Sometimes, when serious fire risks are discovered in a premises, a prohibition notice is issued specifying the particular hazard. This will prevent use of the premises until the hazard is rectified.

Another way in which fire safety in buildings is enforced is through the power that local authorities have when they grant planning permission for new buildings. There are rules that specify that new buildings, and alterations or additions to existing buildings, must be safe against fire hazards.

 # Activity

Find out about the fire safety precautions in your school or college.

- How will you escape if there is a fire?
- Where is the fire-fighting equipment located?
- How is it maintained?
- Is the fire warning system in place?
- Who is trained about what to do in the case of fire?

The Health and Safety at Work Act 1974

The main principles of health and safety law in Great Britain are that:

- employers have to look after the health, safety and welfare of all their employees;
- employees and the self employed have to look after their own health and safety;
- everyone has to take care of the health and safety of others, for example members of the public who may be affected by their work.

These principles were set out in the Health and Safety at Work Act 1974, which gives the framework for health and safety law. It is supported by about 400 sets of regulations that set out the details of the law. (A free leaflet, which summarises the law on health and safety at work, 'Health and safety regulation – a short guide', can be obtained from HSE Books, telephone: 01787 881165.)

The Act includes recommended safety policies, as well as a requirement for safety representatives to be appointed from the workforce. There are also approved codes of practice for every workplace and strong enforcement procedures.

Health and safety regulations

The Health and Safety at Work Act 1974 and the relevant acts outline requirements for health and safety in the workplace. In addition, there are regulations made under these acts which give even more detail about specific aspects of health and safety.

Regulations have the same force in law as the acts themselves, and employers must therefore comply with them to be within the law.

Control of Substances Hazardous to Health 1988 (COSHH) regulations

About 100,000 chemicals are in everyday use, and not all of them have been properly tested for the possibility that they might cause cancer or allergies, or have other toxic effects on the human body. Most workers are regularly exposed to toxic substances.

Substances are classed as hazardous if they cause short- or long-term harm. They include dusts, fumes and gases, liquids, pastes, powders, oils, resins, aerosols and sprays. Inks and toners can be toxic. Liquid chemicals such as cleaning, antiseptic and sterilising fluids and solvents are often potential hazards which may affect care workers. Although micro-organisms are not chemicals in the sense of the rest of the substances covered by the COSHH regulations, they are nonetheless included, and this is of great importance in a care setting for it offers protection to workers.

The COSHH regulations apply to every workplace.

The prevention and control of exposure to hazardous substances

Employers must prevent the exposure of employees to hazardous substances. Sometimes, complete prevention is not reasonably practicable, in which case it is legal to use the hazardous substance providing there are proper control measures.

Preventing exposure involves eliminating the use of the substance or substituting a less hazardous substance. *Controlling*, on the other hand, includes

1 totally enclosing the process;
2 using adequate ventilation;
3 using safe systems of work and handling procedures.

This third option is the most frequently used in hospitals and other care settings, as it is not usually possible to eliminate the hazard totally. As well as making sure all employees are aware of safe working practices and handling procedures, the use of personal protective equipment and clothing is also important. Information must be given to workers about the dangers of their work, and training must take place to ensure that ways of avoiding the dangers are understood.

Enforcing the COSHH regulations

The Health and Safety Commission, which is responsible for the Health and Safety Inspectorate, enforces the COSHH Regulations. When a health-and-safety inspector visits a workplace, they have to find out whether the employer has carried out all that is required. Their checklist is as follows:

- Has a complete audit of substances been carried out?
- Have those substances identified as being hazardous to health been assessed?
- Has the employer provided copies of all relevant information to employees?
- Has a central group been set up to review all the information and agree the assessment?
- Does the evidence used for the assessment include information from all relevant bodies?
- Have all necessary preventative and control measures been implemented?
- Are the procedures being observed, and is all the necessary equipment in good working order?
- Has personal protective clothing and equipment been issued?
- Is airborne monitoring being carried out where necessary, and are the results being made available? Are occupational exposure limits being exceeded?
- Is health surveillance being carried out, and are health records being made available?
- Has full information, instruction and training about the risks of hazardous substances and precautions to be taken been given to employees?

Health and Safety (First Aid) Regulations 1981

All workplaces must have first-aid equipment and arrangements for making sure that injured workers are treated quickly. Employers must:

- provide first-aid equipment, facilities, arrangements and personnel;
- inform all employees of the arrangements for getting first aid.

Self-employed people must provide their own first-aid cover.

The regulations further stipulate that first-aid arrangements must be 'adequate and appropriate'. The employer decides what should be provided, taking into account the following factors:

- the number of employees;
- the nature of the work;
- the size of the workplace;
- the distance of the workplace from outside medical services.

These factors determine what equipment and facilities must be present, such as first-aid rooms, first-aid boxes and eye-wash bottles.

First-aid boxes must be provided in a box marked with a white cross on a green background. Travelling kits should be provided where necessary. First-aid personnel who hold a current first-aid certificate from a training course approved by the Health and Safety Executive must be appointed. Two approved organisations are St John's Ambulance and the Red Cross. Trained first-aiders administer emergency first aid and know how to take charge in an emergency, for example by calling a doctor or ambulance. They should also take responsibility for first-aid equipment and facilities. Even the smallest workplace must have one first-aider on duty at all times when employees are at work. Large employers should ensure that there is one first-aider for every 50 employees. Records should be kept in an accident book of all first-aid cases treated.

Activity

Investigate first-aid provision in your school or college. Where are the first-aid boxes, and what are their contents? Who are the first-aid personnel? What training is provided? Is there an accident-recording book? Prepare a report.

The Reporting of Injuries, Diseases and Dangerous Occurrences Regulations 1985 (RIDDOR)

These regulations are concerned with recording and reporting accidents and ill-health at work.

If there are more than 10 employees, then there must be an **accident book** in which are recorded

- accidents;
- sickness which may have been caused by work;
- dangerous occurrences and 'near misses'.

Employees must tell the employer verbally or in writing as soon as possible of any such problems, and then the employer is legally bound to investigate.

Employers must report to the Health and Safety Executive or the environmental health department of the local authority whenever the following events occur:

- fatal accidents;
- a major injury or condition requiring medical treatment;
- dangerous occurrences;
- accidents causing incapacity for more than three days;
- some work-related diseases;
- gas incidents.

More serious accidents and dangerous occurrences must be reported immediately, and a written report provided within seven days.

There are special forms which must be completed when diseases occur, and there are 28 categories of reportable diseases, including poisoning and skin and lung diseases.

Trade-union safety representatives must have access to all information relating to all these problems in the workplace. The Employment Medical Advisory Service, which is part of the HSE, gives advice and information on the reporting of diseases.

Activity

> Find out about the accident book to be found in your school or college, and also in your work placement. Note the range of incidents reported.

Manual Operations Handling Regulations 1992

More than a quarter of accidents occurring in the workplace each year and reported to the enforcing authorities are associated with manual handling. The vast majority of these result in people being absent from work for over three days. The injuries are commonly sprains and strains, often of the back.

For medical and health services, 55% of all over-three-day injuries are caused by manual-handling accidents. The sprains and strains arise from incorrect ways of lifting and moving loads. Many manual-handling injuries are cumulative, resulting from poor posture and excessive repetition of particular movements. Sometimes the injury is attributable to a single handling incident, but not often. A full recovery is not always made, and physical impairment or even permanent disability can result.

The Manual Operations Handling Regulations 1992 are made under the Health and Safety at Work Act 1974. These implement a European Commission (EC) directive on manual handling. There is now an ergonomic approach to this aspect of work. Ergonomics is sometimes described as 'fitting the job to the person, rather than the person to the job'.

The Regulations require employers to carry out the following measures:

- avoid hazardous manual-handling operations where possible by redesigning the task, or by automating or mechanising the process;
- make an assessment of any hazardous manual-handling operation that cannot be avoided;
- reduce the risk of injury from those operations by improving the task, the load and the working environment.

Accurate records of accidents and ill-health will help identify potentially risky manual-handling operations. When a full assessment of the task has taken place, attention must then be given to reducing the risk of injury. Mechanical assistance may be possible.

Full training should be given to employees to ensure that they know how to safely carry out all the manual-handling operations required of them.

Activity

Find out about how heavy loads are moved around in your school or college. What mechanical assistance is provided?

Health and social care workers associated with environmental health issues

Many people employed in health and social care occupations have roles which include aspects of environmental health. Similarly, many people employed in the sector will face risks associated with their employment.

Environmental health officers (EHO)

The majority of EHOs are employed by local authorities. The job of these EHOs is to make sure that the local area has as safe and healthy an environment for its residents as possible. In order to do this, their responsibilities include:

- checking that food manufactured or sold in the area is produced and stored in hygienic conditions (see pages 255–7);
- investigating potential sources of infectious disease, areas of nuisance, animal welfare, and the licensing of body piercing and tattooing premises;
- maintaining decent living conditions for local people, particularly those in rented private accommodation;
- identifying possible health and safety hazards and investigating accidents;
- monitoring all types of pollution, such as air pollution from industrial processes and transport, and noise pollution.

An increasing number of EHOs are working in the private sector, where they are referred to as environmental health advisors or consultants. They advise companies of their legal duties and help them maintain good standards within the organisation.

Becoming an EHO involves both theoretical and practical training. This is usually undertaken on a four-year degree 'sandwich' course that combines academic studies with a year's practical work. Entry requirements for such a course include Science A Levels or an appropriate AVCE (Health and Social Care or Science). Environmental Health courses cover science, technology, statistics, public administration, law, occupational health and safety, pollution and public health and housing. In addition to a degree, students must pass exams set by the Chartered Institute of Environmental Health (CIEH). Some Science graduates can take postgraduate training.

(Information taken from the Chartered Institute of Environmental Health website, www.cieh.org.uk)

Occupational health nurses

Occupational health nurses may work in industry, health services, commerce and education (Figure 5.15). They may be employed as a member of a large occupational health service team, often attached to a personnel department, or they may be employed as independent practitioners.

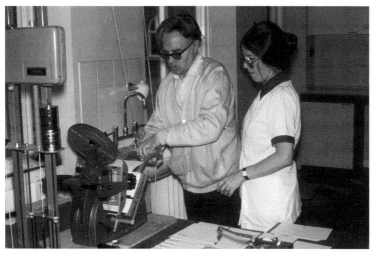

Figure 5.15 Occupational health nurse

Occupational health nurses are often considered to be leaders in public health in the workplace setting. Their responsibilities may include:

• the prevention of health problems, promotion of healthy living and working conditions;

• understanding the effects of work on health and health at work;

• basic first aid and health screening;

• work force and workplace monitoring and health need assessment;

• health promotion;

• education and training;

• counselling and support;

• risk assessment and risk management.

Registered nurses can take a post registration studies programme to become an Occupational health nurse. Useful preliminary experience would include working in an accident and emergency setting and practice nursing, and having an understanding of health promotion and education, health and safety issues, health screening, stress management and basic first aid.

(Information taken from the NHS Careers website, www.nhscareers.nhs.uk)

Housing officers

Housing officers deal with the day-to-day running of rented properties. They are responsible to ensure that clients' housing is healthy and appropriate. The work entails allocating vacant properties and overseeing exchanges between tenants. Housing officers may interview applicants for housing and assess their needs. They may discuss benefits with prospective tenants. They are responsible for visiting properties to check that they are being maintained properly and necessary repairs are being carried out. Housing officers take action when rent is not paid. This may involve giving advice, or in some cases legal action.

Their work involves keeping records, writing reports, attending and conducting meetings and working with statistics.

Housing officers are usually employed by local authorities although employment may also be provided by housing associations, government departments, charitable trusts, voluntary organisations, property companies and private landlords. In their work they may be in contact with social services departments, welfare rights organisations and citizen advice bureaux.

Housing officers may specialise in a particular area of work, such as homelessness, housing finance or welfare benefits.

There are no minimum entry qualifications. People may enter with GCSEs, a degree (there are degrees available in Housing Studies) or a postgraduate qualification. People may study part time or receive training in the workplace.

(Information taken from the national jobs and learning website, www.worktrain.gov.uk)

Social workers

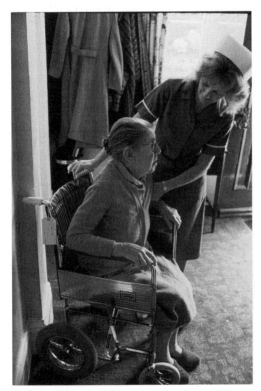

Figure 5.16 Social Worker

Social workers (Figure 5.16) support many kinds of people who need protection. As far as possible, people in need of help are encouraged to continue to live in their own homes, with personal social services organised by social workers. Like housing officers (above) they may have responsibility to ensure that clients' housing is healthy and appropriate.

Social workers are usually responsible for a 'caseload' of clients. They may specialise in a particular area, for example:

- children and families;
- adoption and fostering;
- health care settings;
- care management;
- mental health;
- work with offenders.

Social workers spend much of their time visiting clients. They have to keep case notes and write reports. They liaise with other professionals such as health care staff, housing officers, police, court officials and teachers.

In England and Wales, social workers are employed by local authority social services departments. In Scotland they are employed by social work departments and in Northern Ireland they are employed by area health and social services departments. Other employers include education departments, NHS trusts, national and local voluntary organisations, criminal justice services and private organisations.

(Information taken from the national jobs and learning website, www.worktrain.gov.uk)

Hospital workers

Many hospital workers have roles that include aspects of environmental health. Hospital laboratory workers, for example, have an important role in environmental health. The **Public Health Laboratory Service** (PHLS) covers England and Wales and consists of 49 laboratories, usually located on major hospital sites. Employees include medical staff Medical Laboratory Scientific Officers (MLSOs) and clinical scientists. They may be microbiologists or zoologists. PHLS work is carried out to protect the population from infection. In order to do this it:

- undertakes the diagnosis of disease in hospitalised patients;
- diagnoses illness within the general community;
- is involved in food and environmental microbiology;
- carries out disease surveillance;
- carries out research.

Many specimens sent to the PHSL come from environmental health departments of local authorities.

Activity

For each of the occupations described above:

1 Read the description of the responsibilities each professional has. What risks do you think they may face in carrying out these responsibilities?

2 If possible, interview local professionals and ask them about their responsibilities, the risks they face in carrying out these responsibilities, and precautions they take in order to reduce these risks.

Resources

Visits

Useful places to visit include:

- water treatment plants;
- refuse collection centres;
- sewage plants.

Speakers

It may be possible to invite speakers from local pressure groups, such as Friends of the Earth, or those with occupational health responsibilities.

Written information

- Leaflets and booklets are obtainable from the Health and Safety Executive, trade unions, local organisations, National Society for Clean Air, DEFRA (previously Ministry of Agriculture and Fisheries), Environmental Health Officers, Environment Agency, water companies and local authorities.
- Many legislative regulations are outlined in health and safety publications.
- Local newspapers feature local environmental issues on a regular basis.

Television

There are regular television documentaries on environmental health issues.

Teletext pages 155 and 169 give current hourly pollution levels for each UK region and country and a 24 hour forecast. There is also advice on air pollution and health. (This information is also available on freephone 0800 556677).

Useful websites

The internet will be a valuable resource for accessing information on issues concerning the environment on local, national or international scales. Some examples are given below. Some of these have convenient links to other relevant web sites.

Chartered Institute of Environmental Health
www.cieh.org.uk

Royal Environmental Health Institute of Scotland
www.rehis.org

Climate Action Network
Global network of NGOs working to promote government and individual action to limit human-induced climate change to ecologically sustainable levels.
www.climatenetwork.org

DEFRA (Department for Environment, Food and Rural Affairs)
This government department has taken over responsibility for agriculture, the food industry and fisheries from MAFF. It has taken on the environment , rural development, countryside, wildlife and sustainable development reponsibilities from the former DETR. Their website provides information on energy efficiency schemes.
www.defra.gov.uk

DoH (Department of Health)
www.doh.gov.uk

Department of Trade and Industry (DTI)
This Government department provides information on renewable sources of energy on the following website:
www.dti.gov.uk/renewable/main.html

Department for Transport, Local Government and the Regions (DTLR)

This Government department has responsibilities for transport, local government, housing, planning, regeneration, urban and regional policy. It has responsibility for building regulations and fire protection. The Health and Safety Commission and Executive report to DTLR ministers.

www.dtlr.go.uk

Department for Transport, Local Government and the Regions (Planning Information)

www.planning.dtlr.gov.uk

Environment Agency

A non-departmental public body. The most important environmental adviser and regulator in England and Wales.

www.environment-agency.gov.uk
www.environmentagency.wales.gov.uk

Scottish Environment Protection Agency (SEPA)

www.sepa.org.uk

Friends of the Earth

www.foe.co.uk

Greenpeace UK

wwwgreenpeace.org

Health and Safety Executive

Gives Health and Safety related information and statistics. (Information about Health and Safety at Work in Great Britain can also be obtained from HSE Infoline 08701 545500.)

www.hse.gov.uk

National Air Quality Information Archive Bulletin System

Gives current hourly pollution levels for each UK region and country and a 24-hour forecast.

www.aeat.co.uk/netcen/airqual/forecast.html

To check your local authority's progress on local air quality management and see if your local authority has had to declare an air quality management area:

www.aet.co.uk/netcen/airqual/aqma/home.html

National Society for Clean Air (NSCA)

www.nsca.org.uk

NHS Careers

www.nhscareers.nhs.uk

open.gov.uk

This service provides a first entry point to UK public sector information.

www.ukonline.gov.uk

The Pesticides Safety Dictorate (PSD)

This is an Executive Agency of DEFRA (see above), which administers the regulation of pesticides.

www.pesticides.gov.uk

Pesticides Action Network UK
This is an independent body that works to eliminate the hazards of pesticides.

The Public Health Laboratory Service (PHLS)
www.phls.co.uk

RSPB (Royal Society for the Protection of Birds)
www.rspb.org.uk

WHO (World Health Organisation)
www.who.int/home-page/

Worktrain – The National Jobs and Learning Site
www.worktrain.go.uk

Legislation

Students are expected to consider the relevant aims and objectives of legislation. They are not required to know particular details. Although dates of relevant legislation are provided, new legislation is under continuous development and the latest versions must be used. These can be found on the internet (www.legislation.hmso.gov.uk). This website contains the full text of all Public and Local Acts of the UK Parliament. From July 1999 all new Acts of the Scottish Parliament are found on the 'Scottish Legislation' website. Legislation made by the National Assembly for Wales is published on the 'Wales Legislation' website. The Statutory Publications Office is currently developing a Statute Law Database (SLD) that will comprise an updated version of all Acts of the UK Parliament and the Scottish Parliament, incorporating within any single piece of legislation all the amendments which have been made since its enactment. Further information on this can be found on www.lcd.gov.uk/lawdatfr.htm In the meantime, the Annual Chronological Tables of Statutes and the Chronological Tables of Local and Private Acts provide information as to the status of individual Acts and Measures and references to the Acts and Statutory Instruments by which the Act or Measure has been affected. Copies of these tables are generally available from your local reference library.

Relevant pieces of legislation

- The Building Act 1984
- The Clean Air Act 1956, 1993
- The Dogs (Fouling of Land) Act 1996
- The Environmental Protection Act 1990
- The Food Safety Act 1990
- The Health and Safety at Work Act 1974
- The Home Energy Conservation Act 1995
- The Housing Act 1985
- The Housing Associations Act 1985
- The Local Government and Housing Act 1989

- The Road Traffic Reduction Act 1997
- The Road Traffic Reduction (National Targets) Act 1998
- The Transport Act 1985
- The Waste Minimisation Act 1998
- The Water Industry Act 1991, 1999
- The Water Resources Act 1991

Glossary

Brownfield land   A brownfield site is an area of land that has been previously developed. It is defined as 'an area of land which is or was occupied by a permanent structure (excluding agriculture or forestry buildings), and associated fixed surface infrastructure'.

ELDC   Economically less developed country.

EMDC   Economically more developed country.

Eutrofication   The enrichment of waterways by nitrates and phosphates that can be caused by the leaching of fertiliser from agricultural land or from sewage effluent.

Green Belt land   A zone around a town or city in which there are legal restrictions on the construction of new buildings.

Herbicide   A chemical used to kill weeds.

Intensive agriculture   Food production in which there are high inputs of capital and/or labour per unit area of land.

Organic farming   The production of animals or crops without the use of chemical fertilisers, or pesticides.

Pesticide   A chemical used to kill animal or plant pests.

Urbanisation   The increased number of people living in cities.

Answers

Chapter 5

Air pollution

The number of deaths increases with increasing smoke and sulphur dioxide. It is not clear from the table which of these has the greatest effect.

Chapter 6

Influences on health and disease

This chapter covers:

- the main causes of disease;
- how information is gathered and used to determine the patterns of disease;
- the spread and incidence of some diseases;
- organisms that cause disease;
- how diseases are transmitted;
- the factors that influence disease patterns;
- how diseases are prevented and controlled.

The main types of disease

In order to prevent and control diseases, it is necessary that the ways in which we acquire diseases, and the spread and pattern of diseases in communities, is understood.

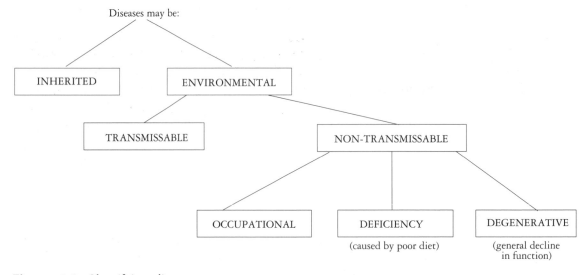

Figure 6.1 Classifying diseases

Diseases can be categorised in different ways. For example, they may be divided into **physical diseases**, which cause damage to any part of the body, and **mental diseases**, which cause changes to the mind.

An alternative way of classifying diseases is shown in Figure 6.1. They may be divided into **inherited diseases**, which are caused by an inherited genetic fault, and **environmental diseases**, which are caused by environmental factors, such as deficiencies in the diet or factors related to a person's occupation. Environmental diseases may be **transmissible**, which are caused by harmful organisms that invade the body (pathogens) and can be passed from one human to another, and **non-transmissible**, which are not caused by pathogens and can not be passed from person to person. **Occupational diseases**, which are diseases to which workers in certain occupations are particularly prone, are examples of non-transmissible diseases.

Inherited diseases

These conditions arise from the genes an individual has (see Chapter 4). They are also known as genetic diseases, or disorders, and may be passed down from one, or both, parents. They may be caused by dominant or recessive genes, or by chromosome abnormalities. Examples of inherited diseases are:

- sickle cell anaemia;
- haemophilia;
- cystic fibrosis;
- Huntingdon's chorea;
- muscular dystrophy.

There is a description of **sickle cell anaemia** and **haemophilia** on pages 206 and 215 in Chapter 4.

Activity

It may be possible to treat children with certain genetic diseases with **gene therapy**. This involves replacing a harmful gene with the correct gene. Find an example of this treatment being used, for example, in the information produced by the charity 'Jeans for Genes' (see 'Resources' in Chapter 4, page 221). In the example you find, what disease was being treated and how was the correct gene added?

Environmental diseases

These are diseases caused by a harmful environment. For example, they may be caused by pathogens in the environment, by poor diet, or by particular hazards in the working environment. Environmental diseases may be transmissible or non-transmissible.

Transmissible diseases

Transmissible diseases are also known as **infectious diseases**, and are the leading cause of global mortality and debility. These diseases are caused by **pathogens**. Pathogens are **parasites**, i.e. they are dependent on a live host for food and shelter. **Ectoparasites** live on the skin, while **endoparasites** are internal.

Pathogens may be:

- bacteria;
- viruses;
- protozoa;
- fungi;
- worms.

(These groups are described in the section on 'Causes of disease' on pages 299–308.)

Influenza

'Flu is an example of a transmissible disease which is caused by a virus (Figure 6.2). Influenza epidemics break out frequently, affecting large numbers of people in a particular area. Sometimes the outbreaks are **pandemic**: they spread across continents. A serious pandemic outbreak occurred in 1918 when 20 million people died worldwide. In 1968 there was an outbreak of 'flu which affected a quarter of the UK population, and killed about 1000 people.

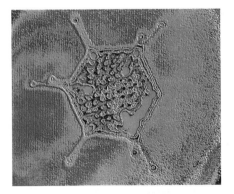

Figure 6.2 Influenza viruses seen with the electron microscope

The 'flu virus enters the respiratory tract in droplets and attacks the epithelial cells lining the air passages. There is an incubation period of two or three days. Then the symptoms appear. The temperature rises to 40°C on the first day, and this is accompanied by shivering, headache, sore throat and nasal congestion. Aches in limbs are common. After three to four days the temperature falls, but a cough may develop because of damage to the trachea and bronchioles. Sometimes pathogenic bacteria invade the damaged air passages and cause bronchitis or pneumonia.

Activity

Vaccination against 'flu is available. Find out, for example, from your community health centre, which members of the population are encouraged to take advantage of this

Non-transmissible diseases

These are diseases that are not caused by pathogens, and cannot be passed from person to person. One of the categories of non-transmissible diseases is occupational diseases.

Occupational diseases

Occupational diseases are caused by a hazardous working environment, and examples include repetitive strain injury and dust diseases, which are described below.

Repetitive strain injury

This is caused by the repetitive movement of part of the body. The strain is felt in joints and muscles. 'Tennis elbow' is an example of a repetitive strain injury. Keyboard workers, assembly-line workers and musicians may all experience pain and stiffness in the affected joints and muscles. Symptoms usually disappear with rest, but can have long term effects.

Dust diseases

Silicosis, asbestosis and farmer's lung are all examples of dust diseases.

- **Silicosis** Caused by particles of silica from rock or stone. The inhaled particles are trapped in the alveoli, and the lungs become fibrous and distorted. This reduces the surface area for gas exchange.
- **Asbestosis** Caused by the inhalation of particles of asbestos. The lower part of the lung becomes fibrous and cancer can result.
- **Farmer's lung** Caused by an allergy to fungal spores that grow in hay and are inhaled. An acute reversible form can occur a few hours after exposure; a chronic form, with the gradual development of irreversible breathlessness, can develop, with or without preceding acute attacks.

Activity

What precautions can be taken to reduce the likelihood of dust diseases developing?

The spread and incidence of disease

The study of the distribution of diseases is **epidemiology**, and sources of information patterns of disease are described on pages 295–9 The incidence of a disease varies from place to place and over time. The spread and incidence of two diseases are described below.

Malaria

Malaria is one of the world's biggest killers. Forty per cent of the world's population live in areas where the disease is endemic. In sub-Saharan Africa, malaria kills between 3000 and 4500 daily.

The World Health Organisation co-ordinated a worldwide eradication programme in the 1950s. They predicted that malaria would be eliminated from endemic areas by 1990. It is estimated that 25 million lives were saved and malaria was cleared from some countries. However, the programme was not the success the WHO predicted. This was because:

- the malarial parasite became resistant to the drugs used;
- the mosquitoes, which are vectors of the malarial parasite, became resistant to the insecticides, such as DDT, which were used against them.

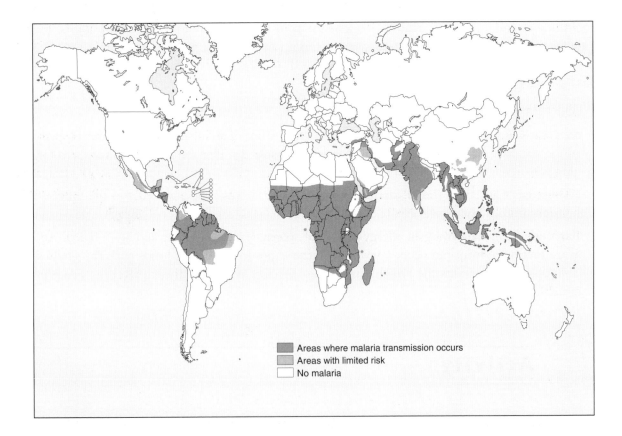

Figure 6.3 The global incidence of malaria

In the past decade the global incidence of malaria has been increasing. This is for a variety of reasons:

- an increase in drug-resistant forms of the malarial parasite;
- an increase in the proportion of cases caused by the most harmful form of the malarial parasite;
- climatic and environmental changes that favour the spread of mosquitoes;
- the migration of people because of war and civil unrest;
- the failure to develop a vaccine.

Figure 6.3 shows the global distribution of malaria.

Malaria was common in Britain from the sixteenth century until the end of the eighteenth century. It was known as 'marsh fever', and in some marshy areas such as the Somerset Levels, the Essex and Kent coasts and the Severn estuary, the disease was responsible for tripling the rate of infant mortality.

Scientists have suggested that malaria could return to Britain as an endemic disease. It is thought that with global warming it will become easier for mosquitoes to breed in the UK. Millions of people from the UK visit the malaria-infected regions of the world and the malarial parasites are becoming more drug resistant.

Every year a number of people in the UK develop malaria as a result of picking up the parasite abroad. There are also a number of cases of malaria that occur in people who have not been abroad, but who live near an airport. These are caused by malaria-carrying mosquitoes that are brought back on aeroplanes from tropical regions where the disease is endemic. Although aircraft are routinely sprayed with insecticide a few mosquitoes still survive.

Meningitis

Meningitis can be caused by bacterial or viral infection. The only form of bacterial meningitis that occurs in epidemics is **meningococcal meningitis**. The bacteria which cause this are present in about 10% of people but rarely cause disease. When a person does develop the disease, the lining of the brain – the meninges – become inflamed and death can occur within a few hours. Survivors can be left with both mental and physical disabilities.

The symptoms of meningococcal meningitis include:

- fever;
- stiff neck;
- severe headache;
- dislike of bright lights;
- vomiting;
- drowsiness;
- a rash that does *not* turn white when pressed with a glass (Figure 6.4).

In the UK there are about 2000 cases of the disease a year. One in 10 of the people who develop the disease, die. People with the disease are now more than twice as likely to survive the disease than they were a decade ago. This is because both the detection and the treatment of meningitis

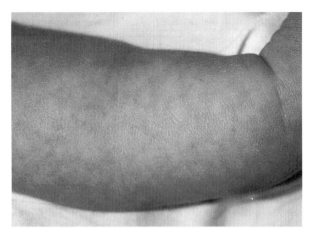

Figure 6.4 Rash caused by meningitis

have improved. In recent years a vaccine has become available that protects against the meningitis C form. This has almost eradicated this form of the disease from the UK.

Other forms of the disease cannot be controlled by vaccination, for example, the form of the disease which can cause septicaemia (blood poisoning) which leads to gangrene and organ failure. Survivors may require organ transplants or amputations. The incidence of this form of the disease in the UK has risen from 229 cases in 1989, to 1822 in 2000. There is now better detection of the disease, but it is not yet understood why there has been this increase in incidence.

Meningitis occurs globally. It is endemic in temperate climates. There is generally a steady number of sporadic cases with a seasonal increase in winter and spring.

WHO facts on the global incidence of meningitis

• 1.2 million cases of bacterial meningitis are estimated to occur each year; 135 000 of them are fatal.

• Approximately 500,000 of these cases and 50,000 of the deaths are due to meningococcal meningitis.

• The largest epidemics of meningococcal meningitis are experienced by sub-Saharan African countries in a 'meningitis belt' extending from Ethiopia in the east to Senegal in the west.

• A large widespread epidemic can follow on from a localised outbreak the previous year, and rates remain high in the following one to two years unless measures such as mass immunisation are used.

Activity

Find out about the change in the incidence of tuberculosis (TB) in the UK. What factors have contributed to the change?

(See page 336 for the answers.)

Sources of information on patterns of disease

In order to reduce the incidence of disease and to assist with health planning, it is important that there is information available on **patterns** of disease. In other words, information is needed on both the **incidence** (frequency of **occurrence**) and the **distribution** (on a local, national and global scale).

There is a wide range of sources of information available for students and health professionals.

Government statistics

The **Office for National Statistics (ONS)** is the government department that provides statistical and registration services. The ONS is responsible for producing a wide range of economic and social statistics. The Office was formed in 1996 when the Central Statistical Office merged with the Office for Population, Censuses and Surveys. Statistics are provided on the following themes: agriculture, fishing and forestry; health and care; education and training; commerce, energy and industry; economy; natural and built environment; transport, travel and tourism; labour market; crime and justice; population and migration and social and welfare. This information can be found on the ONS website (see 'Resources').

The social and health information gathered by the ONS comes from a variety of sources:

1 Registration

The ONS also incorporates the **General Register Office for England and Wales (GRO)**. The GRO is responsible for ensuring the registration of all births, marriages and deaths in England and Wales. Scotland and Northern Ireland have their own GROs.

At birth, the only information collected about the baby is its name, sex, place and date of birth (other information refers to the baby's parents). In death registration more information is gathered. The age and occupation of the dead person and where they lived are recorded, as well as the cause of death. This information usually comes from a death certificate completed by a doctor.

2 Surveys of the population

The **census** is the only survey that samples every member of the population (Figure 6.5). This survey has been completed every 10 years in the UK since 1801. In 2001 the Census form contained 40 questions in England and 41 questions in Wales. In an average household, the form took about 30 minutes for completion. The first set of questions were about accommodation and relationships within the household, and were answered by the householder or joint householder on behalf of all the people in the household. The remaining questions were addressed to each individual within the household. These questions covered:

- demographics (e.g., age, sex);
- cultural characteristics (e.g., ethnic group);
- state of health/long-term illness;
- qualifications;

IL1

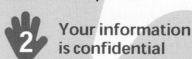

count me in
Census2001

This is
your Census!

Put yourself in the picture

The Census is a count of the whole UK population that only takes place every 10 years. Census information will be used to share out billions of pounds of public money in years to come. To make sure everyone benefits, we need the whole picture.

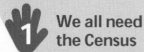

1 We all need
the Census

Census information is used to benefit us all
— we all need to be included so we can get
the services we need in the future.

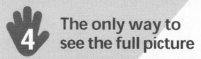

2 Your information
is confidential

Census forms are held in the strictest confidence — and are not released for 100 years!

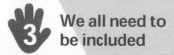

3 We all need to
be included

The Census is the only complete picture of the nation we have — it is impossible to plan services for invisible people.

4 The only way to
see the full picture

The Census is a unique set of facts and figures because it counts everyone in the country at the same time — there is no other way of capturing a complete picture of the nation.

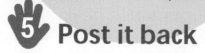

5 Post it back

Simply fill in the Census form on 29 April
and post it back in the reply-paid envelope.

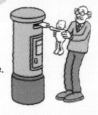

Remember

Sunday
29
April

is Census Day

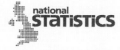

national
STATISTICS

'Crown copyright 2000: National Statistics

Figure 6.5 Publicity material produced for the 2001 Census

- employment/economic activity;
- workplace and journey to work.

The information given is confidential by law. After 100 years the information is released to the Public Record Office. There is a fine of £1000 for the failure to complete a form. The 2001 Census cost £255 million for the UK as a whole. The results will be available, mainly on the internet, from Summer 2003.

Usually in surveys, however, only a representative sample of the population is taken. The **Social Survey Division (SSD)** of the Office for National Statistics carries out survey research for the government departments and other public bodies on a range of social issues. They carry out eight continuous surveys throughout the year, every year. For example the General Household Survey has collected data from a number of families who fill in an extensive questionnaire, since 1971. In addition the SSD carry out surveys, which are commissioned, to give information on particular topics. They collect information from more than half a million people each year through:

- personal interviews, mainly in people's own homes;
- telephone interviews;
- postal surveys.

A number of the surveys carried out by the SSD provide information on health and care. Questions on health are included in many of the surveys on other topics, but a number of surveys are carried out that focus particularly on health. Recent examples include:

- survey of smoking, drinking and drug use among secondary school children;
- national diet and nutrition surveys;
- health education monitoring survey;
- adult dental health survey.

The Health Survey for England is a series of annual surveys about the health of people in England. The survey was first carried out in 1991 by the Office for Population Censuses and Surveys, which is now part of the Office for National Statistics. From 1994 onwards the survey has been carried out by the Joint Survey Unit of the National Centre of Social Research and the Department of Epidemiology and Public Health at University College London. The survey aims:

- to provide annual data about the nations health;
- to estimate the proportion of the population with specific health conditions;
- to estimate the prevalence of risk factors associated with these conditions;
- to examine differences between population sub-groups;
- to monitor targets in health strategy;
- (since 1995) to measure the height of children at different ages, replacing the national study of health and growth.

The survey combines questionnaire answers and physical measurements such as ECG readings, lung functions, and blood and saliva analysis. Further information and findings can be found on the website listed in 'Resources' at the end of the chapter.

3 Special notification

Data is gathered from certificates for sickness and notifiable diseases, and from the hospital records of patients.

District and regional health authority reports

There are eight **Regional Health Authorities (RHAs)** in England. The RHAs are involved in identifying and managing local research programmes. At five year intervals, data from the Health Survey for England is combined. This gives information on core topics at Regional Health Authority level. Core topics include:

- general health and psycho-social indicators;
- smoking;
- alcohol;
- demographic and socio-economic indicators;
- use of health services and prescribed medicines;
- blood pressure.

RHAs are divided into **District Health Authorities**. Each of these serves a population of about half a million people. They have to produce an annual report. This may be available at your local library, or you can phone your DHA and ask for a copy to be sent to you. In a typical report you will find information about the following:

- numbers of GPs and dentists in the area;
- numbers of community pharmacists;
- number of ophthalmic opticians and practitioners;
- a list of the main hospital and community health providers;
- a review of the year including new developments;
- financial information;
- plans for the future.

World Health Organisation (WHO) statistics

Various WHO publications contain useful epidemiological information, for example, the *World Health Statistics Quarterly* and the *Weekly Epidemiological Record (WER)*. Details of WHO publications can be found on the WHO website.

The WHO have created a global surveillance system for infectious diseases. Once a communicable disease outbreak has been confirmed, information is placed on the World Wide Web.

The WHO Statistical Information System (WHOSIS) has a website that describes and, where possible, provides access to, statistical and epidemiological data.

Addresses for these websites are given at the end of the chapter. See page 266, Chapter 5 for a description of the WHO.

Academic studies

Universities carry out a considerable amount of medical research. This may be funded by the Medical Research Council, the Department of Health and the Higher Education Funding Council for England. Medical charities and industry are also major funders of medical research. The findings of this research are published in academic journals, some of which are available on line. Examples of journals with a focus on patterns of disease include the *International Journal of Epidemiology* and the *Journal of Clinical Epidemiology*. Details of these, and a full list of similar journals can be found on www.mednets.com/epidemiojournals.htm Mainstream medical and health journals, such as *The Lancet* and the *British Medical Journal* also publish a number of articles with an epidemiological content.

The causes of disease

It is important to know about the micro-organisms responsible for causing disease, the behaviour of the micro-organisms and examples of the diseases they cause, in order to prevent disease.

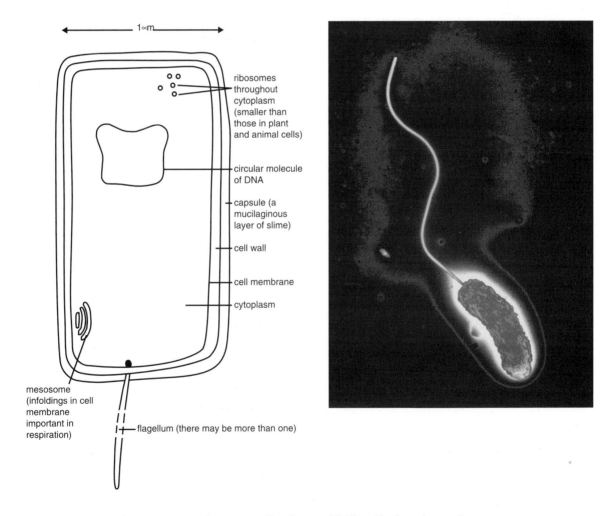

Figure 6.6 a) The structure of a generalised bacterium

b) The Cholera bacterium

Bacteria

Bacteria are the smallest organisms that have a cellular structure. They can be found in many environments, including in and on humans. Table 6.1 shows the four main bacterial shapes.

Activity

Bacteria have a very different cell structure from the cell structure of plants and animals. Compare the structure of a bacterial cell (shown in Figure 6.6a, above) with the structure of an animal cell (Figure 4.4 on page 165).

Conditions necessary for the growth of bacteria

If conditions are suitable, bacteria reproduce very rapidly. They divide into two identical daughter cells (**binary fission**). This may happen every 20 minutes, which means huge numbers may be formed. The conditions that affect the growth rate of bacteria include:

* temperature (see activity below);
* nutrient availability;
* pH;
* oxygen availability.

Most bacteria require oxygen for their respiration and are known as **aerobic**. Some bacteria do not use oxygen and are known as **anaerobic**. **Facultative anaerobes** can use oxygen if it is available, but **obligate anaerobes** cannot use oxygen for respiration. The bacterium that causes tetanus (see page 302) is an example of an anaerobic bacterium.

Activity

1 If a single bacterium is placed in a fresh medium, and divisions take place every 20 minutes, how many bacteria will there be after 10 hours? You may be surprised by the answer!

(See page 336 for the answer.)

2 Experiment to investigate the effect of temperature on bacterial growth.

You will need five petri dishes of nutrient agar.

1 Leave the petri dishes uncovered in the laboratory for about 30 minutes.

2   Replace the lids and treat as follows:

Plate 1:   Leave at room temperature (20–25°C)

Plate 2:   Leave in a refrigerator (3–5°C)

Plate 3:   Leave in the freezing compartment of a refrigerator (below 0°C)

Plate 4:   Leave in an incubator (37°C)

Plate 5:   Heat in a hot oven or place in a pressure cooker for 15 minutes (121°C+) and then at room temperature (20–25°C)

Label each plate.

3   After two or three days, tape the two halves of each plate together for safety reasons, and then examine. Make a table to show your observations.

4   To dispose of the plates safely, place in a disposable autoclave bag and autoclave for 15 minutes.

a   At what temperature did bacteria grow quickest?

b   What implications do your results have for food storage?

Behaviour under adverse conditions

Some bacteria can produce spores as survival structures in adverse conditions. Spores are very resistant to drought, heat and ultraviolet radiation and can remain viable for years. They develop inside the bacterial cell, which splits open to release them. Because they are so difficult to destroy, bacterial spores can be a problem in food production and storage. The pathogen that causes anthrax, *Bacillus anthracis*, is an example of a spore forming bacterium.

Shape	Example	Disease caused	Shape	Example	Disease caused
spherical (cocci) ○ ○ ○ single			**rod-shapedl (baccilli)** ▭ single	Clostridium terani	teranus
⊙⊙⊙⊙⊙ chains	Streptocous pyrogen	scarlet fever	▭▭▭▭ chains	Bacillus anthracis	anthrax
⊙⊙⊙ clumps	Staphylocous aureus	boils Pneumonia	flagellate	Salmonella typhi	typhoid fever
◎ pairs in a capsule	Diplococus pneumon	Pneumonia	**spiral-shaped (spirollum)**	Treponemia pallidum	syphilis
∞ pairs	Neisser gonorno	gonorrhoea	**comma-shaped (vibro)**	Vibrio cholerae	cholera

Table 6.1 Forms of bacteria

Examples of diseases caused by bacteria

Although some bacteria are pathogenic (cause disease), most are not harmful and some are beneficial to humans. For example, they are important in the breakdown of dead organisms and the recycling of nutrients and bacteria are used to produce antibiotics. Examples of pathogenic bacteria are shown in Table 6.1. There are bacteria that colonise and affect every part of the human body. Most bacterial diseases can be successfully treated, providing adequate medical resources are available. Three examples of disease causing bacteria are described below:

Boils

Staphylococci bacteria cause pus-forming infections such as boils (Figure 6.7) and abscesses. The toxin formed by these bacteria can cause food poisoning.

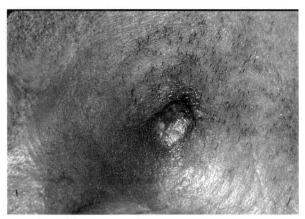

Figure 6.7 A boil caused by Staphylocci bacteria

Sore throats

Streptococci bacteria cause 'strep throat', a form of sore throat. The bacterium has a toxin that affects blood cells by breaking down the haemoglobin. There are a range of other diseases caused by *Streptococci* bacteria such as bacterial pneumonia, meningitis and scarlet fever.

Tetanus

Tetanus is caused by the bacterium *Clostridium tetani*. These are not spread from person to person like many bacterial infections. Instead they enter a wound, particularly a deep puncture wound, such as one made with a nail or knife. The bacteria are found everywhere, usually in soil, dust and manure, and they can form spores to survive adverse conditions (see above). These spores may enter the body and, because the bacterium is anaerobic, they germinate if oxygen is deficient, for example, in a deep cut, and the bacteria multiply rapidly. They produce a toxin that spreads throughout the body. The first symptoms are usually a headache and spasms of the jaw muscle. This is why tetanus is also called 'lockjaw'. These spasms spread to other muscles of the body and convulsions may be severe enough to cause broken bones. Prolonged infection eventually leads to respiratory failure and 60% of cases are fatal.

The disease can be treated with antibiotics and surgery to remove the bacteria. An antitoxin can be used to neutralise the toxin, and drugs can be used to reduce the muscle spasms. Vaccination against tetanus is available (see page 324).

Viruses

Viruses are, on average, about 50 times smaller than bacteria. They cannot be seen with a light microscope, and can only reproduce inside the living cells of a host. Viruses have a very simple, non-cellular structure. They contain a core of DNA or RNA surrounded by a protein coat.

(Photographs of viruses can be seen on 'The Big Picture Book of Viruses' website – details are given in 'Resources' at the end of the chapter.)

Examples of diseases caused by viruses

Influenza

See page 290.

HIV/AIDS

Acquired Immune Deficiency Syndrome (**AIDS**) is caused by the **human immunodeficiency virus (HIV)**. The structure of this virus is shown in Figures 6.8. The virus attacks certain cells of the immune system known as helper T-cells. This means that the entire immune system can no longer defend the body against the invasion of pathogens. AIDS is not itself a disease. Instead it describes the collection of diseases a person may develop because of having an impaired immune system. A number of these diseases, such as types of cancer and pneumonia, would otherwise be rare.

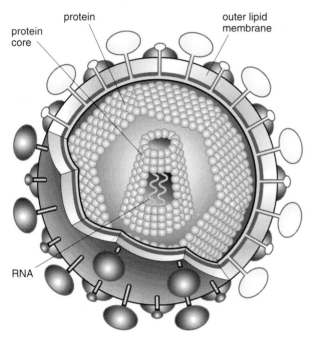

Figure 6.8 Diagram of human immunodeficiency virus (HIV)

The virus is spread from one person to another in bodily fluids. It is a very fragile virus and can only survive outside the body for a very short time. The virus can be transmitted by:

- sexual intercourse;
- sharing intravenous needles (for example in drug abuse);
- blood transfusions;
- crossing the placenta from mother to foetus.

It may take years between a person becoming infected with the virus (becoming **HIV positive**) and the development of symptoms. There is no cure for AIDS but drugs can be used to slow down the onset of symptoms. However, these drugs are expensive and so are not widely available in poor areas of the world such as Sub-Saharan Africa where AIDS is most common. The drugs also have a number of side effects. It is difficult to develop a vaccine for AIDS because the outer protein coat of the virus changes.

Currently, the best option is to prevent the spread of the virus. This can be helped by:

- educating people about the spread of the virus;
- the use of condoms;

- changes in sexual behaviour, for example, having fewer sexual partners;
- schemes to reduce the sharing of needles for drug use;
- the screening and treatment of blood used in transfusions.

Protozoa

Protozoa are single-celled organisms, some of which are parasitic. Many diseases are caused by these parasites, particularly in developing countries.

Examples of diseases caused by protozoa

Amoebic dysentery

Amoebic dysentery is caused by the protozoan *Entamoeba histolytica*. An infection of the intestinal tract with this organism leads to severe diarrhoea that contains blood and mucus. Sufferers of the disease develop a fever and abdominal pain. Amoebic dysentery is mainly confined to tropical and sub-tropical countries. The disease is spread by eating contaminated food or using contaminated water. Epidemics are common in overcrowded insanitary conditions, (although there are about 1000 cases a year reported in the UK).

The faeces of an infected person contain amoebic cysts. If these are swallowed by another person, they attach themselves to the lining of the gut. The amoebae reproduce and damage the walls of the large intestine. If the walls become perforated, the person may die.

Plasmodium

Plasmodium is the protozoan that causes malaria. It is carried from human to human by a mosquito **vector**. It is probably responsible for more human deaths in the tropics than any other organism. It is estimated that about 100 million cases of malaria occur in the world each year. It has been estimated that in tropical Africa alone, malaria accounts for 750,000 deaths each year, mainly among young children. In some developing areas, up to 5% of the children under the age of five die from malaria each year. In a number of areas the situation has been becoming worse since the late 1970s. This is largely due to the increased resistance of the mosquito vector to insecticides, and of Plasmodium parasites to anti-malarial drugs.

When the Plasmodium first enters the human, it goes to the liver where it feeds and reproduces for about two weeks. During this time the person will start to feel ill, and there will be a rise in body temperature. A fever then develops as the parasite leaves the liver and enters the bloodstream. The fever subsides as the parasites enter the red blood

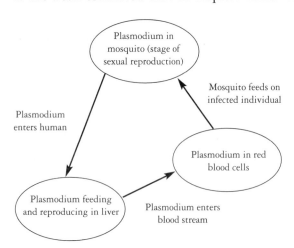

Figure 6.9 Simplified life cycle of Plasmodium

cells. A few days later the fever returns as the red blood cells burst, releasing many more parasites and their waste products into the blood.

When the female mosquito feeds on the blood of an infected person, the protozoa enter her blood. The parasite undergoes sexual reproduction in the stomach of the mosquito and the offspring make their way to the salivary glands. When the mosquito feeds again, the parasites are injected into a new host.

Activity

1 Can you suggest methods to prevent malaria, that could be used at different stages in the life cycle.

2 How is susceptibility to malaria affected in carriers of sickle cell anaemia? (See page 214)?

(See page 337 for the answers.)

Nematodes (roundworms)

Nematodes are elongated, round 'worms' with pointed ends. They are found in very large numbers in a wide range of habitats. It is estimated that the 10,000 known species represent only about 2% of their full number. Most are free-living, although it is the parasitic ones that are best well known.

Examples of diseases caused by roundworms

Threadworms

These are the most common bowel parasites in children in the UK, and are described in the article below:

River blindness

A well-known example of a disease caused by nematodes, is **river blindness** or **onchocerciasis**. The condition is endemic in 30 African and six Latin American countries. Figure 6.10 describes the disease and the work carried out by the charity Sight Savers International to prevent the disease.

Fungi

The group of fungi includes moulds and yeasts. Unlike bacteria, fungi are more likely to infect plants than animals, and few are human parasites.

Some tips to keep out those unwelcome creepy-crawlies

by Jean Waterworth, health visitor

Of all the creepy-crawlies that from time to time take up residence in or on us – and there are quite a few – worms seem to cause the most distress.

Head lice, for example, have almost achieved social respectability (not many young children escape them altogether) whereas threadworms are still a taboo subject, despite the fact that they are surprisingly common, specially in children.

Threadworms look, as their name implies, just like thin white cotton threads and can sometimes be seen in the bowel motion.

The worms live in the lower part of the bowel and emerge at night to lay eggs on the skin around the anus (back passage). This causes irritation so the child scratches himself and contaminates his fingernails with the eggs.

If he subsequently puts his fingers in his mouth he will be re-infested; likewise if he touches food, whoever eats it will become infected.

The eggs than pass through to the bowel, and the whole process starts all over again.

The good news is that although threadworms are a nuisance they aren't harmful. They seldom have any effect other than keeping children awake with itching or possibly making them wet the bed.

Doctors will prescribe a medicine to get rid of the worms and will probably advise the whole family to be treated – adults as well as children.

This is important as symptomless infection is common and if one member of the family is left untreated he could re-infect the rest.

Other measures should include making sure everyone uses their own flannel and towel, changing the child's pyjamas or nightie and sheets as often as possible and vacuuming the carpet frequently.

To prevent threadworms keep your children's fingernails short and clean and teach them to wash their hands after using the toilet and before eating.

If your family is affected take comfort from the fact that so are plenty of others – it's just that nobody talks about it.

And a final tip – if you floss your teeth, don't throw your used bits of floss down the toilet, it might cause unnecessary panic!

(*Okehampton Times*, 3 February 1994)

Examples of diseases caused by fungi

Oral and vaginal thrush

Thrush is caused by infection with a yeast-like fungus, *Candida albicans*. The fungus grows on moist areas of the body and can cause oral or vaginal thrush. The skin has red or white inflamed patches, and is sore and itchy. Thrush tends to develop if the skin is already damaged or if the normal bacteria found on skin have been destroyed by antibiotics. Oral thrush is a characteristic infection in people who develop AIDS (see above). Antifungal drugs can be used to treat thrush.

Athlete's foot

This is an infection of the skin between the toes caused by the fungus *Tinea* (Figure 6.11). Spores of the fungus can be picked up by bare feet. The spores will germinate in moist, warm conditions. The fungus digests the surface of the skin, and, if left untreated, can cause raw, painful areas on the feet. It can be treated with anti-fungal powders or creams.

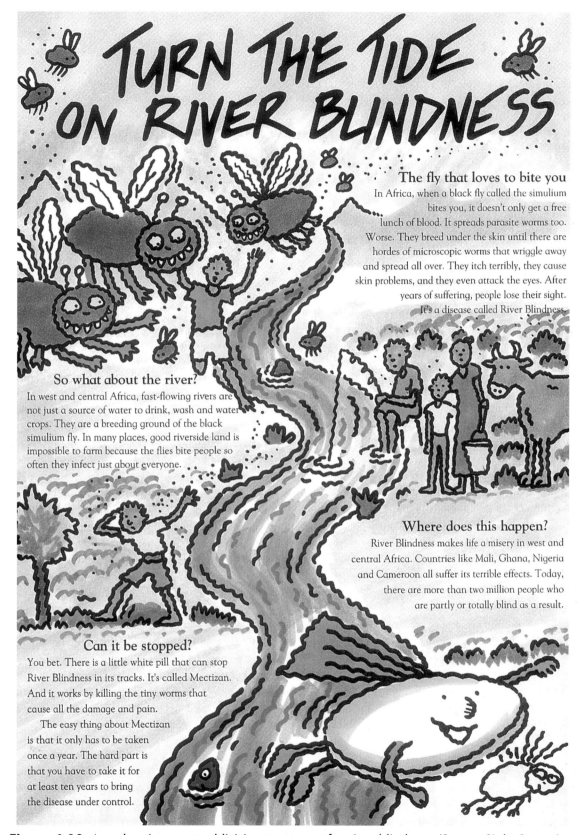

Figure 6.10 An advertisement publicising treatment for river blindness (Source Sight Savers)

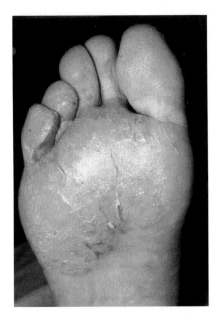

Figure 6.11 Athlete's foot

Table 6.2 The classification of major infectious diseases by mode of transmission

Airborne respiratory diseases	Intestinal discharge diseases (includes water- and food-borne)	Open sores or lesion diseases (direct contact)	Vector-borne diseases	Droplet spread diseases
Chicken pox	Amoebic dysentery	Aids	African sleeping sickness	Anthrax
Common colds	Bacterial dysentery (shigellosis) (staphylococcal)	Anthrax		Chicken pox
Diphtheria		Erysipelas	Encephalitis	Common colds
Influenza		Gonorrhoea	Lyme disease	Diphtheria
Measles	Cholera	Scarlet fever	Malaria	Influenza
Meningitis	Giardiasis	Small pox	Rocky Mountain spotted fever	Meningitis
Pneumonia	Hookworm	Syphilis		Poliomyelitis
Poliomyelitis	Poliomyelitis	Tuberculosis	Tularemia	Rubella
Rubella	Salmonellosis	Tularemia	Typhus fever	Scarlet fever
Scarlet fever	Typhoid fever		Yellow fever	Streptococcal throat infections
Small pox	Hepatitis			
Throat infections				
Tuberculosis				Tuberculosis
Whooping cough				

The transmission of infectious diseases

A key principle involved in the prevention of disease is recognising how people become infected by disease-causing organisms, and relating infection to the clinical stages of the disease process. Table 6.2 summarises the modes of transmission of a number of major infectious diseases.

Infection through contamination

Air

If an agar plate is left open to the air, within a few days fungi and bacteria will be growing. This is because bacteria and their spores, and fungal spores, settle on the plate from the air. In this way pathogens can infect their hosts, for example, through wounds or the respiratory pathway.

Water

Typhoid fever is an example of a disease in which the pathogen can be water-borne. It is most common where sanitation is poor and water purification is inadequate. Faeces of the infected individuals contain the pathogenic bacilli. If there are inadequate means of sewage disposal, the water supplies become contaminated, and healthy individuals drinking the water become infected. In 1937 there were 43 deaths and over 300 cases of typhoid fever in Croydon, in the south of England, arising from contaminated drinking water.

Food

Salmonella and botulism are examples of diseases that can only spread in food but many of the bacteria that are found in faeces and are water-borne (see above), can also be food-borne, for example, cholera, typhoid, and dysentery. The diseases caused by these bacteria tend to have very specific symptoms, and a long incubation period. They are very dangerous and may be referred to as food poisoning, but they are most commonly referred to by their actual names.

Usually, the term *'food poisoning'* is used to describe acute attacks of an explosive nature. Abdominal pain, diarrhoea and vomiting are associated with food-poisoning episodes, and these symptoms usually arise between two and 36 hours after eating contaminated food.

Food-poisoning bacteria divide very rapidly in conditions that are favourable to their growth. These include a warm temperature, humidity and a good food supply. Most bacteria usually require oxygen, but some, on the other hand, can only multiply when oxygen is absent; this latter condition is described as 'anaerobic'. The bacterium *Clostridium welchii* (*perfringens*) is a common cause of food poisoning. This is a bacteria organism which is also the most common cause of **gas gangrene** (the breakdown of skin and muscle tissue by toxins and gas production). The organism is resistant to heat and may survive in pre-cooked foods such as stews and pies, which are not correctly stored.

Some food-poisoning bacteria produce heat-resistant spores. These form when conditions are unfavourable for growth. They survive heat treatment, then start to grow again when favourable conditions return. Some food-poisoning organisms produce toxins, which can be very dangerous, for example *Clostridium botulinum*.

Infection through contact

Direct physical contact with people

Diseases that are spread by direct physical contact are known as **contagious diseases**. Relatively few diseases are spread through direct physical contact with an infected person. Examples include sexually transmitted diseases; the tropical disease **yaws**; **trachoma** (a common eye disease); the common wart; impetigo; and herpes simplex, which causes 'cold sores'.

Direct physical contact with infected materials

Infected materials can spread pathogens from one person to another. Examples of such materials include towels, sheets and cosmetics. Inanimate objects that spread pathogens are known as **fomites**. *Staphylococcus* infections can be spread in this way.

Droplet infection

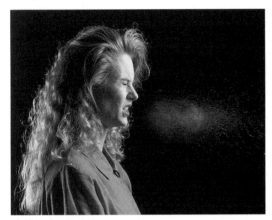

Figure 6.12 A photograph of a sneeze

Respiratory infections in particular are usually spread by droplet infection. Sneezing, coughing or even talking can result in a spray of droplets containing viruses or bacteria (Figure 6.12). These can then be inhaled by other people.

Infection by vectors

An organism that transmits a pathogen is known as a vector. It may actually contain the pathogen that multiplies within it – for example, the Plasmodium parasite in the mosquito (see the section on 'Malaria' on pages 292–3); or it may carry the pathogen on the outside of its body – for example, a housefly might transfer cholera from faeces to food where it may be ingested.

Rodents

Rodents such as rats may transmit pathogens to humans, either from themselves, or from the fleas that live on them:

1 Leptospirosis (Wiel's disease)

A disease caused by bacteria that are transmitted from rodents and other mammals to humans. It can be picked up from water that has been contaminated by these animals. The disease begins with a fever that could easily be mistaken for 'flu. It may affect the liver causing jaundice, it may cause meningitis or it may affect the kidneys.

2 Bubonic plague

A disease caused by a bacterium that is transmitted from rats and other wild rodents to humans by rat fleas. Painful swellings develop in the lymph nodes in the groin and armpits. These may burst and then heal or they may bleed under the skin, which can lead to ulcers and may be fatal.

Dogs

Dogs may transmit a number of diseases to humans. Examples of these include **toxocariasis** (see Chapter 5), page 259 on 'Dog fouling penalties') and **leptospirosis** (see above).

Incubation period

The incubation period is the interval between the pathogen being picked up and the appearance of the first symptoms. During this time, the pathogen will be increasing in numbers in the body. Diseases have specific incubation periods. Examples of these are given in Table 6.3.

Table 6.3 Incubation periods of some common diseases

Disease	Incubation period
Cholera	1–5 days
Meningococcal meningitis	2–10 days, usually 3–4 days
Influenza	2 or 3 days
Tuberculosis	A few weeks to a few months
Amoebic dysentery	A few days to several weeks
Tetanus	Usually about two weeks, but can be several months
HIV/AIDS	Initial incubation a few weeks, but up to ten years or more before the symptoms of AIDS may develop
Malaria	From a week to a year

Acute illness

An acute illness has a rapid onset, severe symptoms and a brief duration. Diseases have specific **signs** and **symptoms**. Signs are indications of a particular disorder that are observed by a health professional, but not apparent to the patient. For example, if a doctor suspected a patient had measles, he would look for white lesions inside the patient's mouth (Koplik's spots). Symptoms are indications of a particular disorder that are noticed by the patient. For example, a person with measles would notice the fever, cough and rash. Chapter 3 gives the signs and symptoms of a number of diseases.

Crisis is the turning point of a disease, after which the patient either improves or deteriorates. Since the advent of antibiotics, infections seldom reach the point of crisis.

Recovery and remission period

If the severity of symptoms lessens, or temporally disappears, this is known as **remission**. It is often used to describe the reduction in the size of a cancer and the symptoms it is causing.

Influences on disease

Diseases affect some individuals and not others, and the difference may arise because of other influencing factors. Examples of these factors are described below.

Social and economic circumstances

In 1997 the Government ordered an independent inquiry into inequalities in health. It confirmed that a person's social and economic circumstances will influence the likelihood that they will suffer from certain diseases. Social and economic factors that are known to have an effect on health include:

- income and expenditure;
- social class;
- unemployment;
- housing;
- diet;
- education;
- health;
- culture.

Diet

Many diseases arise as a result of malnutrition. This is any disorder of nutrition resulting from eating an unbalanced diet. It includes both dietary deficiencies and overeating. Examples of diseases caused by malnutrition are given in Table 6.5, page 326.

Culture

The Independent Inquiry into Inequalities in Health Report published in 1998 confirmed that there were many indications of poorer health among the minority ethnic groups in England. For example, certain ethnic minority women may not attend clinics unless they are staffed by women.

Lifestyle choices

It is recognised that people's lifestyles and behaviour are causative factors in many diseases. Important factors include:

- diet;
- exercise and maintaining mobility;
- stress;

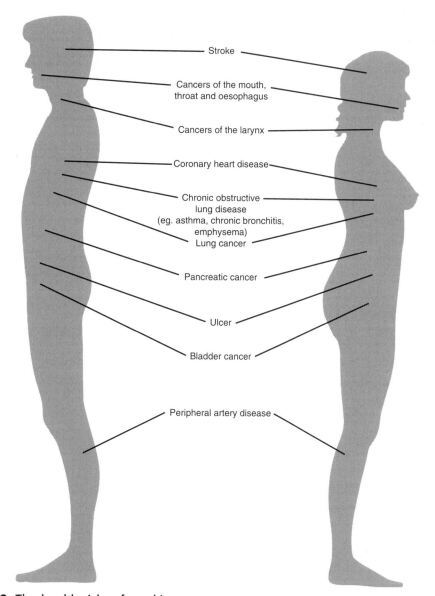

Figure 6.13 The health risks of smoking

- recreation and leisure activities;
- smoking;
- alcohol and substance abuse;
- sexual behaviour.

Drug abuse

Table 6.4 shows that a variety of diseases are associated with illegal drug use. Particular problems are associated with intravenous drug use. AIDS, hepatitis C and other bloodborne diseases are spread through the use of previously-used needles. In an effort to prevent drug abusers using these dirty needles, there are a number of needle exchange programmes, which make sterile needles available in exchange for used needles.

Table 6.4 Examples of diseases associated with particular illegal drugs

Drug	Diseases and conditions associated with use
cocaine	depression, heart disease
PCP (also know as 'angel dust')	heart problems, acute renal failure
marijuana	bronchitis, asthma, sinusitis
injected drugs (e.g. heroin)	HIV, AIDS, hepatitis

Smoking

Smoking is the biggest single cause of preventable disease and premature death. There are five times more people killed by smoking than by road accidents, suicide, murder, AIDS and illegal drugs put together. About 13 million people in the UK smoke. More cigarettes are smoked per person in the UK than the European average, and more deaths are caused by smoking than in other countries. Passive smoking (breathing other people's smoke) kills hundreds of people every year. Figure 6.13 shows the diseases that are caused by smoking. Smoking is a key factor in deaths from coronary heart disease (CHD) and strokes. A third of all cancer deaths and between 80% and 90% of deaths from lung cancer are caused by smoking.

The main components of cigarette smoke that cause harm are:

Nicotine

A powerful drug in tobacco that causes physical and psychological addiction to smoking. It increases heart rate and blood pressure, and the risk of blood clots.

Tar

A black sticky substance that contains cancer-causing chemicals (carcinogens). It clogs up the lungs and the chemicals are gradually absorbed, causing irritation and damage.

Carbon monoxide

A harmful gas that combines with haemoglobin in the red blood cells, reducing the amount of oxygen the blood carries. A reduction of oxygen to the muscles of the heart is particularly harmful.

Environment

The environment a person lives in affects their chances of suffering from certain diseases.

Living close to nuclear waste establishments

Radioactive waste comes from a number of sources, and ranges from paper towels used in hospitals to acid solution from irradiated nuclear fuel. It is classified into four categories:

High level waste (HLW)

This is also known as heat-generating waste, and consists mainly of nitric acid solution containing fission products separated from irradiated nuclear fuel during reprocessing.

Intermediate level waste (ILW)

This consists mainly of metals, with smaller quantities of organic materials, inorganic sludges, cement, graphite glass and ceramics. ILW mainly arises from the dismantling and reprocessing of spent fuel, and from the general operation of nuclear plants.

Low level waste (LLW)

This includes metals (redundant equipment) and organic materials (laboratory equipment, clothing and paper towels). The organic materials come mainly from areas where radioactive materials are used, for example, hospitals and research establishments.

Very low level waste (VLLW)

This covers waste with very low concentrations of radioactivity, and mainly arises from hospitals and non-nuclear industry sources.

These nuclear wastes are disposed of in a variety of ways, depending on their level of radioactivity.

1 VLLW is disposed of by various means such as domestic refuse at landfill sites or by incineration.

2 LLW is disposed of inside a concrete vault at Drigg, near Sellafield, Cumbria.

3 ILW and HLW are currently stored. ILW is contained in cement and put inside steel drums, which are then placed in an above-ground concrete store. HLW is concentrated by evaporation and then stored inside double-walled stainless steel tanks inside thick concrete walls. A small quantity of HLW is immobilised in glass.

In September 2001 the Government launched a sixth-month consultation which aimed to initiate a nationwide debate on the issue.

We know about the harmful effects of radiation on human health from accidents in nuclear power plants, and from testing and using nuclear weapons. Radioactive chemicals, such as strontium-90, iodine and caesium, can be released into air or water as a result of accidents in nuclear power stations. This happened in the UK in 1957 at Sellafield, and there was a far worse accident at Chernobyl in the USSR in 1986. More than 200 people suffered radiation sickness and 31 were killed. Birth defects are still very common in the area. The radioactivity content in the muscles of sheep was so high in Scotland, Cumbria and Wales after Chernobyl that slaughter was not permitted for two months. The radioactive wastes are carried into the air and then absorbed into grass, and from there into cattle or sheep. Humans may be contaminated from eating the affected meat or milk.

Radioactive iodine affects the thyroid, and strontium-90 accumulates in bone adjacent to the marrow where blood cells are made. A nuclear bomb was dropped on Hiroshima and Nagasaki in 1945 and strontium-90 was among the radioactive materials released. This radiation had very many effects, including a high incidence of leukaemia (see Figure 6.14).

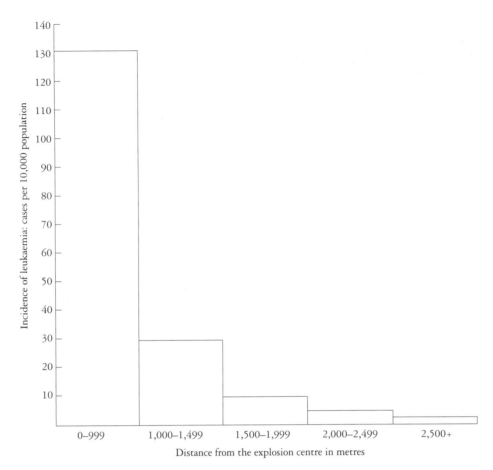

Figure 6.14 The relationship between the incidence of leukemia and the distance from the centre of the atomic explosion in Hiroshima

The report from *The Guardian* (21 October 1993), below, describes a link found between childhood cancers and radiation doses received by fathers who worked at the Sellafield nuclear plant

Activity

Find out about the advantages and disadvantages of using nuclear power stations to provide electricity.

Racial and cultural differences

Some inherited diseases only affect people from certain racial groups. Examples of these are given below.

Study finds limited Sellafield cancer link

In the widest and most detailed study so far, a government agency has found a statistical link between children with leukaemia and non-Hodgkin's lymphoma and radiation doses received by fathers who worked at the Sellafield nuclear plant in Cumbria.

However, the study published yesterday by the Health and Safety Executive also said that radiation alone does not explain the link.

The news comes two weeks after a High Court judge ruled that there was insufficient evidence to allow a suit by the families of two children whose fathers had worked at Sellafield. And a week ago two papers in the *British Medical Journal* suggested that a link between paternal exposure and childhood leukaemia was unlikely.

A 'cluster' of unexpected leukaemia incidence near the nuclear complex was first identified 10 years ago, and since then there has been a heated debate over its significance.

However, the latest study by the health executive does not resolve the confusion. It reported that a 'strong statistical association' appeared to exist only for children born to employees who lived in Seascale itself, and only for those who started work before 1965.

Many of Sellafield's workers live beyond the parish. 'For West Cumbria as a whole, we found little evidence to suggest a father's high pre-conception radiation dose increases the risk of leukaemia and lymphoma for his children,' said Eddie Varney, the executive's deputy chief inspector of nuclear installations.

Later he added: 'We cannot find any single factor which satisfactorily explains what we have seen in West Cumbria. We can't find any causal links to workplace practices. All we have is statistical associations.' ...

The research – the first to confirm findings three years ago by the late Professor Martin Gardner – covered not just cases of leukaemia in children born and diagnosed in West Cumbria, but in children born there and diagnosed elsewhere. The study also covered a wider timespan, and concerned itself with all other cancers.

Confusingly, the latest findings also appeared to support – but not confirm – another hypothesis, 'biological mixing', proposing that when settled communities are 'invaded' by people from outside there is likely to be a greater incidence of leukaemia.

'When you try to attach a cause,' said Mr Varney 'you run into difficulties. About 90 per cent of the Sellafield working population live outside Seascale, and a lot of those people have had very high radiation doses, and you don't see the same association.'

British Nuclear Fuels, which operates Sellafield, said in a statement yesterday that the executive had produced 'yet further evidence' that the father–child association 'does not work'.

Dr Patrick Green, of Friends of the Earth, said: 'Despite spending millions of pounds in a desperate attempt to get Sellafield off the hook, BNFL cannot explain away the radiation excess.' ...

(The Guardian, 21 October 1993)

Thalassaemia

Thalassaemia is an inherited blood disorder that affects mainly affects people of Mediterranean and South Asian descent. This disease is described on pages 202–4 in Chapter 4.

Malaria and sickle cell anaemia

Malaria is described on pages 292–3 and sickle cell anaemia is described on page 215 in Chapter 4.

Sickle cell anaemia is most common in people of African or African-Caribbean descent, but it may also occur in people from India, Pakistan, the Middle East or the Eastern Mediterranean. This distribution has probably come about because the disease can give some resistance to malaria. People who carry a gene for sickle cell disorder, but who do not actually have the disease, are said to have **sickle cell trait**.

Individuals who have sickle cell trait are less likely to catch malaria because the malarial parasite does not reproduce in affected red blood cells. This advantage now explains why sickle cell anaemia affects people who originated from areas where malaria is endemic, but not people who originated from areas where there is no malaria.

In Britain there are about 6000 cases of sickle cell disease, which is a similar figure to the number of patients with cystic fibrosis and haemophilia.

Lack of sanitation and quality of water supplies

A clean water supply and efficient sewage disposal are both important in maintaining a healthy population and keeping it free of disease. A description of these water treatments is described below in Chapter 5. See 'A clean water supply' on page 250, and 'Sewage treatment' on pages 251–2.

The prevention and control of disease

Scales of mechanisms to control disease range from the activity of individual cells of the body to international co-operation. The prevention of disease needs to be understood at a personal, local, national and international level.

How the body protects itself against disease

There are a number of mechanisms that the body deploys in an effort to control and prevent disease. They begin with the prevention of invasion by pathogens.

Natural barriers

The skin

The skin covers the body and provides a physical barrier that protects underlying tissue from physical abrasion, bacterial invasion, dehydration and ultraviolet radiation.

See Figure 6.15, which shows the human skin structure. The epidermis contains **keratin**, a waterproof protein that serves as an effective barrier against bacteria. The ability of the skin to detect temperature, touch, pressure and pain also helps in the avoidance of physical damage, and hence of the entry of bacteria.

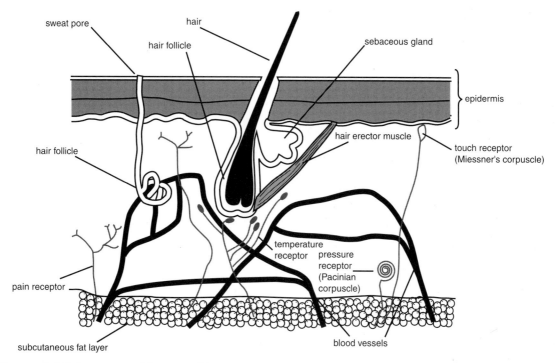

Figure 6.15 Structure of human skin

Mucus membranes

Mucus membranes also line the digestive, respiratory, excretory and reproductive tracts. These membranes secrete mucus, which prevents the cavities from drying out and traps dust particles and microbes. In the respiratory tract, cilia sweep these particles away.

Repair mechanisms

Even though the skin is such an effective barrier to micro-organisms, it is still essential that any damage be rapidly repaired. Repair consists of the following stages:

- clotting;
- an inflammatory response;
- phagocytosis;
- the production of scar tissue;
- the creation of a new skin surface;
- the scab sloughing off.

Clotting

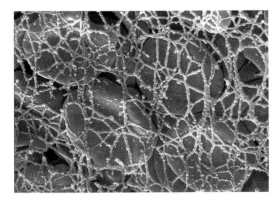

Figure 6.16 Red blood cells enmeshed in fibrin in a blood clot

A clot forms for two main reasons:

• to prevent further blood loss;

• to block the entry of micro-organisms.

Because blood circulation is pressurised, speed is vital in dealing with any leaks. Within the first few seconds of bleeding, the platelets react. They stick to the damaged tissues and send out biochemical messages to soluble clotting proteins in the plasma. This causes them to change into solid gel-like and fibrous clots.

If a clot forms in undamaged blood vessels, it can have very serious consequences. To prevent blood clots accidentally forming when they are not needed, the clotting process takes place through a highly complex series of reactions dependent on at least 12 clotting factors (see Figure 6.18).

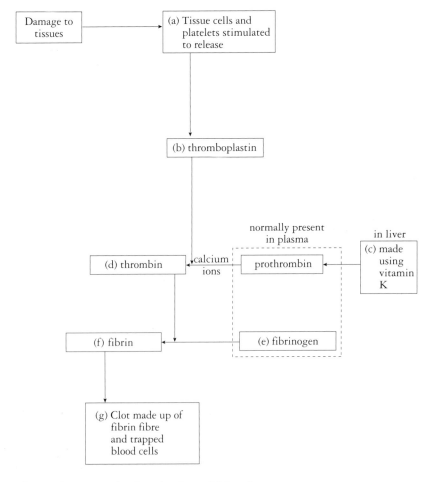

Figure 6.17 The main stages in the clotting of blood

Inflammatory response

The inflammatory response is both protective and defensive. It attempts to neutralise and destroy toxic agents and to prevent their spread, and is characterised by the tissue that surrounds a wound becoming red, swollen, hot and painful. Think, for example, of the response to a rusty nail scratching the skin, or to a sore throat caused by bacteria. Figure 6.18 shows the main steps involved in the inflammatory response. The immune response and phagocytosis mentioned are explained below.

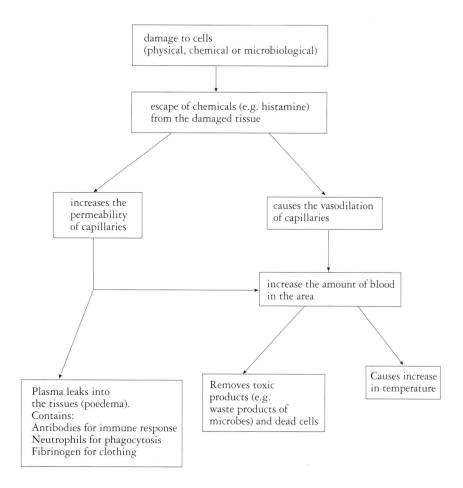

Figure 6.18 The main stages of the inflamatory response

In all but the mildest inflammation, **pus formation** occurs. Pus contains living and non-living white blood cells and debris from other dead tissue. If it does not drain it becomes an **abscess**, and if inflamed tissue is shed several times an **ulcer** forms.

Phagocytosis

Phagocytosis is a non-specific form of resistance against micro-organisms or other foreign particles of matter. It involves the ingestion and destruction of these by **phagocytes**. The white blood cells, **neutrophils**, are a type of phagocyte. In response to chemicals released by damaged cells, they may leave the blood vessels and migrate to the site of the infection (see the

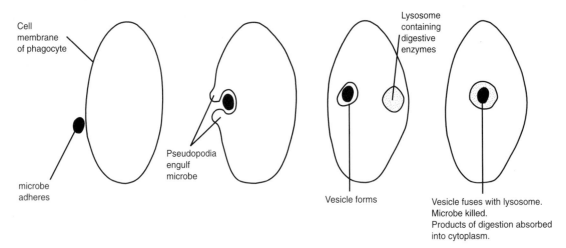

Figure 6.19 The mechanics of phagocytosis

'Inflammatory response' section above). Non-migratory or **fixed** phagocytes are found in many organs, for example liver, lungs, brain, spleen and lymph nodes.

Both types of phagocyte function in the same way, with the first step involving attachment of the bacteria and the second step involving its ingestion.

Antibacterial secretions

Many of the body fluids produced on the exterior of the body contain antimicrobial substances. For example:

- **tears** produce a enzyme that kills bacteria.
- **sebum**, an oily fluid produced by the sebaceous glands in the skin, inhibits the growth of certain bacteria.

The hydrochloric acid produced in the stomach lowers the pH to 2. This is acidic enough to kill off many potentially harmful bacteria. The natural pH of the skin, which is between 3 and 5, is also acidic enough to discourage the growth of many of the microbes with which it comes into contact.

Immunity

If pathogens overcome the barriers described above and invade the body, there are various coping mechanisms which can be used to eliminate them, or at least prevent harmful symptoms they may cause.

Natural immunity

Antibodies are protein molecules produced by white blood cells known as **lymphocytes**. They are produced in response to **antigens** – proteins or polysaccharides that coat foreign material such as bacteria. Antibodies are produced that are each specific to a single antigen. The production of antibodies is not restricted to the blood: they also occur on mucus surfaces – for example in the respiratory system – and in the alimentary canal.

There are two types of lymphocyte, the **T cells** and **B cells**, which develop in different ways and have different functions.

- T cells have membranes in which there are receptors for antigens. When one of these cells recognises a complementary antigen, it attaches itself to it and destroys it.
- B cells recognise antigens in a similar way to T cells, but respond differently. They are stimulated to produce many **plasma cells**, each of which synthesises and liberates identical antibodies at a rate of nearly 2,000 molecules per second.

There are many different ways in which antibodies prevent the replication and harmful effects of micro-organisms. These include:

- causing the foreign particles to stick together;
- neutralising the toxins produced by the pathogen;
- breaking down foreign material;
- stimulating phagocytosis (see above).

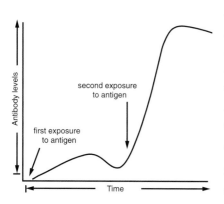

Figure 6.20 The primary and secondary response to antigen

As well as forming antibody-producing plasma cells, the B lymphocytes also produce **memory cells**. These enable an individual who has been exposed to an antigen once to respond more promptly and rigorously in a subsequent encounter (see Figure 6.20). This is called the **secondary response**, and is what gives an individual **immunity** to a disease that they have already encountered.

The type of immunity described above is known as **active immunity**. This is because the individual makes their own antibodies. **Passive immunity** involves the *acquisition*, not synthesis, of antibodies. Babies have passive immunity because they acquire antibodies which have passed across the placenta from their mother (Figure 6.21).

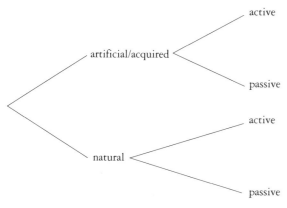

Figure 6.21 A summary of types of immune status

Artificial immunity

The immune response can be artificially induced by **vaccination**. When the vaccine is introduced into the bloodstream, the antigens it contains stimulate the production of antibodies without causing the disease itself.

There are a number of different types of vaccine:

- **Living attenuated micro-organisms.**
  These are living pathogens which multiply but have been weakened, e.g., by heating or by culturing them outside the

human body, so that they are unable to cause the symptoms of the disease. Examples include the vaccines against measles, tuberculosis, poliomyelitis and rubella (German measles).

- **Dead micro-organisms**. Although harmless, these still induce antibody production. Examples include vaccines against typhoid, influenza and whooping cough.
- **Toxoids**. In some cases the toxin alone will cause antibody production. The toxin can be made harmless and used as a vaccine.
- **Extracted antigens**. The antigens can be taken from the pathogens and used as a vaccine. For example, the influenza vaccine can be prepared in this way.
- **Artificial antigens**. The genes responsible for antigen production in a pathogen can be transferred to a non-pathogen. This harmless organism can be grown in a fermenter where it will produce the antigen which can be harvested and used in a vaccine.

All the above methods produce what is known as **active** immunity because they cause the individual to synthesise their own antibodies. **Passive** immunity involves the acquisition or synthesis of antibodies. These can be acquired artificially. Antibodies from other mammals, e.g., horses, are injected in the form of a **serum**. For example, tetanus and diphtheria can be prevented in this way.

Activity

1 Which type of immunity acts most immediately, active or passive?

2 Which type of immunity would be the longest-lasting, active or passive?

3 Suggest a situation in which passive immunisation would be more useful than active immunisation.

(See page 337 for the answers.)

Factors that reduce the ability to resist infection

Malnutrition

(See table 6.5)

As we have seen, the antibodies produced in the immune response are proteins. This explains why a person with a diet deficient in protein is likely to have reduced immunity – they do not have enough protein in the body to make an adequate amount of antibodies. Two conditions seen in starving people who have extreme protein deficiency are **kwashiorkor** and **marasmus**. People with both these conditions have reduced immunity. The condition **anorexia nervosa** (Figure 6.23), a wasting disease that develops from severe dieting also causes a reduction in immunity.

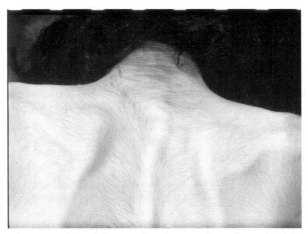

Figure 6.22 Anorexics have reduced immunity that makes them highly susceptible to infections

Stress

Stress occurs when there is a change in a person's life that they find difficult to cope with.

Stress, and how we manage our stress levels, is linked directly to our health. A constant unmanageable level of stress will lead to physical and mental ill health.

Activity

Factors that cause stress are known as **stressors**. Examples of stressors include:

- bereavement;
- the birth of a child;
- moving house.

Can you think of other examples of stressors?

Table 6.5 Diseases caused by malnutrition

Nature of malnutrition	Disease
Lack of	
Iron	Anaemia
Calcium	Rickets, osteoporosis
Vitamin A	Scarring of the cornea
Vitamin D	Rickets in children, ostoemalacia in adults
Vitamin B$_1$	Beri-beri
Vitamin C	Scurvy
Protein	Kwashiorkor, marasmus
Fibre	Cancer, coronary heart disease
Surplus	
Fats	Cancer, coronary heart disease
Sodium	High blood pressure
Nitrates	Stomach cancer

When a person is under stress, the hormone adrenaline is produced. Some effects of adrenaline include:

- an increased heart rate;
- less blood flowing through the skin, which may make a person appear pale;
- less blood flowing around the gut, which leads to the feeling of butterflies;
- increased sweating.

If the stress continues, eventually the adrenal gland, which produces adrenaline, will no longer function properly and the person will become ill. More than a quarter of a million British people are absent from work each day because of stress-related illnesses, and it is estimated that these cost £7 billion per year in sick pay, lost production and health service provision. There are various disorders that are triggered by stress. For example:

1 **Physical health problems,** such as stomach ulcers, heart attacks, skin disorders such as eczema and psoriasis, myalgic encephalomyelitis (ME). The function of the immune system is reduced, resulting in an increased number of infections.

2 **Emotional effects,** such as anxiety, insomnia and depression.

3 **Behavioural effects,** such as increased smoking or consumption of alcohol.

Table 6.6 shows many of the short and long term symptoms of stress.

Table 6.6 Symptoms associated with stress

Behavioural short term	Physical short term	Emotional short term
Over indulgence in smoking, alcohol or drugs	Headaches	Tiredness
Accidents	Back aches	Anxiety
Impulsive, emotional behaviour	Sleeping badly	Boredom
Poor relationships with others at home and at work	Indigestion	Irritability
Poor work performance	Nausea	Depression
Emotional withdrawal	Dizziness	Inability to concentrate
	Excessive sweating	Apathy
	Trembling	
Behavioural long term	**Physical long term**	**Emotional long term**
Marital and family breakdown	Heart disease	Insomnia
Social isolation	Hypertension	Chronic depression and anxiety
	Ulcers	
	Poor general health	

Medication

One of the most obvious cases in which medication reduces the ability to resist infection is the use of **immunosuppression**. This is where drugs are used to reduce the functioning of the immune system. It is used to stop the rejection of organs or tissues in transplants. Without these drugs, the immune system of the recipient will recognise the donated tissue or organ as 'foreign', and attack it. The drugs suppress the immune system, then this leaves the person who received the transplant, vulnerable to infection.

Case study

Helen is now six. When she was born she was often very unwell and at 18 months she was diagnosed as having the inherited condition, SCID (severe combined immune deficiency). Twenty years ago, children like Helen would have had to live their short life in a sealed environment to prevent them coming into contact with germs. Now, however, bone marrow transplants are available, but first the child's own immune system must be destroyed in order to prevent the rejection of the donated bone marrow. Helen was lucky because her sister, Clare, had bone marrow which was suitable for donation. When she was two she went to hospital for the transplant. Before she received the donated bone marrow, immunosuppression drugs were used to destroy Helen's immune system. This meant that she was even more susceptible to infections than she ever had been until the donated bone marrow started working. In the hospital she was kept in a sealed room in which the air was filtered to prevent the entry of pathogens. Back at home everything had to be kept very clean. Her family had to remove their shoes outside and wash their hands in an antibacterial solution and for a year, friends were not allowed to visit. Keeping the home free of germs really was a matter of life and death. Four years on, Helen is fine and living life to the full.

Chronic diseases

The ability to resist infection is reduced in those suffering from chronic diseases. **Diabetes** was described in Chapter 3, pages 135–7. Diabetics can suffer damage to their blood vessels and nerves, as well as a decreased ability to fight infection. Because of their poor blood flow and damage to injuries going unnoticed, infections may develop, particularly in the feet.

Prevention and control of diseases within care settings by care workers

Health professionals have important roles to play in preventing and controlling the spread of diseases.

Staff awareness and training

Cross-infection is the transfer of infection from one patient to another in hospital or other care setting. It is a major problem. At any one time, nine percent of hospital in-patients are suffering from an infection acquired following their admission to hospital. The emergence of micro-organisms that are resistant to antibiotics, increases the threat to patients who acquire infections. The Department of Health suggests that about 30% of Hospital Acquired Infections (HAIs) are preventable. It is important that all staff are made aware of how infection can spread and are given training in how to prevent it. There are a number of different sources of information available to health professionals:

- **Governmental guidelines** are provided, for example, for hospital environmental hygiene; hand hygiene; the use of personal protective equipment gowns, masks, gloves etc.) and the use and disposal of sharps (needles and blades).

- **Specialist publications**, such as the *Journal of Hospital Infection* and the *British Journal of Infection Control*.

- **Articles** in more general medical journals, such as the *British Medical Journal* (*BMJ*) and *Journal of Infectious Diseases*.

- **Internet**, for example the *BMJ* and *Journal of Infectious Diseases* are available on-line.

- **Organisations**, such as the Hospital Infection Society, Infection Control Nurses Association and Association of Domestic Management.

- **Conferences and workshops**, for example, the Infection Control Nurses Association holds an annual conference.

- **Training courses.**

- **Posters** and **leaflets** (Figure 6.24).
- **CD Rom** produced by the Infection Control Nurses Association for all levels of health care workers within a hospital environment.

Cross-infection control staff

Community Infection Control Nurses (CICNs) are employed to help prevent and control infections and communicable diseases. Their work may be targeted to:

- the NHS;
- statutory services;
- voluntary agencies;
- the private sector;
- the general public.

The first infection control nurse was appointed in the 1950s when *Staphylococcal* infections (see page 302) were common in hospitals, despite the use of antibiotics. In 1970 the Infection Control Nurses Association (ICNA) was formed. The ICNA provides information for both health professionals, and for parents, children and informal carers (website details are provided in 'Resources' at the end of the chapter).

A survey of community infection control nurses carried out in 1998, showed that CICNs provide a comprehensive community infection control service that includes:

- advice and support;
- training and education;
- policy and guideline development;
- audit (collecting evidence on infection control, and assessing quality).

Infection Control Doctors (ICDs) are doctors who specialise in the prevention of communicable diseases in hospitals and the community. In 1997 a Diploma in Hospital Infection Control was established to help formalise their training .

The **Hospital Infection Research Laboratory** was set up by the Medical Research Council (MRC) in 1964. It employs research scientists to investigate all aspects of infection in hospitals. Particular interests include the assessment of new disinfectants and evaluation of automatic washer disinfectors for endoscopes.

Activity

Go to the ICNA website (www.icna.co.uk) and read the advice leaflet given to health professionals on how to wash hands correctly. Effective hand washing is thought to contribute more than any other procedure to the control of hospital acquired infection. (Figure 6.24)

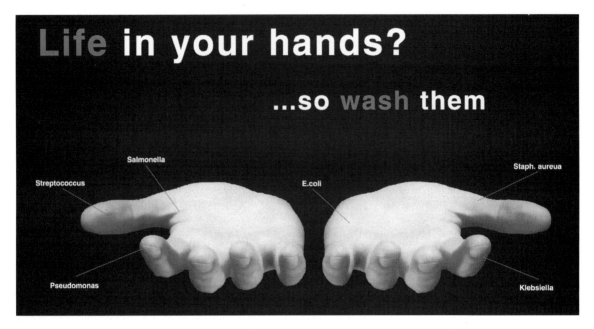

Figure 6.23 Poster aimed at health professionals to help prevent cross infection

Regulations on reporting illness

Legislation exists to ensure that diseases are reported to the relevant authority. Employers have a duty to report accidents, injuries, and work-related diseases to the Health and Safety Executive. Examples of **reportable diseases** include tuberculosis and hepatitis. The Reporting of Injuries, Diseases and Dangerous Occurrences Regulations 1985 (RIDDOR) is described on pages 278–9 in Chapter 5.

Doctors are required by law to report to the local health authority, the name, sex and address of any patient suffering from a **notifiable disease** including the following:

- mumps
- rubella
- dysentery
- whooping cough
- scarlet fever
- malaria
- tuberculosis
- food poisoning or suspected food poisoning
- meningitis
- ophthalmia neonatorum
- tetanus
- leptosporosis
- meningococcal septicaemia (without meningitis)
- viral hepatitis

- typhoid fever
- paratyphoid fever
- acute poliomyelitis
- acute encephalitis
- cholera
- plague
- anthrax
- diphtheria
- yellow fever
- typhus
- relapsing fever
- rabies
- viral haemorrhagic fever.

(**Note** HIV/AIDS is not a notifiable disease, although there is an anonymous, confidential reporting system for the purpose of national statistics.)

The aims of the notification procedures are:

- to keep records of numbers and types of infections in the community at any given time;
- to allow preventative measures to be introduced immediately;
- to allow doctors to be informed and reminded of symptoms;
- to allow the provision of adequate treatment facilities;
- to allow research to be carried out;
- to keep track of the success of national immunisation strategies.

Monitoring of clients' health

Observations and measurements ◇ (see pages 189–201 in *Vocational A Level Health and Social Care*) can be used to spot signs and symptoms of disease, or the potential for disease, in clients. This enables the necessary steps to be taken:

- to prevent disease occurring;
- to allow steps to be taken to control a disease already present;
- to give an opportunity to curb the spread of disease.

Routine **observations** commonly used in a care setting include:

- facial expression and posture;
- skin colour and texture;
- breathing quality.

Routine physiological **measurements** commonly used in a care setting include:

- pulse;
- blood pressure;

- temperature;
- peak flow;
- lung volume;
- weight;
- urine and blood analysis (see Chapter 3).

The role of public bodies

World Health Organisation (WHO)

The WHO have an important role in the prevention and control of disease on a global scale.

(See page 266, Chapter 5 for a description of the WHO and its roles, and page 298 earlier in this chapter for a description of the information on patterns of disease provided by the WHO.)

As mentioned earlier in the chapter, the WHO have created a Global Outbreak Alert and Response Network. Its aim is to:

- combat the international spread of outbreaks;
- ensure that appropriate technical assistance reaches affected states rapidly;
- contribute to preparing for long-term epidemics;
- evaluate international efforts to contain outbreaks.

European Parliament

- The European Parliament represents 375 million people in 15 European countries.
- The first elections to the European Parliament took place in 1979.
- There are 625 representatives in the European Parliament who are elected every five years.

The European Parliament produces legislation, and it has been agreed that 'a high level of human health protection must be ensured in the definition and implementation of all European Community policies and activities.' The European Parliament provides incentive measures designed to protect and improve human health. Areas that the European Parliament have been involved in include:

- cancer;
- AIDS and other communicable diseases;
- drug dependence;
- drug use in sport;
- mental health.

In 2000 the health strategy of the European Community included an action plan which aims to:

- improve health information;
- establish a rapid-reaction mechanism to respond to major health threats;
- tackle the determining factors for health.

Environmental and public health departments

Environmental health is concerned with housing, sanitation, food, clean air and water supplies. Public health is concerned with assessing the needs and trends in health and disease of populations as distinct from individuals. It includes epidemiology, health promotion, health service planning and evaluation, control of transmissible diseases and environmental hazards.

2MT:The government departments (for websites see 'Resources' on pages 284–6 at the end of Chapter 5) that have a role in environmental and public health include:

DEFRA (Department for Environment, Food and Rural Affairs)

This government department has taken over responsibility for agriculture, the food industry and fisheries from MAFF. It has taken on the environment , rural development, countryside, wildlife and sustainable development responsibilities from the former DETR.

DoH (Department of Health)

Within this department, the Public Health Group has responsibility for protecting and improving the nation's health. It develops and implements policies to prevent disease, prolong life and identify any factors which might affect or threaten the health of the public.

Department for Transport, Local Government and the Regions (DTLR)

This Government department has responsibilities for transport, local government, housing, planning, regeneration, urban and regional policy. It has responsibility for building regulations and fire protection. The Health and Safety Commission and Executive (see pages 273–4 in Chapter 5) report to DTLR ministers.

Inspection agencies

Inspection agencies (for websites see 'Resources' on pages 284–6 at the end of Chapter 5) that have a role in the prevention of disease include:

Environment Agency

This is the most important environmental regulator in England and Wales. It is described on page 249 in Chapter 5. In Scotland this work is carried out by the Scottish Environment Protection Agency (SEPA).

Health and Safety Executive

This works with local authorities to ensure that health and safety law is put into practice. It is described on pages 273–4 in Chapter 5.

Health education and promotion units

There are a number of different definitions of health promotion, and one that is often used is the WHO definition: 'Health promotion is the process of enabling people to increase control over, and to improve, their health.'

The **Health Development Agency (HDA)**, which replaced the Health Education Authority, aims to boost the status of public health by advising on good practice and commissioning new research. Chapter 2, gives more information on the HDA and other organisations concerned with health education and promotion.

Glossary

Aerobic bacteria   Bacteria that require oxygen for their respiration.

Anaerobic bacteria   Bacteria that do not use oxygen for their respiration.

Candida   Fungus that causes oral and vaginal thrush.

Clostridia   Bacteria that cause tetanus.

Congenital disease   A disease that is present at birth. It may have been inherited, or may have occurred as a result of injury or infection in the womb or at birth.

Cross-infection   The transfer of infection from one patient to another in hospital.

Diabetes   Any disorder of the metabolism causing excessive thirst and the production of large volumes of urine. An example is *diabetes mellitus* in which a lack of the hormone insulin prevents the correct control of blood sugar level.

Disease   A form of ill health or illness with a particular set of symptoms.

Endemic   A disease that is always present in the population.

Environmental disease   A disease caused by the environment (i.e. not inherited).

Environmental health medicine   The branch of medicine concerned with housing, sanitation, food, clean air and water supplies.

Epidemic   Rapid rise in the incidence of a disease, so that a large proportion of the population suffer from it.

Epidemiology   The study of factors that determine the spread of disease, and the patterns of disease in populations.

Haemophilia   A hereditary disorder in which blood clots very slowly.

Immunosuppression   The reduction in the functioning of the immune system, for example, by drugs used in organ transplants.

Incubation period   The interval between the pathogen being picked up and the appearance of the first symptoms.

Influenza   A highly contagious viral infection that affects the respiratory system.

Inherited disease   A disease that is transmitted through genetic mechanisms.

Malaria   An infectious disease caused by a protozoan that is transmitted from person to person by mosquitoes.

Meningitis   An inflammation of the lining of the brain caused by viral or bacterial infection.

Non-transmissible disease   A disease that cannot be passed from one person to another.

Occupational disease   A disease caused by a hazardous working environment such as repetitive strain injury and dust diseases.

Parasites   Organisms that live on, or in, a living organism.

Pathogens   Organisms that cause a disease, for example, some bacteria and fungi.

Public health medicine   The branch of medicine concerned with assessing the needs and trends in health and disease of populations as distinct from individuals. It includes epidemiology, health promotion, health service planning and evaluation, control of transmissible diseases and environmental hazards.

Protozoa   Single celled organisms, some of which are parasitic.

Remission period   A period during which the severity of the symptoms of a disease lessens, or temporarily disappears.

Repetitive strain injury   Pain caused by the repetitive movement of part of the body.

Sickle cell anaemia   An inherited blood disorder that affects people of African origin. Carriers of the disease have some resistance to malaria.

Signs   Indications of a particular disorder that are observed by a health professional, but not apparent to the patient.

Staphylococci   Bacteria that cause boils.

Streptococci   Bacteria that cause sore throats.

Symptoms Indications of a particular disorder that are noticed by the patient.

Thalassaemia   An inherited blood disorder, widespread in Mediterranean countries, Asia and Africa.

Tinea   Fungus that causes athlete's foot.

Transmissible disease   A disease that can be passed from one person to another.

Vector   An organism that transmits a pathogen.

Viruses   Have a very simple, non-cellular structure. They contain a core of DNA or RNA surrounded by a protein coat and can only reproduce inside the living cells of a host.

Resources

Information sources could include:

- community health centres;
- health authority departments;
- health promotion units;
- Internet websites;
- World Health Organisation;
- UNICEF;
- local and national media reports;
- CD-ROMS;
- environmental health officers and organisations;
- health and social care workers, including health visitors.

Useful websites

The European Parliament
www.europarl.eu.int

The Health Development Agency (this has replaced the Health Education Authority)
www.hda-online.org.uk

The Hospital Infection Society
www.his.org.uk

The Hospital Infection Research Laboratory
www.bham.ar.uk

The Infection Control Nurses Association
www.icna.co.uk

A full list of such journals with results of research into patterns of disease
www.mednets.com/epidemiojournals.htm

The Meningitis Trust
www.meningitis-trust.org.uk

The Meningitis Research Foundation
www.meningitis.org

The National Statistics website, which contains a vast range of official UK statistics and information about statistics
www.statistics.go.uk

Information from the Social Survey Division
www.statistics.gov.uk/ssd

Information on the Health Survey for England
www.doh.gov.uk/public/hthsurep.htm

'The Big Picture Book of Viruses', which gives images and other information on viruses
www.virology.net/Big_ Virology/BVHomepage.html

Information on the World Health Organisation including details of their publications on patterns of disease
www.who.int

Information on communicable disease outbreaks from WHO Global Infectious Disease Surveillance
www.who.ch/emc/outbreak-news/

The WHO Statistical Information System website which describes and, where possible, provides access to, statistical and epidemiological data.
www.who.int/whosis/

Answers

Chapter 6

The spread and incidence of disease

Cases of TB have risen more than one fifth in a decade in England and Wales. The number of cases in London has risen by nearly one third since 1993. TB rates in the capital are four times higher than in the rest of the country.

Homelessness, poverty, overcrowding and drug resistant strains of the bacteria have contributed to the increase.

Bacteria

After 10 hours there would be 67,108,864 bacteria.

Malaria

1 The number of mosquitoes can be reduced by reducing areas of water where they breed, using fish to feed on the larvae, or with the use of insecticides.

People can avoid being bitten by mosquitoes by the use of nets and screens and insect repellent.

Drugs can be used to kill the Plasmodium parasite.

2 Carriers of a gene for sickle cell anaemia are less susceptible to malaria.

Artificial immunity

1 Passive immunity acts more immediately than active immunity because the antibodies are already present.

2 Active immunity is longer lasting because memory cells are formed which give a rapid immune response if there is a subsequent exposure to the pathogen.

3 An example of a situation in which passive immunisation would be more useful would be in the prevention of tetanus if a person was cut. This is because passive immunisation has a more immediate effect.

Chapter 7

Sociological aspects of health and illness

This chapter covers:

- sociological perspectives
- sociological concepts
- sociology of health
- sociological influences on policy making and practice
- sociological research methods
- assessment guidance

Introduction

How we think about and respond to health and illness is strongly influenced by factors such as social status, gender, age and the norms and values we share with others. Health care professionals need to be able to understand the influence of such social factors on individual experiences of health and illness. Policy makers also need to take these factors into account when they are attempting to predict health care needs and plan services for communities. In this chapter we explore:

- the nature of sociology and review some of the main themes and perspectives
- some important sociological concepts relevant to health and illness
- sociological approaches to the study of health and illness
- sociological influences on policy making and practice
- sociological research methods and their application in the study of health and illness.

The assessment for this unit requires you to carry out an investigation into a health care issue or topic. Some suggestions for suitable investigations are given throughout the chapter and guidance on planning your investigation is given at the end.

Sociological perspectives

The nature of sociology

Sociology is one of a range of academic disciplines called the **social sciences**. These also include economics, politics, history, psychology and anthropology. The social sciences are concerned with understanding human behaviour. There is often overlap between the interests of different disciplines within the social sciences which can at times be confusing. In particular there is an overlap in the areas of social life studied by psychologists and sociologists.

Both disciplines are interested in how we learn, how we construct or make sense of the world and how social conditions affect our behaviour and life experiences. Yet there remain differences in approach. Psychologists, for the most part, focus on the individual response to social conditions, reasoning processes and factors that influence individual human behaviour. Sociologists, on the other hand, are most often concerned with exploring the relationships between different aspects of social life, social conventions, institutions, group experiences and their impact on individuals and societies. Sociologists aim to understand, classify and explain different social conditions, their origins and causes and their influence on people's lives.

Like other academic disciplines, sociologists have developed their own special terms to describe how societies are organised and how our lives are shaped by our social experiences. In some cases, depending on the particular emphasis of the sociologist, different terms may be used to refer to the same thing. Many of the terms used in sociology are broad **concepts** that are used to indicate

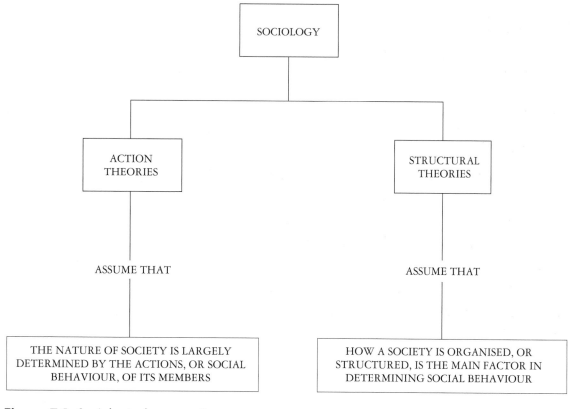

Figure 7.1 Sociological perspectives

a general way of thinking about some aspect of society. For example most sociologists will agree that the concept of health can be understood in a variety of ways depending on the perspective of the person using the term. For doctors 'a healthy person' may mean that the person has no known medical condition. For psychologists a healthy person may be someone who has a 'positive psychological response' to illness or disease. We will explore some concepts of health later in the chapter.

Sociological perspectives

Sociologists tend to approach the study of society from two broad perspectives. Some argue that the way society is organised or 'structured' is the most important factor influencing our life experiences. Social structures, such as membership of gender or social class groups, are said to be most important in determining individual life experiences. For this group of **structuralists** the main aim is to understand how the formal and informal organisation of society influences our lives.

Others argue that the way a society is organised is really a consequence, not a cause, of social behaviour and experience. Understanding how interactions, personal views and values shape our life experiences is the main aim of **Social Action** theories.

Structural theories

Structuralist approaches to sociology focus on the way society is organised and examine how this affects social behaviour and life chances. Within the Structuralist approach to sociology we can identify two distinctive sociological perspectives.

Consensus theories

Consensus means agreement and consensus theorists argue that societies exist because people agree to abide by common sets of values and codes of conduct. Humans, they argue, are essentially social beings. We depend on each other (interdependence) and naturally form social relationships with each other and, as a consequence, form societies. We are born into social institutions such as the family and go on to form and join other social institutions such as schools, universities and work places. These social institutions provide us with stability and security but they also reinforce certain forms of social behaviour.

These social institutions perform vital social functions by creating and maintaining social conditions that shape and determine what life will be like for us. They contribute to the overall stability and harmony of society and, as a consequence, the well-being of its members. Sociologists who emphasise the social function of different social conditions and behaviours are known as **Functionalists**. Functionalists argue that even apparently undesirable conditions such as poverty and ill health can have important positive influences on how well society operates. For example poverty can be seen to contribute positively to society because it enables manufacturers of cheap and shoddy goods to sell their products. Removing poverty, it is argued, would lead to more unemployment for workers in these industries.

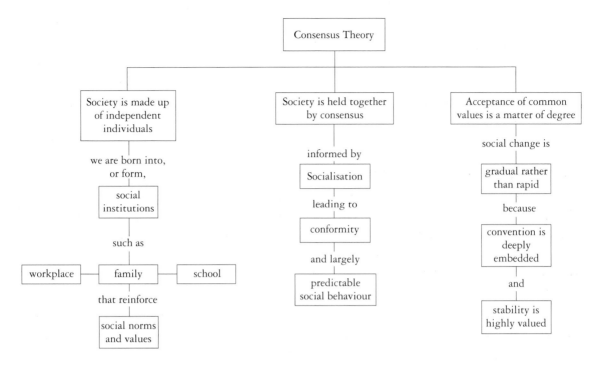

Figure 7.2 Consensus theories

Activity

Make a list of the ways ill health might be said to serve a useful social function.

Make another list of the negative influences of ill health on society.

Do you think that ill health is, on balance, performing a useful social function?

Conflict theories

Unlike the Consensus Theorists, who emphasise agreement, stability, social harmony and a process of gradual change within society, Conflict Theorists argue that a more detailed examination will reveal that society is made up of groups of people who have different and conflicting interests. Social institutions and the way they operate reflect this ongoing conflict. For Marxists the main reason for this conflict lies in the different economic interests of the middle and working classes. From this point of view the interests of the middle class are often opposed to those of the working class. For example middle class families often value higher education, academic qualifications and professional status because they reinforce the kinds of ideas and attitudes that they value. Middle class children are more likely to go to university, are less likely to be unemployed, earn higher salaries and usually have better working conditions than their working class contemporaries. As a consequence they will also benefit from better health and increased life expectancy.

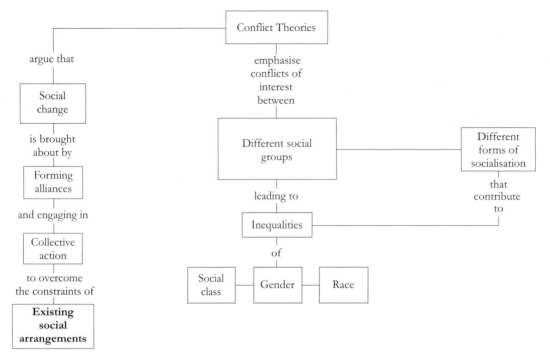

Figure 7.3 Conflict theories

Sociological concepts

In this section we will examine some important sociological concepts.

Socialisation

Socialisation is the term used by sociologists to describe how we learn about how to behave with other people in different social situations. The process of socialisation begins as soon as we are born and is ongoing throughout our lives. The values, conventions and social expectations that are introduced and reinforced within social institutions, such as the family or school play an important part in determining how we live our lives. This process of socialisation will, in turn, influence our experience of health and illness.

 Activity

Often the informal reactions of family members to ill health will influence the way we react to our own ill health. Think about your own family life. Consider how your parents, older brother or sisters or other family members' experiences of ill health have influenced your way of thinking about health and illness.

For example if someone in your family feels ill and complains of having a headache and a high temperature how do the family react?

Do they:

Use painkillers such as paracetamol as soon as the pain begins?

Immediately make an appointment with the GP?

Ignore it and hope it will go away soon because 'it's probably just a virus that's going around'?

Say 'there's always something wrong with you,' and carry on watching TV?

How have responses such as these influenced your thinking about illness?

Social stratification

Social stratification refers to the way that societies tend to develop hierarchical divisions between different groups of people. These divisions usually involve differences in access to power, wealth and favourable life experiences. Social stratification normally leads to inequalities between different groups within society.

Social class

There are different ways of understanding social class. We can think of class in terms of economic groups. For example Karl Marx (1818–83) thought society could be divided up into the 'bourgeoisie' – those who owned the means of production (the factory owners and other wealthy groups) and the 'proletariat' – those who produced the goods that created wealth. The terms bourgeoisie and proletariat are rarely used outside of Marxist circles today but many sociologists still see the differences between middle class and working class groups as largely economic.

For others the situation is much more complex. Max Weber (1864–1920) argued that society could not simply be polarised into two opposing social classes. For example neither the Senior Consultant nor the Hospital Porter own the means of production but this doesn't mean that they belong to the same social class. In many situations it is social status, the importance given to a person's role, which is important. The status of the Consultant is higher than that of the Hospital Porter and, as a consequence, the Consultant can demand a higher salary, better working conditions and a greater say in what happens within the hospital than the Porter. Social class is also an indicator of relative power within society. The generally high regard that is given to some groups, such as doctors, within our society means that, even outside of the hospital, the consultant is likely to be able to exercise more power in many social situations than the porter.

Defined in these ways social class membership is determined by wealth, social status and access to social power for different groups in society. Members of the same social class will tend to share similar values, have distinctive patterns of consumption and lifestyle and usually have a sense of belonging to their own social class group.

Social role

Society is made up of individuals relating to each other according to assumed roles. Depending on the social context we may have a number of different social roles. In families these might include father, son, brother, cousin etc. In the work place these might be employee, manager, colleague, friend etc. Sometimes these roles may come into conflict and the person has to try to balance one against the other.

Activity

Make a list of your own social roles. What conflicts can arise between these different roles?

Sex and gender

Society may also be divided by sex. Although on the surface this might appear to be a simple division between men and women, sociologists use the terms **sex** and **gender** to emphasise the need to distinguish between the **biological differences** and **social role differences**. A person's sex is the biological category to which they belong, i.e. male or female. Gender, on the other hand, describes the social role characteristics seen to be appropriate to men and women. These vary over time, in different settings and according to the expectations, values and norms of society.

We use the terms **masculine** and **feminine** to describe gender attributes for each sex. Although it is common to link masculine characteristics with men and feminine characteristics with women, this practice reflects cultural expectations rather than the biological characteristics of women and men. In different cultures the role expectations for men and women will be different to those that are common in our culture.

Assumptions about appropriate social roles can lead to discrimination and disadvantage. Differences in health status between men and women may be the result of sex (biological) differences or gender (social role) differences

Activity

Men and women often have different ways of responding to ill health. Women often find it easier to express their emotions while men have a tendency to keep things 'bottled up'. This can influence the way they deal with emotional stress in everyday life and may account for differing patterns of mental illness between women and men.

Can you think of other health conditions where stress is a contributing factor? Does sex or gender play any part in these health conditions?

Equality

Sociologists look at equality in three basic ways.

1 **Formal equality** – where people are treated equally according to set criteria. Criteria for medical aid following an accident or in health emergencies are based on judgements about medical need rather than economic or social criteria. Anyone, including visitors to this country, who is injured in an accident has a right of access to emergency medical treatment irrespective of income, age, or other criteria.

2 **Equality of Opportunity** – many social resources are allocated on a competitive basis (i.e. educational qualifications, jobs, salaries). Some people argue that everyone should have an equal opportunity to compete. All unnecessary barriers to access health, educational or social services should be removed.

3 **Equality of Outcome** – being treated as an equal, or being able to compete with everyone else is not always enough to ensure that resources are fairly distributed. In a competitive society there will be winners and losers. The winners are typically those who are already advantaged whilst the losers are typically those who are already disadvantaged. One response is to measure equality in terms of where people end up rather than where they start. This form of equality emphasises the need to think in terms of more equal outcomes. In terms of health we find that the poorest groups within society are more likely to have the worst health outcomes.

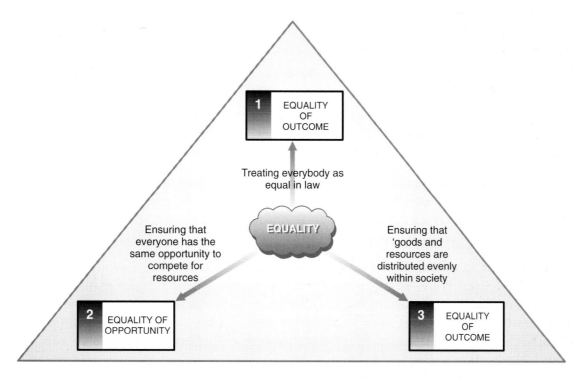

Figure 7.4 Equality

Inequality

It is important to begin by stressing that being 'equal' does not mean that everyone is the same. Clearly there are many differences between us and it is inevitable that we all have different chances of being ill. Sometimes this is an unavoidable consequence of biology or personal circumstance. Where differences arise because of avoidable circumstances we may judge these to be unfair. These differences are inequalities, implying that the causes could and should be avoided. It is clear that, even when biological factors are taken into account, social influences are important in determining a person's health status. For example when we find differences between the health of people from professional groups and unemployed groups we may argue that one contributory factor is uneven distribution of wealth. A possible response might be to increase levels of financial support to the worst affected groups.

Activity

Find out about differences in health and illness in your area. (You can gather this information from your local health authority website, annual report or the National Statistics web site www.statistics.gov.uk)

What factors do you think contribute to the differences you found between groups?

Are these the result of biological or social factors?

Could changing social conditions such as income, education or access to services reduce differences?

Race and ethnicity

In a similar way to the way that sociologists think about sex and gender they also distinguish between the concepts of **race** and **ethnicity**. Race refers to our biological origins and may have some influence on genetically determined diseases.

Ethnicity refers to shared cultural factors related to racial group that influence people's lives. These include such things as religion, values, beliefs, traditions and norms of behaviour. The importance of cultural factors in determining health is variable rather than fixed. Not all members of the same ethnic group share exactly the same values, attitudes or traditions. For example an Irish child growing up in England will share a common biological ancestry with other Irish people in Ireland but, because the child is also exposed to English culture, the norms and values that influence behaviour will be different to those of a child growing up in Ireland. The child is, of course, also exposed to a variety of other cultural viewpoints and these also influence the way the child perceives the world.

Activity

What ethnic group do you belong to?

Try to identify some of the key beliefs, values and behavioural norms that you associate with your ethnic group.

How might some of these influence lifestyle-related health conditions?

Culture

Within different societies, communities, and groups, expectations about normal behaviour vary. The different expectations, traditions and behavioural patterns that arise are a consequence of culture. Culture refers to the beliefs, values and ways of behaving shared by members of particular groups, communities and societies.

Beliefs are the general feelings or viewpoints we hold about the social world. They make up the general framework that comprises a culture. For example in western European culture most people believe that we are (or ought to be) free, independent and able to control our own destinies. But being free or independent is difficult to define and although we may share a general belief in freedom we may not agree what it means in practice.

Values are the opinions that we hold about how people ought to behave, what is important in everyday life and what the overall goals of life are about. For many people in our society having a high status job is seen as important although some may feel that earning large amounts of money is more important than status. For others being able to spend time with family and friends is more important than earning lots of money or advancing a career.

Norms are the expected patterns of behaviour of everyday life such as shaking hands when we meet someone for the first time. Students in a classroom almost always behave according to the expected norms bringing pens and notebooks, making notes, and answering questions when asked by the teacher.

Deviancy is a term used when behaviour differs, or deviates, from the accepted norms. When someone commits a criminal act this is clearly at odds with accepted social norms, but deviancy may also be used to describe the way that society, or professions such as medicine and social work intervene to control the behaviour of people who deviate from the behaviours of 'normal' mentally well people. From some sociological perspectives, health and social care services represent attempts to control deviant behaviour rather than as purely benevolent services intended to ease suffering or reduce inequalities.

Activity

Think about a GP's waiting room. What are the normal patterns of behaviour that you would expect to see amongst patients? How do people communicate with each other? What normally happens when you get in to see the doctor?

The sociology of health and illness

One of the key insights of sociology has been to show that health and illness are not simply a consequence of biology. Our health, or the ill health we experience, is closely linked to the social conditions that we live in. This view has been around for many years and it can be traced back to the originators of sociology in the 19th century. The early concerns of medical sociology, now more often called 'the sociology of health and illness', centered on the extent to which social and economic structures determined people's experiences of ill health. Later on sociologists became interested in exploring how individual or collective social actions influenced people's control over their lives and health status.

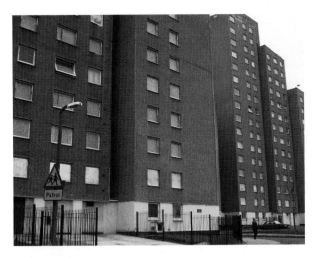

Where we live can have a dramatic influence on our health

Contemporary sociological interest is dominated by research into the range of social inequalities in health and illness. There is also great interest in determining the degree to which inequalities in health can be reduced by interventions to change the structure of society, such as the application of social policies to reduce economic inequality.

Another growing area of research focuses on meanings, perceptions and effects of social interactions around health and illness. Sociologists are also concerned to understand interactions about health and illness between people in families, between doctors and patients and between people in the wider community. Some of this work has concentrated on how health professions define, control, organise, classify and respond to perceived health problems. Sociologists are particularly interested in how disease categories change as the role of medicine changes, and the way that 'new diseases' are incorporated into medical practice.

Individual and community health is strongly influenced by social conditions. Factors such as income level, gender, ethnic group, housing conditions and educational achievement play an important part in determining our health status. In simple terms the sociology of health and illness aims to analyse, explain and evaluate the relationships between social conditions and health.

What is health?

Concepts are broad generalisations that we use to help us to think about abstract ideas such as justice, equality and health. Sometimes there are attempts to provide accurate definitions of these concepts but, although there is often agreement about some points it seems impossible to provide complete and accurate definitions to suit all possible applications. Even so it is useful to try to understand what sorts of ways people talk about and apply concepts of health. One place to start is to look at the different ways that people use and understand the term 'health'.

Attempts to define health can be divided into two main types **professional definitions**, those used by doctors, nurses and other health care professionals, and **lay beliefs**, the everyday popular views that ordinary people have about health. Professional definitions are obviously important because they help us to understand how doctors, nurses and others think about health and illness. But lay beliefs are also important because they influence the way that ordinary people think about and respond to issues of health and illness.

Some professional definitions define health in terms of the absence of disease or illness. These are called 'negative definitions' of health because they focus on ill health rather than health. One example is the medical model of health.

The medical model of health

The medical model of health emerged, alongside germ theory, towards the end of the 19th century. According to the medical model, health is present when there is an absence of disease. The medical model also proposes that:

- All disease is caused by a specific disease agent such as a virus, bacterium, toxin or genetic factor.
- The patient's body is a kind of machine – rather than a person living in a complex social environment.
- Patients are the passive recipients of medical intervention designed to repair the dysfunctional machine.
- Medical technology, medicines, surgery and science are the appropriate responses to ill health.

Social models of health

In contrast to the medical model of health with its emphasis on ill health and disease as an isolated personal experience, social models place health and illness within a complex, constantly changing social environment. Social models emphasise the important influence of factors such as lifestyle, poverty, education, housing and social support on health and illness.

Health may also be defined in positive terms. In his book, *Health: The Foundations for Achievement* the philosopher David Seedhouse, identifies five perspectives on health that emphasise health as a positive condition:

1 **Health as an ideal state** – in 1946 the World Health Organisation defined health as 'a state of complete physical, mental and social well being and not merely the absence of disease or infirmity' One problem with this definition is that its emphasis on complete well-being seems to make health impossible to achieve.

2 **Health as fitness for 'normal' social function** – this kind of definition emphasises the need for individuals to fit in with the expectations of society. It is possible to have some degree of illness, disability or disease and remain healthy, as long as you can continue to perform your 'normal social role'. One problem is how do we decide what is a normal social role?

3 **Health as a commodity** – from this point of view health is something that can be supplied – by providing medical care services – or bought, e.g. by purchasing 'healthy' foods. The difficulty with this approach is that it sees health as external to the person and their social circumstances. Health becomes a matter of supplying appropriate technologies and services. In many ways provision of health care services has simply changed patterns of ill health and disease within modern society so that instead of death occurring as a consequence of infectious disease it often arises as a consequence of degenerative changes associated with lifestyle and ageing.

4 **Health as a personal or spiritual strength** – from this perspective a person's personal physical, emotional or spiritual strength, even during illness or disease, is viewed as a measure of their health. The ability to recover from illness, or adapt well to changing circumstances, is the measure of a healthy person. The main problem with this approach is the individuality and vagueness of the definition. It is difficult to see how this kind of definition could be used to improve health within a society because interpretation of adaptability and personal resourcefulness is very subjective.

5 **Health as the basis for personal potential** – Seedhouse proposes the view that health is having a sound foundation (including things such as adequate financial, physical, intellectual and emotional resources) on which to make the most of our capacity to determine our own future. As a philosopher Seedhouse is concerned with ethical issues such as autonomy and self-determination. This approach presumes that we share some agreement about the desirability of individuality, independence and self-determination as valuable qualities. This works well in western cultures where these are strong values but may be less useful in societies where individual needs are of less importance.

Activity

Assignment suggestion

An investigation into the way magazines report, inform and present images of health and illness.

Possible research questions:

What similarities and difference is there between the ways that men's and women's magazine deal with health related issues?

What kinds of health related issues are raised in problem pages in magazines?

Do approaches vary according to target readership age, gender or social class groups?

How can concepts and definitions of health described above be applied to magazine articles and advertising?

Illness

When you feel unwell you may have a number of signs and symptoms that, when subjected to medical examination, can be given a name. On most occasions, however, we feel unwell and yet no known disease is present. Illness is the subjective feeling that the patient has when they feel unwell.

Disease

Medical examination involves an exploration of the patient's symptoms – how the patient says she feels – and medical signs such as raised blood pressure, skin rash, abnormal changes in blood chemistry etc. The doctor then compares her findings with medically agreed signs and symptoms for a range of possible conditions and diagnoses the most appropriate disease. The medical naming of an illness defines it as a disease. It is of course possible to have a disease and not feel ill. Many people with conditions such as diabetes, epilepsy or asthma will have a clear medical diagnosis but this doesn't mean that they always feel ill.

Impairment

Refers to the loss or abnormality of a physiological structure or function. So an abnormality of the bones in the lower leg may lead to an impaired gait – the way a person walks. Impairment refers to the physical condition of a person.

Disability

Disability can be defined as a restriction or lack of ability to perform certain physical or mental functions within a range of accepted standards of normal function. Impairment may cause disability if the impairment reduces a person's ability to function within normal levels. Disability refers to restricted ability to perform physical or mental functions to a 'normal' standard.

Handicap

A person may also be disadvantaged because they have certain impairments or disabilities. The disadvantage they suffer is called a handicap. The degree to which a person with an impairment or disability may suffer handicap will depend on their social circumstances, their personal response to their disability and the response of society to people with similar disabilities. Handicap is essentially about the way that we respond to impairment and disability. Changing social perceptions of disability can significantly reduce handicap even without changing the nature of the disability.

Social structure and health

There are well-established links between factors such as socioeconomic status, gender, ethnicity, level of education and health. One of the key areas of interest for sociologists is the existence of significant differences in the distribution of health and illness within the population. Evidence for an association between poverty and ill health is well established. Factors such as where you live, your gender, ethnic group, living and working conditions also play an important role in determining your health.

Activity

Social determinants of health and illness

Diseases of the circulatory system such as coronary heart disease and strokes are amongst the main reasons for ill health and premature death in the UK. Carry out a literature review to find out the main social factors that contribute to the development of these conditions.

There are clear differences between the health of some groups within the population. Mortality (death) and morbidity (illness) rates in the population are strongly influenced by socioeconomic, gender and ethnic groupings. For many years sociologists have argued that differences in health between these groups cannot be adequately explained by biological factors. A large number of studies have shown that differences in health exist between social groups and many researchers have argued that, because social conditions are so important in determining the health, we should regard these differences as inequalities in health.

Recent government policy on health acknowledges these views and aims to bring about improvements in the health of the population by improving social conditions, particularly amongst the worst off groups within society. Government departments and agencies now place strong emphasis on reducing inequalities in health through various public health and social policy measures.

Extract 1 Our Healthier Nation Website www.ohn.gov.uk

Reducing Health Inequalities: an Action Report

- 44% of men in unskilled manual households smoke compared to 15% of men in professional households. Among women, 32% smoke in unskilled households and semi-skilled households compared with 14% in professional households.

Source ONS, 1998 General Household Survey, GB

Inequalities in health

Measuring inequalities in health

Sociologists use a variety of different ways to measure inequalities in health but one common method has been to explore the differences in mortality and morbidity between socioeconomic groups within society. Sir Douglas Black's Working Party on Inequalities in Health (*The Black Report*, 1980) and *The Health Divide* (1987 and 1992) found that the risk of mortality and morbidity was significantly higher within lower occupational groups. Where statistically significant differences occur across different socioeconomic groups, with worsening health occurring within poorer groups, sociologists use the term 'social class gradient'.

Extract 2 Reducing Health Inequalities: an Action Report Our Healthier Nation Website www.ohn.gov.uk

The death rate from coronary heart disease in people under 65 is almost three times higher in Manchester than in Oxfordshire.

A boy in Manchester can expect to live more than seven years fewer than his contemporary in Barnet. A girl in Manchester can expect to live six years fewer than her contemporary in Kensington, Chelsea and Westminster.

It is important to note that the terms 'social class' and 'socioeconomic group' are not necessarily used to mean the same thing. The concept of social class as we have seen earlier, is made up of a number of related elements, including:

- Economic characteristics such as wealth, income and occupation.
- Political characteristics such as social status and power.
- Cultural characteristics such as lifestyle, values, beliefs and level of education.

Definitions of socio-economic groups used in statistical studies may use some of these factors to determine membership of socioeconomic groups but there are many different classification systems in use. The use of different classification systems can make health data based on socioeconomic groups difficult to compare across different studies. Two examples of classification systems in current use are set out in the tables below.

Activity

Many studies have shown that inequalities in health also occur across different ethnic and gender groups. Carry out an Internet search to identify sources of data on inequalities in health according to Social Class, Gender and Ethnicity. You should aim to find at least three examples for each.

Table 7.1 Registrar General's classification of social class

Social class	Occupation type	Examples
I	Professional	Doctors, Accountants, Engineers
II	Managerial and Technical/ Intermediate	Marketing and Sales Managers, Teachers, Journalists.
III NM	Skilled Non-manual	Clerks, cashiers, retail staff.
III M	Skilled Manual	Carpenters, Goods van drivers, Joiners.
IV	Partly Skilled	Warehousemen, Security Guards, machine tool operators.
V	Unskilled	Building and Civil Engineering Labourers, other Labourers, Cleaners.

Table 7.2 New Criteria Socio-Economic Class (NC-SEC)

Class	Example
1	Higher managerial and professional occupations
1.1	Employers and managers in large organisations
1.2	Higher professionals
2	Lower managerial and professional occupations
3	Intermediate occupations
4	Small employers and own account workers
5	Lower supervisory, craft and related occupations
6	Semi-routine occupations
7	Routine occupations
8	Never worked and long term unemployed
9	Unclassified

Useful websites

Department of Health	www.doh.gov.uk
Health Action Zones on The Internet	www.haznet.org.uk
Health Development Agency	www.hda-online.org.uk
National Institute for Clinical Excellence	www.nice.org.uk
Office for National Statistics	www.statistics.gov.uk
Our Healthier Nation	www.ohn.gov.uk

One common measure of health used by statisticians is the Standardised Mortality Rate (SMR). The SMR enables us to estimate the increased or decreased likelihood of mortality amongst different groups. The 'expected' death rate in the general population is assigned an SMR of 100. Higher than expected rates within the groups or areas studied will have an SMR above 100, whilst lower than expected death rates will have an SMR below 100.

Activity

Find out what the SMRs for deaths from such things as cancer, coronary heart disease, suicide or accidents are in your area. (You can find this information published in *Regional Trends* or on the national statistics web site at www.statistics.gov.uk)

Are the rates higher or lower than the nationally expected levels?

Why do you think this is so?

Sex and gender differences

Men and women use health care services in different ways. From the tables below we can see that the overall use of Inpatient and GP services is higher amongst women than it is amongst men. In the 16–24 age group women are more than twice as likely to use GP services than men (Table 7.4). The percentage of men over 74 using hospital inpatient services is significantly higher than amongst women in the same age group (Table 7.3).

Table 7.3 Use of hospital inpatient services (%) by sex and age group 1998–99

	16–24	25–34	35–44	45–54	55–64	65–74	74+	All 16 and over
Men	4	5	5	7	11	15	21	8
Women	11	15	8	8	10	10	15	11

Source General Household Survey, Office for National Statistics

Table 7.4 Use of GP services (%)by sex and age group 1998–99

	16–24	25–34	35–44	45–54	55–64	65–74	74+	All 16 and over
Men	7	9	10	12	16	17	21	12
Women	15	18	16	19	17	19	21	18

Source General Household Survey, Office for National Statistics

Activity

The tables above illustrate the different ways that men and women make use of health care services. Make a list of possible reasons for differences in use of NHS services between men and women.

Ethnicity and health

People from ethnic minority groups in Britain are more likely to suffer ill health than the host population. According to studies carried out for the Commission for Racial Equality infant mortality is 100% higher for the children of African-Caribbean or Pakistani mothers than it is for white mothers. Pakistani and Bangladeshi people are five times more likely to be diagnosed with diabetes and 50% more likely to have coronary heart disease than white people. African-Caribbean women have 80% higher rates for diagnosed hypertension (high blood pressure) than whites. Irish-born men are the only immigrant group whose mortality is higher in Britain than in their country of origin

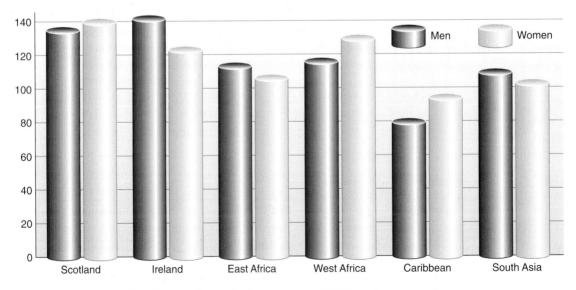

Figure 7.5 Standardised mortality ratio by country of birth: all causes

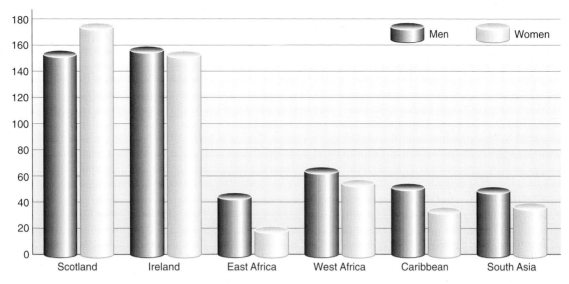

Figure 7.6 Standardised mortality ratio by country of birth: lung cancer

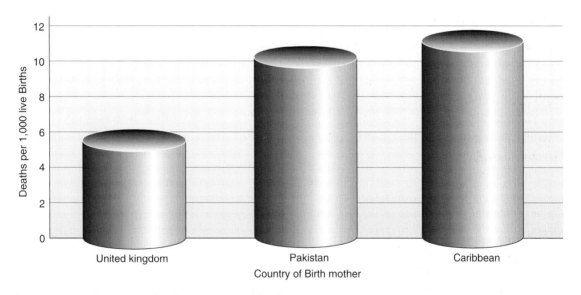

Figure 7.7 Infant mortality by country of birth

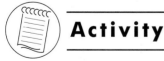

Activity

The charts above show how mortality rates are influenced by country of birth. Make a list of possible reasons for these differences.

Sociological influences on policy making and practice

Sociological research and theory provides a basis for much of current thinking on health care policy and practice. Current health policies, as we have seen, aim to reduce inequalities in health and local providers use evidence gathered from surveys to help them to plan services. Sociology now plays an important role in the education and training of health care professionals encouraging a broader awareness of the need to take into account the social context of health and illness.

Activity

Assignment suggestion

Investigate health inequalities in your area.

Possible research questions:

What are the main inequalities in health that have been identified by your local health agencies? (Health Authorities, Health Action Zones and Regional Public Health Observatories will publish information about this on their website).

What explanations can be given to explain these inequalities?

How are policy makers and service providers attempting to reduce these inequalities?

Social construction and health

The influence of sociology on health policy and practice extends beyond the provision of statistical data and includes a critical analysis of social behaviour, carer–client and interprofessional relationships. Many sociologists argue that our view of the world – our sense of what is real, true or false – is dependent on our social experience. Everything we see, think or believe is dependent to some degree on our existing knowledge and the social context in which we live. Our perceptions of health develop from these experiences and, as a consequence, our notions of illness and disease follow from these underlying assumptions. In this sense the world is 'socially constructed.'

The problem of measurement

In the West ill health is most often measured in terms of disease and death. Improvements in health are measured in terms of increases in life expectancy and rely on medical definitions of health. Medical emphasis on illness and disease distorts the wider picture of health and has resulted in an expansion of medical services rather than health services. Social construction theories argue that this approach does not properly represent how people think about health in their everyday lives. For social constructionists notions of health and ill health change over time in line with the dominant ideologies of society. Many medical diagnoses, they argue, are simply representations of cultural and professional preferences.

Evidence based health care

Evidence based health care is the practice of providing health care in accordance with systematically reviewed scientific studies intended to measure the effectiveness of different treatment options. Based on the assumption that medicine is an objective science that lies at the heart of health care, the government set up the National Institute for Clinical Excellence (NICE). The institute is responsible for researching treatments for health conditions and developing National Frameworks for health care. (You can look at some of the work that NICE does on their website www.nice.org.uk).

Medicine claims a scientific and objective base and this, coupled with particular cultural and political values in the late 20th century, has led to the dominance of evidence-based medicine. A closer look at medical practice reveals a different picture. Diagnostic criteria for many conditions are often vague and subjective. Conditions such as depression, dementia, asthma, epilepsy, anorexia nervosa, and hypertension are notoriously difficult to diagnose with accuracy. Although there are standardised diagnostic criteria, diagnosis relies heavily on doctors' previous experience, interpretation and personal judgement about the significance of a patient's signs and symptoms. Coupled with the fact that doctors often have to make quick decisions in difficult situations medicine is often more about experience and good judgement than it is about reliable scientific evidence. In this sense it is more interpretive than objective.

The reliability and practical application of evidence drawn from scientific studies can also be questioned. Medical research is commonly funded by drug manufacturers and is carried out in controlled conditions using relatively small sample populations. Researchers tend to follow funding and this has led to an over reliance on scientific studies focusing on comparisons of drug therapies or medical interventions. Funding for research into social influences on health and illness is much less widely available. Drug companies have little interest in sponsoring projects with no clear link to their products and traditional scientific research methodologies are difficult to apply in 'real life' situations. The interpretive nature of these studies is less appealing to medical elites and policy makers who often place a higher value on the 'objective' scientific studies more common in medical research. As a consequence emphasis within the drive towards evidence based health care favours scientific rather than interpretive research, missing the point that health care practice is interpretive rather than scientific.

Professionals, patients and power

Another key concern within the sociology of health is the relationship between professionals and their clients. How health workers interact with each other and with their clients has an important effect on how we perceive, and respond to health and illness.

Traditionally sociologists have looked at relationships in health care in terms of structural theories – conflict or consensus – or in terms of social action theories such as symbolic interaction or labelling theory. Usually this is characterised as a meeting between the knowledgeable professional and the ignorant patient. More recently it is argued that the professional patient relationship has changed and is now more typically one in which the participants are each expert, although with different areas of expertise. Professional knowledge centres around categories of disease, treatment options etc. while the patient's expertise is more concerned with personal experience, expectations and demands to be made on the professional. For example patients visiting their GP often have expectations that a diagnosis will be made, treatment offered and improved health will be the result. The GP may be unable to make a clear diagnosis because signs and symptoms are vague or inconsistent with diagnostic criteria, or the patient's expected treatment options – for example antibiotic therapy – may not be appropriate.

In addition patients are increasingly encouraged to find out as much as they can about medical conditions, treatment options, service entitlements and lifestyle factors influencing their own health. Better education, the use of drop-in health centres, well-women clinics, along with telephone and Internet services such as NHS Direct are changing the balance of power within professional-patient relationships. The relationship between the patient and the doctor is not just a matter of the doctor making decisions and then applying them to the patient but will also include the patient's expectations of appropriate medical responses and their impact on lifestyle and social behaviour.

Activity

Assignment suggestion

Carry out a survey of Internet based health services around the world.

Possible research questions:

Who are the services directed at?

What kinds of information and support are available for people accessing sites?

How might the Internet aid people with disabilities, mobility problems or those who live in rural locations to get access to appropriate health care support?

Activity

Make a list of the kind of responses that patients might expect from a visit to their GP. For example do we expect to:

Always undergo a physical examination?

Come away with a prescription for drug therapy?

Feel better after undergoing a course of treatment?

How do you think these expectations might influence interactions between doctors and patients?

Activity

Assignment suggestion

An investigation into patients' expectations of health care interactions.

Some possible research questions:

What kinds of expectations do patients have of GP services?

Do expectations vary according to the patient's age, gender or social group?

Does the gender of the health care professional influence the patient's expectations?

Sociologist have typically approached issues of power in health settings in terms of a top down approach, often explaining power relationships as a conflict between the interests of dominant and oppressed groups. Early studies suggested that the medical profession, dominated by male doctors, exercised a gender influenced power over their mainly female patients typical of other power relationships within a patriarchal (male-dominated) society. Women's behaviour was more likely to be viewed as neurotic by male doctors and one effect of this was the over-representation of women prescribed treatment for anxiety and neurotic disorders. In the late 1960s this resulted in over prescribing of tranquilisers and sedatives to women whose principle problems were the result of family problems, domestic violence, poverty, poor housing or lack of adequate social support with child care. Ann Oakley in *Women Confined* (1980) drew attention to the impact of male domination of obstetric medicine and the displacement of midwives from their role in supporting women during pregnancy and childbirth. This medicalisation of an otherwise normal social and cultural experience led to the practice of hospital births and reduced women's control over their own bodies during childbirth.

The development of medical science, with its emphasis on technology and scientific explanations of health and illness in the 19th and 20th centuries focused attention on the role of scientific thinking in changing power relationships within society. The French philosopher Michel Foucault (1926–1984) examined the way that knowledge contributed to the development of new techniques of control (technologies of power) that arose alongside the development of schools, hospitals and prisons during the 19th century. His work shows how the changing ideas about human behaviour that came about with the birth of these institutions, along with the emerging disciplines of social science and medicine, generated new techniques of observation, classification and control that relied on notions of normality and deviance developed within the disciplines.

Foucault argued that the hospitals, (along with prisons, schools and asylums) are effectively laboratories for the study of human behaviour. The new professions developed and expanded beyond the confines of the institution, emerging as powerful and dominant forces within society. In the process they have displaced other ways of thinking about human behaviour.

Foucault identified five 'technologies of power' or ways of changing the individual that can be seen in action in health care settings.

Spatialisation: This is represented by the practice of creating unique categories and spaces for different categories of illness (or deviance). There is a strong emphasis on individuality and a focus on the body of the individual. The practice of assigning patients to medical specialisms, wards and categories of disease on admission to hospital, is one way that we can see spatialisation operating in health care.

Spatialisation also helps professionals (and patients) to reduce complex personal health issues to a more manageable disease classification. Treatment regimes can then be selected and applied to restore or reform the patient's physical, social or psychological dysfunction. Terms such as 'diabetic', 'schizophrenic' and 'epileptic' focus on the disease rather than the person and provide a simplistic basis for understanding the person and their perceived needs.

Activity

Make a list of terms that are sometimes applied by health professionals when referring to clients or patients. What kind of ideas and images do these terms generate? Think about terms such as geriatric patient, neurotic, psychosomatic disorder, drug addict and cancer.

Are some terms more favourable than others?

Control of 'Micro-activities': Controlling and measuring the detailed events of physical and social life (micro-activities) is common in medicine and health care. When a person enters a health care setting a series of observations, measurements, tests and recordings are initiated. These include observation and recording of physical characteristics such as height, weight, complexion, skin condition etc. They often involve intimate examination of bodily functions such as analysis of urine, faeces, blood and body chemistry. The purpose of these investigations is to classify, categorise, diagnose and establish the appropriate diagnosis, and therefore the location for the patient within the health care framework.

Activity

Ask some of your family or friends about their experiences of admission to hospital, school or college.

Try to identify ways in which people are observed, measured and categorised in these kinds of settings

Repetitive Exercises: Once an initial diagnosis has been developed the patient is subjected to a treatment plan. This includes standardised and repetitive exercises that have been previously determined as appropriate to treat the patient's condition. E.g. medication, blood test, monitoring of emotional, social and physical functioning etc. Treatment may also include prescription or restriction of certain patterns of social activity according to the professional's perception of the 'problem'. If the patient does not respond as expected a more specific, individualised programme may be initiated.

Activity

Repetitive exercises and individualised programmes are also common in social work, education and other personal support settings.

Can you think of examples of how these practices are used in educational settings?

Detailed Hierarchies: Institutional practices and professional activities are strongly influenced by hierarchal relationships between individuals. Hierarchies also exist between competing forms of knowledge and professional groups. Each person knows his or her position within the hierarchy and this influences their thinking, decision-making and behaviour.

Hierarchies are not always fixed and relationships may change according to the context. For example the dominant professional in a health care setting is often the medical practitioner, but sometimes, for example if there are social conditions to consider, the dominant role may pass to a social worker. Where issues of rehabilitation arise then the dominant role may be assigned to a physiotherapist, psychologist or occupational therapist.

In some settings there are strong visual and symbolic signs that are used to communicate the hierarchical order. These include the use of uniforms, formal titles and forms of address, architecture and furnishings. More subtle interpersonal factors such as use of specialist terminology, tone of voice and gesture also indicate a person's place within a hierarchy.

 Activity

> Think about an institutional setting such as a school, hospital or doctor's surgery. Brainstorm a list of physical and interpersonal clues that indicate hierarchal relationships.

Normalising Judgements: The fifth disciplinary technique that Foucault describes is the development and application of approved definitions of normal and abnormal behaviour. In medicine observed signs and symptoms are measured against accepted standards of normality. In some cases normality may be relatively easy to establish – percentage of oxygen or other chemicals in the blood for example. In other cases, assessments of psychological or behavioural norms are more open to question.

Foucault points out that the observer's 'normalising judgements' are also understood and internalised by the subject providing a further psychological reinforcement of 'normal' behaviour. In other words patients often make their own judgements about what the doctor is looking for, or consider normal. Patients may exaggerate symptoms in order to get help or under report symptoms if they wish to avoid further intervention. These normalising judgements constitute strong psychological pressures to conform to prevailing social norms and values.

Approaches to sociological research

Positivism

For some social scientists, the logic methods and procedures of the physical sciences can be applied to the study of society. Auguste Comte (1798–1857) believed that applying the methods and reasoning strategies of natural science to the study of society would produce a positive science of society. It would show that there were laws that governed social behaviour just as there were laws of physics or chemistry.

Advocates of this approach believe that it is possible to observe, define and measure social facts. From this, they argue, it will be possible to discover sociological laws and make reliable predictions about human behaviour. These social scientists tend to favour research methods that will result in quantitative, or numerically measurable, data.

Interpretivism

Unlike the subject of the physical sciences – matter – humans are not simply objects. We interpret our environment and change our behaviour according to our experiences and their meanings. We construct our own sense of reality from these experiences and meanings.

For interpretivists the key research task is to discover what health and illness means and how these meanings are constructed and what the influence of different meanings is on our lives. Interpretivists tend to favour qualitative research methods that provide information to show how people understand or give meaning to their experiences of health and illness.

Sociologists from both perspectives may use similar research methods but their research questions and emphasis on the importance of achieving statistically quantifiable results will vary. The Positivist will seek to uncover and measure social facts and emphasise those that are seen to be statistically significant. The Interpretivist will focus on what health and illness means to a society and its members.

Levels of sociological analysis

One way to understand the differing approaches to the sociology of health is to consider the levels of analysis applied by researchers. Sociologists studying health and illness approach their subject from three levels of analysis:

Individual

At the individual level the focus is on personal perceptions of health and illness. Sarah Nettleton in her book *The Sociology of Health and Illness* (1995) points out that studies into lay perceptions of health and illness show that non-manual workers tended to have more positive perceptions of health than manual workers. Non-manual workers tended to believe that health could be influenced by their own lifestyle choices. Manual workers, by contrast, were more likely to focus on ill health and feel that ill health is largely a consequence of external or biological conditions.

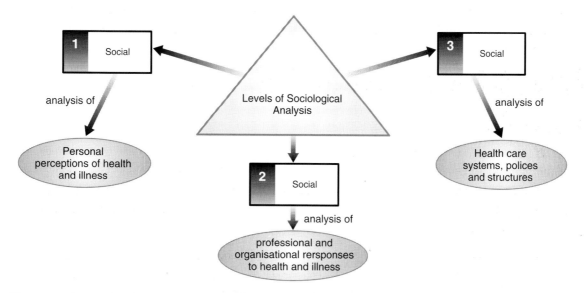

Figure 7.8 Levels of sociological analysis

Social

Analysis at the social level involves exploration of the ways that health care professions and organisations develop and act in relation to health and illness. Some sociologists focus on the professional and organisational factors that shape our thinking and responses to health and illness. Analysis at this level may include studies of professional power, organisational culture and professional-client interactions.

Societal

At this level the sociologist examines how political, social and health care structures influence health and illness. This may involve research into the impact of social policies on health and illness, or explorations of the role of powerful groups in shaping the nature of health care provision.

Research methods

Social research may be carried out in a variety of ways using a range of different research methods. In this chapter we provide a very brief outline of some common research techniques but you should refer to the chapter on research in health and social care in the core textbook, Health and Social Care for Vocational A-level for a more detailed exploration of research methods in health and social care.

Common approaches to social research in health care include:

Surveys – used for researching large populations often using questionnaires or structured interview techniques.

Fieldwork studies – are of value when researchers want to study smaller populations in their normal environment. Fieldwork studies are particularly useful for studying complex social settings where there are small numbers of participants. Examples of typical fieldwork research include studies of professional relationships in an operating theatre, or patients' perceptions of care in a hospice. Fieldwork research often involves a variety of research techniques such as reflective journals, focus group discussions, interviews and unstructured observation.

Experiments – these are used in the natural sciences to control and test out the effects of specific variables on organisms or objects. Sociologists wishing to test out the effects of changes in social conditions on social behaviour rarely use experiments as variables influencing human behaviour are complex, and the aim of sociology is usually to study human behaviour in its normal social context. However some situations such as communal living, or changes to the physical environment may lend themselves to experimental research methods.

Non-reactive research – many forms of social research involve interaction between researchers and subjects of research. When we interact with each other we usually use both verbal and nonverbal forms of communication and often try to anticipate what the other person is trying to communicate. In fieldwork and survey research this can mean that the subject tries to anticipate what the researcher wants to know and responds not only to the questions but also assumptions about the nature of the research. This can lead to unintentional researcher influence, resulting in biased or misleading results. In order to reduce the amount of researcher influence on the subject's responses, some researchers carry out 'non-reactive' research studies. These studies involve non-intrusive observation, analysis of archive materials, letters, administrative records, policy documents and official statistics. By reducing contact between the researcher and her target population the researcher aims to minimize the amount of observer influence on the project's findings.

Discourse analysis – this kind of research explores the way that we talk about, communicate and express views on different social issues. Discourse analysis may involve detailed analysis of the language, images, gestures and shared understanding that form the way we communicate about issues such as ill health. An analysis of visual representation of health in magazines could be seen as a form of discourse analysis.

Sampling – researchers using social survey methods often make use of questionnaires or structured interviews. Surveys consist of a series of simple questions that are asked to a cross section of a group of people that the sociologist wishes to study. The group you wish to study is called the **population**. The population is the general group, such as people who use health care services in a given area, or patients seen in an outpatient clinic. Where the population being studied is small it may be possible to survey the whole population – for example in a study of patient satisfaction with pain relief treatment in a hospital ward. In most cases the population is too large to be surveyed and the researcher needs to survey a sample of the whole population.

Samples are taken from a **sample frame** e.g. the names of all the patients seen in a GP surgery during the previous 12 months. The researcher then selects which patients to survey and develops a survey sample. There are a number of different ways to develop a sample depending on the purpose of the survey.

Random Samples are sometimes used when the researcher wants to try to avoid bias in selecting subjects for the survey. Selecting every third name from the sample frame or picking names out of a hat might be useful for this kind of sample.

Sometimes it is important to ensure that special groups are included in a survey. In a survey of GP patients it might be important to include representatives from all age and gender groups. The sample frame would be divided into age and gender sub groups and a random sample drawn up from each category. This is known as **stratified sampling**.

Sometimes interviewers are asked to survey set numbers of people in each group e.g. 10 men between 16–25, 20 men between 25–35 etc. where the researchers are trying to match the age and gender groups against known use of a service. This is called **quota sampling** and is often used by market researchers.

Activity

Imagine that you have been asked to research the exercise patterns of girls and boys in a large school. The population, 1500+ male and female students, is very large and it is unlikely that you would be able to survey every student. You need to develop a sample for your study.

How would you go about devising your **sampling frame** for your study?

How would you develop a random quota sample from your sample frame to ensure that your study is representative of different gender and age groups?

What actions would you take to try to minimise researcher influence on subject responses?

Assessment guidance

For this unit you are required to carry out an investigation into a health care issue or topic. You will need to begin by brainstorming possible research topics. You will need to take into account a number of practical and ethical issues such as:

- The amount of time you have available to carry out the study
- The sensitivity of the topic area and the need to get permission from appropriate people connected to your study
- Suitable research techniques – such as interview, observations, or questionnaires – and your ability to use them within the time available
- The willingness of subjects to participate in your study
- The amount of time you will need to develop research tools (e.g. questionnaires) and analyse results.

You should ensure that you discuss your proposed investigation with your tutor on a regular basis and take into account the need for a clear research plan. Think carefully about the research methods you will use. A common student error is to opt for questionnaires, as they seem straightforward and easy to carry out. In practice questionnaires are probably one of the most difficult research tools to design. Analysis of results is time consuming and may result in little information of value to the researcher. This is particularly so when questionnaires contain large amounts of questions designed to place the subject within a sample group (age group, gender, etc.).

One useful alternative is to use **structured interviews** for large samples or **semi-structured interviews** for smaller sample groups. Structured interviews are similar to questionnaires but allow the researcher to explain ambiguous questions and relieve the respondent from the effort required to read and fill in large numbers of questions. Semi-structured interviews limit the scope of the interview to pre-determined topics but allow the respondent opportunities to provide a wider range of responses. Interviews can be time consuming but, if they are well planned, they allow the researcher to gather more detailed information by rephrasing or asking additional questions when unexpected issues arise.

Planning your investigation

Some suggestions have been provided during the chapter to help you to think about suitable topics for your assessed work. You should also discuss your plans with your tutor. Health care research may sometimes involve complex and confidential information that some people are reluctant to share with you. You should give this serious consideration when you select a topic. Try to avoid obviously sensitive areas such as investigations of personal experiences of ill health. Your task is to show your understanding of the contribution of sociology to our understanding of health and illness not to gather personal information about people with 'interesting' health problems!

It is important to take time to think about and plan your investigation taking into account practical and ethical issues. Try to focus on realistic, achievable research goals that will allow you to make the best use of your everyday access to suitable subject groups. Remember that health care professionals are busy providing health care support to people in need. It is not a good idea to turn up at your local hospital and expect to be allowed to interview patients, or health care staff.

There are a great many ways that you can investigate how social behaviour influences health and illness drawing on examples from your everyday life. You could begin by developing some research questions. For example:

- Do girls and boys have different patterns of participation in exercise?
- Do boys take more risks than girls?
- Why do some people give up smoking while others don't?
- Why do some people dislike school sports and games activities?

Remember to take into account the assessment requirements for this unit. During your investigation you need to be able to show that you have:

- Used an appropriate sociological research method for your chosen area of study
- Identified and explained relevant sociological theory and perspectives that are linked to your study (for example theories of socialisation may be used to explain gender differences in risk taking behaviour)
- Given examples of relevant policy responses (these are likely to include health education campaigns, availability of health related services such as hospitals, sports centres and youth advice services)
- Discussed factors that influence service design and delivery and their relationship to the sociological perspective
- Shown how the activities of the services reflect sociological approaches to health and illness.

Glossary

beliefs   the feelings or viewpoints which a person holds about the world

concensus theories   the idea that society exists because humans are social creatures and agree to live by a set of common rules

concept   a general way of thinking about some aspect of society

conflict theorists   people who believe that society is really made up of groups of people whose interests are in direct conflict

culture   the beliefs, values and behaviour shared by members of any particular group, community or society

deviancy   a term to describe someone whose behaviour differs from the expected norm

disease   the name given to an illness which corresponds to a previously defined set of medical symptoms

disability   a restriction in someone's ability to perform functions to the normal accepted standard

equality of opportunity   where people have an equal chance of gaining access to the same level of all social resources – like education, health care etc.

equality of outcome   where the emphasis is on where people 'end up' rather than where they began

ethnicity   cultural background shared by members of the same racial group

formal equality   where people are treated equally according to a set of specific criteria

functionalists   sociologists who emphasise the social function of social conditions and behaviour, even if those functions are generally thought to be negative

gender   the social roles appropriate to either sex – this can change over time and between different cultures

handicap   the disadvantage someone with a disability or impairment suffers

illness   the subjective feeling a patient has when they feel unwell

impairment   the loss or abnormality of a physiological function

inequality   a measure of the differences between people that could have been avoided and may be viewed to be unfair

interpretivism   in contrast to positivism, attempts to understand the influence human interpretation has on events; normally more associated with qualitative research

medical models of health   a 19th century model which says that health is the absence of disease

norms   the expected patterns of behaviour within a particular culture

positivism   application of the methods of natural science to social science to formulate social laws; normally based on quantitative methods

race   the biological origins of a human

sex   the biological category to which a human belongs, male or female

social action theories   the idea that society is organised in the way it is due to social interactions between members of that society – the opposing view to that held by structuralists

social models of health   in contrast to the medical model, these models place health within wider sociological context, acknowledging the importance of factors such as lifestyle and education

social sciences   a range of academic disciplines concerned with understanding human behaviour

sociologists   people who are interested in exploring the relationships between groups of people and how this then impacts on individuals within the group and the group as a whole.

structuralists   sociologists who believe that social structures are the most important factors in determining individual life experiences

values   opinions about how people ought to behave, what is important in life and what the goals of life are

Resources

Internet websites

National statistics website
www.statistics.gov.uk

Our Healthier Nation website
www.ohn.gov.uk

Department of health
www.doh.gov.uk

National Institute for Clinical Excellence
www.nice.org.uk

Health Development Agency
www.hda-online.org.uk

Health Action Zones on the Internet
www.haznet.org.uk

www.careandhealth.com

Find out about the Government's strategy for tackling drugs.
www.official-documents.co.uk/document/cm39/3945/contents.htm

Release
Information and advice about drugs.
388 Old Street, London, EC1V 9LT
Tel: 0171 729 5255
Fax: 0171 729 2599

St. John Ambulance
First aid and advice and details of local courses.
1 Grosvenor Crescent, London, SW1X 7EJ
Tel: 0207 235 5231
Fax: 0207 235 0796

Drinkline
For advice on alcohol problems.
Tel: 0800 917 8282

Wrecked
A website exploring alcohol issues in a fun and interesting way.
www.wrecked.co.uk

Check it!
A website with drug facts, where to go for help and a drugs-related quiz.
http://drugs.ort.org

Health Education Authority
For information on national drugs campaigns.
Trevelyan House, 30 Great Peter Street, London SW1P 2HW
www.heaorg.uk/campaigns/drugs/index.htm

Department of Health
Information about the 'Our Healthier Nation' strategy and how you can help prevent accidents.
http://www.doh.gov.uk

Health and Safety Executive
Working to reduce hazards at work.
www.open.gov.uk/hse/hsehome.htm

Royal Society for the Prevention of Accidents
Accident prevention resources and background information.
Edgbaston Park, 353 Bristol Road, Birmingham, B5 7ST
Tel: 0121 248 2000

Eating Disorder Association
Offers help, a listening ear and understanding of eating problems to both sufferers and their families.
www.gurney.org.uk/eda

Mind
Provides information on all aspects of mental distress.
Tel: 0181 522 1728 (London only) 0345 660 163 (outside London) 9:15am–4:45pm Monday to Friday.
Email: contact@mind.org.uk
www.mind.org.uk

Uzone
Expert advice and helplines, specifically about mental health.
www.uzone.org.uk

Tel: 0171 222 5300
Fax: 0171 413 8900
www.hea.org.uk/campaigns/mental_health

Young Minds
Advice and information on a range of mental health issues such as depression
www.youngminds.org.uk/index.young.html

ASH (Action on Smoking and Health)
Provides information on all aspects of tobacco campaigning
http://www.ash.org.uk

British Heart Foundation
Working to prevent heart disease.
14 Fitzhardinge Street, London, W1H 4DH
Tel: 0171 935 0185
Fax: 0171 486 5820
http://bhf.org.uk

Cancer Research Campaign
Produce a booklet 'Q&A Children and Smoking: your questions answered'. They raise
medical, social and political issues related to the dangers of smoking.
10 Cambridge Terrace, London, NW1 4JL
Tel: 0171 224 1333
Fax: 0171 487 4302
http://www.crc.org.uk

Health Education Authority
For advice, support and motivation to give up smoking.

Trevelyan House, 30 Great Peter Street, London, SW1P 2HW
Tel: 0171 222 5300
Fax: 0171 413 8900
www.lifesaver.co.uk

No Smoking Day
Information about the No Smoking Day campaign
Unit 203, 16 Baldwin Gardens, London, EC1 7RJ
Tel: 0207 916 8070
Fax 0207 916 7556
http://www.no-smoking-day.org.uk/main.htm

Index

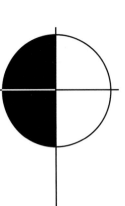